Isolation and Utilization of Essential Oils: As Antimicrobials and Boosters of Antimicrobial Drug Activity

Isolation and Utilization of Essential Oils: As Antimicrobials and Boosters of Antimicrobial Drug Activity

Editors

Elwira Sieniawska
Greige-Gerges Helene
Adriana Trifan

MDPI • Basel • Beijing • Wuhan • Barcelona • Belgrade • Manchester • Tokyo • Cluj • Tianjin

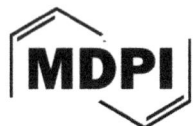

Editors
Elwira Sieniawska
Medical University of Lublin
Poland

Greige-Gerges Helene
Lebanese University
Lebanon

Adriana Trifan
Grigore T. Popa University of
Medicine and Pharmacy Iasi
Romania

Editorial Office
MDPI
St. Alban-Anlage 66
4052 Basel, Switzerland

This is a reprint of articles from the Special Issue published online in the open access journal *Processes* (ISSN 2227-9717) (available at: https://www.mdpi.com/journal/processes/special_issues/Essential_Oils_Antimicrobials).

For citation purposes, cite each article independently as indicated on the article page online and as indicated below:

LastName, A.A.; LastName, B.B.; LastName, C.C. Article Title. *Journal Name* **Year**, *Volume Number*, Page Range.

ISBN 978-3-0365-3999-7 (Hbk)
ISBN 978-3-0365-4000-9 (PDF)

Cover image courtesy of Elwira Sieniawska

© 2022 by the authors. Articles in this book are Open Access and distributed under the Creative Commons Attribution (CC BY) license, which allows users to download, copy and build upon published articles, as long as the author and publisher are properly credited, which ensures maximum dissemination and a wider impact of our publications.
The book as a whole is distributed by MDPI under the terms and conditions of the Creative Commons license CC BY-NC-ND.

Contents

About the Editors vii

Preface to "Isolation and Utilization of Essential Oils: As Antimicrobials and Boosters of Antimicrobial Drug Activity" ix

Elwira Sieniawska, Adriana Trifan and Hélène Greige-Gerges
Special Issue: Isolation and Utilization of Essential Oils: As Antimicrobials and Boosters of Antimicrobial Drug Activity
Reprinted from: *Processes* **2022**, *10*, 309, doi:10.3390/pr10020309 1

Mariana M. B. Azevedo, Catia A. Almeida, Francisco C. M. Chaves, Eduardo Ricci-Júnior, Andreza R. Garcia, Igor A. Rodrigues, Celuta S. Alviano and Daniela S. Alviano
Croton cajucara Essential Oil Nanoemulsion and Its Antifungal Activities
Reprinted from: *Processes* **2021**, *9*, 1872, doi:10.3390/pr9111872 5

Jaroslaw Widelski, Konstantia Graikou, Christos Ganos, Krystyna Skalicka-Wozniak and Ioanna Chinou
Volatiles from Selected Apiaceae Species Cultivated in Poland—Antimicrobial Activities
Reprinted from: *Processes* **2021**, *9*, 695, doi:10.3390/pr9040695 19

Vasiliki K. Pachi, Eleni V. Mikropoulou, Sofia Dimou, Mariangela Dionysopoulou, Aikaterini Argyropoulou, George Diallinas and Maria Halabalaki
Chemical Profiling of *Pistacia lentiscus* var. *Chia* Resin and Essential Oil: Ageing Markers and Antimicrobial Activity
Reprinted from: *Processes* **2021**, *9*, 418, doi:10.3390/pr9030418 31

Dolores Peruč, Dalibor Broznić, Željka Maglica, Zvonimir Marijanović, Ljerka Karleuša and Ivana Gobin
Biofilm Degradation of Nontuberculous Mycobacteria Formed on Stainless Steel Following Treatment with Immortelle (*Helichrysum italicum*) and Common Juniper (*Juniperus communis*) Essential Oils
Reprinted from: *Processes* **2021**, *9*, 362, doi:10.3390/pr9020362 51

Carine Sebaaly, Adriana Trifan, Elwira Sieniawska and Hélène Greige-Gerges
Chitosan-Coating Effect on the Characteristics of Liposomes: A Focus on Bioactive Compounds and Essential Oils: A Review
Reprinted from: *Processes* **2021**, *9*, 445, doi:10.3390/pr9030445 69

Diana Camelia Nuță, Carmen Limban, Cornel Chiriță, Mariana Carmen Chifiriuc, Teodora Costea, Petre Ioniță, Ioana Nicolau and Irina Zarafu
Contribution of Essential Oils to the Fight against Microbial Biofilms—A Review
Reprinted from: *Processes* **2021**, *9*, 537, doi:10.3390/pr9030537 117

Wye-Hong Leong, Kok-Song Lai and Swee-Hua Erin Lim
Combination Therapy Involving *Lavandula angustifolia* and Its Derivatives in Exhibiting Antimicrobial Properties and Combatting Antimicrobial Resistance: Current Challenges and Future Prospects
Reprinted from: *Processes* **2021**, *9*, 609, doi:10.3390/pr9040609 137

About the Editors

Elwira Sieniawska received her Ph.D. in pharmaceutical sciences from the Medical University of Lublin in 2012. She works at the Department of Natural Products Chemistry, Medical University of Lublin. Her scientific experience is based on phytochemistry. She has worked on the isolation and utilization of components of essential oils as antimicrobials and boosters of antimicrobial drug activity; however, the liquid chromatography—mass spectrometry analysis of bacterial metabolites produced under stress conditions is her current interest.

Greige-Gerges Helene obtained her Ph.D. in sciences of drugs from Henri Poincaré University, Nancy I, France in 1999. She is professor at the Faculty of Sciences at the Lebanese University. She has founded the Bioactive Molecules Research Laboratory at the Lebanese University in 2010. She has authored more than 100 peer-reviewed papers. Her research interest includes metabolism of drugs, drug delivery and green solvents.

Adriana Trifan received her Ph.D in Pharmacy from Grigore T. Popa University of Medicine and Pharmacy Iasi in 2012. She is a Lecturer in the Department of Pharmacognosy, Faculty of Pharmacy, Grigore T. Popa University of Medicine and Pharmacy Iasi. She is working on metabolite profiling and the bioactivity of plant extractives. Her current research interest includes the identification of natural compounds that are able to boost the activity of conventional antifungal drugs against dermatophytes.

Preface to "Isolation and Utilization of Essential Oils: As Antimicrobials and Boosters of Antimicrobial Drug Activity"

In the search for new antimicrobial lead compounds, there has been a renewed interest in natural-product-based screening, driven by the fact that plants present a unique pool of compounds. The volatiles produced by plants and present in essential oils possess a broad spectrum of biological properties with applications in many revenue-generating sectors, such as the pharmaceutical, nutraceutical, cosmetic, perfume, agronomy, and sanitary industries. Essential oils are a complex blend of small volatile molecules that play an important role in plant-defensive responses to various attacks, including microbial attacks, and their broad-spectrum antimicrobial activities have generated impressive scientific reports. Furthermore, due to their multicomponent nature, essential oils have a low potential for the development of microbial resistance. The combination of antimicrobial agents with natural products has recently become a research priority. The synergistic interactions between essential oil constituents and antimicrobials are very promising approaches to overcome microbial resistance. The combinations of essential oil constituents and antimicrobial drugs can exert a multitarget activity, being effective in reducing or reversing microbial resistance. Additionally, such combinations have the advantage of reducing the effective doses of both antimicrobial and essential oils, being consequently less toxic than the separated components. The encapsulation of essential oils in nano- and micro-delivery systems (molecular inclusion complexes, polymeric and colloidal systems) is another promising antimicrobial strategy that is currently being extensively investigated. The formulation of essential oils is an efficient approach to boost their antimicrobial activity against different pathogens; it allows overcoming some limitations that result from their physicochemical properties, such as low water solubility, high volatility, and chemical instability.

Elwira Sieniawska, Greige-Gerges Helene, and Adriana Trifan
Editors

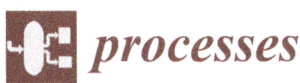

Editorial

Special Issue: Isolation and Utilization of Essential Oils: As Antimicrobials and Boosters of Antimicrobial Drug Activity

Elwira Sieniawska [1,*], Adriana Trifan [2] and Hélène Greige-Gerges [3]

[1] Department of Natural Products Chemistry, Medical University of Lublin, 20-093 Lublin, Poland
[2] Department of Pharmacognosy, Faculty of Pharmacy, Grigore T. Popa University of Medicine and Pharmacy Iasi, 700115 Iasi, Romania; adriana_trifan@yahoo.com
[3] Bioactive Molecules Research Laboratory, Department of Chemistry and Biochemistry, Faculty of Sciences, Section II, Lebanese University, Jdaidet el-Matn B.P. 90656, Lebanon; helenegreige73@gmail.com
* Correspondence: esieniawska@pharmacognosy.org

In the search for new antimicrobial lead compounds, interest in natural-product-based screening has enjoyed a renaissance, driven by the fact that plants present a unique pool of compounds. Volatiles produced by plants and present in essential oils possess a broad spectrum of biological properties with applications in many revenue-generating sectors, such as the pharmaceutical, nutraceutical, cosmetic, perfume, agronomy, and sanitary industries. Essential oils are a complex blend of small volatile molecules playing an important role in plant-defensive response to various insults, including microbial attacks, and their broad-spectrum antimicrobial activities have generated impressive scientific reports. Furthermore, due to their multicomponent nature, essential oils have low potential for the development of microbial resistance. The combination of antimicrobial agents with natural products have recently become a research priority. Synergistic interactions between essential oil constituents and antimicrobials are very promising approaches to overcome microbial resistance. The combinations of essential oil constituents and antimicrobial drugs can exert a multitarget activity, being effective in reducing or reversing microbial resistance. Additionally, such combinations have the advantage of reduced effective doses of both antimicrobial and essential oils, being consequently less toxic than separated components. The encapsulation of essential oils in nano- and micro-delivery systems (molecular inclusion complexes, polymeric and colloidal systems) is another promising antimicrobial strategy that is currently extensively investigated. The formulation of essential oils is an efficient approach to boost their antimicrobial activity against different pathogens; it allows overcoming some limitations that result from their physicochemical properties, such as low water solubility, high volatility, and chemical instability.

The main focus of this thematic collection was placed on the antimicrobial activity of essential oils and their combinations, including the eradication of the existing biofilms; the explanation of mechanisms underlying antimicrobial activity; and the preparation of stable formulations with essential oils boosting their antimicrobial activity and providing greater stability. These issues were addressed in four research papers and three reviews, which present novel advances in the development and application of essential oils as antimicrobial agents via combinatorial and nano-based approaches.

Azevedo et al. [1] developed a stable nanoemulsion (NE) containing *Croton cajucara* 7-hydroxycalamenene-rich essential oil (NECC) with antifungal activity. The authors found the best NECC antifungal activities against *Mucor ramosissimus* (MIC = 12.2 µg/mL) and *Candida albicans* (MIC = 25.6 µg/mL). The formulation totally inhibited extracellular proteases secreted by both studied species and showed no hemolytic effect at the highest tested concentration (2 mg/mL).

Widelski et al. [2] analyzed a panel of essential oils obtained from selected Apiaceae species cultivated in Poland. Eos obtained from *Heracleum dulce*, *Seseli devenyense*, and

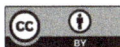

Seseli libanotis exerted the strongest antimicrobial activity, mostly against Gram-positive bacterial strains.

Pachi et al. [3] tested the antimicrobial activities of Chios Mastic Gums (CMGs) with their respective Chios Mastic Oils against fungi and bacteria. They found a moderate antimicrobial activity of mastic and its essential oil and proposed an HPTLC method for the standardization and assessment of the ageing effect on the oil's composition.

Peruč et al. [4] investigated the biofilm degradation ability of *Juniperus communis* and *Helichrysum italicum* EOs against nontuberculous mycobacteria found in plumbing systems, including pipes, tanks, and fittings. They found that *H. italicum* EO showed the strongest biofilm degradation ability against tested strains. Additionally, synergistic combinations of both EOs were effective against investigated mycobacterial strains and can be regarded as potential biofilm degradation agents for use in small water systems such as baths or hot tubs.

Sebaaly et al. [5] discussed the chitosomal encapsulation of EOs in order to ensure targeted delivery and boosted antimicrobial efficacy. Chitosomes, chitosan-coated liposomes, were shown to be a promising strategy overcoming major drawbacks related to the chemical properties of EOs (low water solubility, sensitivity to oxygen, light, heat, and humidity) and their poor bioavailability. The high biocompatibility and biodegradability of chitosan forming polymeric layers on conventional liposomes opens new potential applications as drug delivery systems in the pharmaceutic, cosmetic, and food industries.

Nuță et al. [6] targeted the rising problem related to the occurrence of biofilm-associated ailments. They presented the current literature data on the applications of EOs in chronic wounds and biofilm-mediated infections treatment, alongside the mechanisms of the microbicidal and antibiofilm activity of EOs. The synergistic activity of EO and other antimicrobials, as well as the use of EOs in food industry and as air disinfectants, were also discussed. The same authors raised an issue of difficulties in testing antimicrobial activity of EOs due to their lipophilicity and volatility, and several methods to overcome such challenges were proposed.

Leong et al. [7] provided an insight into the different aspects of antimicrobial activity exhibited by lavender essential oil and its constituents, which are known for their wound healing effects. The authors discussed the synergistic effects displayed by combinatory therapy involving this EO and explored the significance of nano-encapsulation in boosting its antimicrobial effects.

Author Contributions: Conceptualization, E.S., A.T., H.G.-G.; writing—original draft preparation, E.S., A.T., H.G.-G.; writing—review and editing, E.S., A.T., H.G.-G.; project administration, E.S. All authors have read and agreed to the published version of the manuscript.

Institutional Review Board Statement: Not applicable.

Informed Consent Statement: Not applicable.

Data Availability Statement: Not applicable.

Conflicts of Interest: The authors declare no conflict of interest.

References

1. Azevedo, M.M.B.; Almeida, C.A.; Chaves, F.C.M.; Ricci-Júnior, E.; Garcia, A.R.; Rodrigues, I.A.; Alviano, C.S.; Alviano, D.S. *Croton cajucara* Essential Oil Nanoemulsion and Its Antifungal Activities. *Processes* **2021**, *9*, 1872. [CrossRef]
2. Widelski, J.; Graikou, K.; Ganos, C.; Skalicka-Wozniak, K.; Chinou, I. Volatiles from Selected Apiaceae Species Cultivated in Poland—Antimicrobial Activities. *Processes* **2021**, *9*, 695. [CrossRef]
3. Pachi, V.K.; Mikropoulou, E.V.; Dimou, S.; Dionysopoulou, M.; Argyropoulou, A.; Diallinas, G.; Halabalaki, M. Chemical Profiling of *Pistacia lentiscus* var. *Chia* Resin and Essential Oil: Ageing Markers and Antimicrobial Activity. *Processes* **2021**, *9*, 418. [CrossRef]
4. Peruč, D.; Broznić, D.; Maglica, Z.; Marijanović, Z.; Karleuša, L.; Gobin, I. Biofilm Degradation of *Nontuberculous Mycobacteria* Formed on Stainless Steel Following Treatment with Immortelle (*Helichrysum italicum*) and Common Juniper (*Juniperus communis*) Essential Oils. *Processes* **2021**, *9*, 362. [CrossRef]
5. Sebaaly, C.; Trifan, A.; Sieniawska, E.; Greige-Gerges, H. Chitosan-Coating Effect on the Characteristics of Liposomes: A Focus on Bioactive Compounds and Essential Oils: A Review. *Processes* **2021**, *9*, 445. [CrossRef]

6. Nuță, D.C.; Limban, C.; Chiriță, C.; Chifiriuc, M.C.; Costea, T.; Ioniță, P.; Nicolau, I.; Zarafu, I. Contribution of Essential Oils to the Fight against Microbial Biofilms—A Review. *Processes* **2021**, *9*, 537. [CrossRef]
7. Leong, W.H.; Lai, K.S.; Erin Lim, S.H. Combination Therapy Involving *Lavandula angustifolia* and Its Derivatives in Exhibiting Antimicrobial Properties and Combatting Antimicrobial Resistance: Current Challenges and Future Prospects. *Processes* **2021**, *9*, 609. [CrossRef]

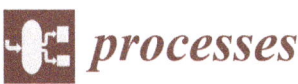

Article

Croton cajucara Essential Oil Nanoemulsion and Its Antifungal Activities

Mariana M. B. Azevedo [1,*], Catia A. Almeida [1], Francisco C. M. Chaves [2], Eduardo Ricci-Júnior [3], Andreza R. Garcia [4], Igor A. Rodrigues [4], Celuta S. Alviano [1] and Daniela S. Alviano [1,*]

[1] Institute of Microbiology Paulo de Góes, General Microbiology Department, Federal University of Rio de Janeiro (IMPG-UFRJ), CCS, Rio de Janeiro 21941-902, RJ, Brazil; catiamancio@yahoo.com.br (C.A.A.); alviano@micro.ufrj.br (C.S.A.)
[2] EMBRAPA Western Amazon AM 10 Highway, Km 29, Manaus 69010-970, AM, Brazil; celio.chaves@embrapa.br
[3] LADEG—Galenic Development Laboratory, School of Pharmacy, Federal University of Rio de Janeiro, CCS, Rio de Janeiro 21941-590, RJ, Brazil; ricci@pharma.ufrj.br
[4] Department of Natural Products and Food, School of Pharmacy, Federal University of Rio de Janeiro, CCS, Rio de Janeiro 21941-590, RJ, Brazil; deh.raposo@yahoo.com.br (A.R.G.); igor@pharma.ufrj.br (I.A.R.)
* Correspondence: maribarros@micro.ufrj.br (M.M.B.A.); danialviano@micro.ufrj.br (D.S.A.)

Abstract: The purpose of this study was to develop a stable nanoemulsion (NE) containing *Croton cajucara* 7-hydroxycalamenene-rich essential oil (NECC) with antifungal activity. The NECCs were prepared using an ultrasonic processor with Pluronic® F-127 as the aqueous phase. In order to evaluate the NECCs, the droplet size, polydispersity index (PdI), percentage of emulsification, and pH were determined along with a stability study. The NECC selected for the study had 15% surfactant, showed 100% emulsification, PdI of 0.249, neutral pH, droplet diameters of about 40 nm, and remained stable over 150 days at room temperature. In addition, the NECC activity against some species of Zygomycetes and Candida, as well as the potential to inhibit fungal extracellular proteases, were assessed, and, finally, the hemolytic activity was evaluated. The best NECC antifungal activities were against *Mucor ramosissimus* (Minimal inhibitory concentration (MIC) = 12.2 µg/mL) and *Candida albicans* (MIC = 25.6 µg/mL). The highest extracellular protease activities of *M. ramosissimus* and *C. albicans* were detected at pH 3 and 4, respectively, which were totally inhibited after NECC treatment. The NECC showed no hemolytic effect at the highest concentration tested (2 mg/mL).

Keywords: nanoemulsion; *Croton cajucara*; essential oil; antifungal activity

1. Introduction

Nanoemulsions, unlike microemulsions, are metastable submicron oil-in-water dispersions with droplet diameters in the range of 10–100 nm, though they can also be described between 20 and 200 nm. They are produced by high-energy methods such as ultrasound generators, high shear agitation, and high-pressure homogenizers. Potential advantages of nanoemulsions over conventional emulsions such as good physical stability, sterilization by filtration, high bioavailability, and low turbidity make them attractive systems for use in the food, cosmetics, and pharmaceutical industries. Nanoemulsions serve as delivery agents for lipophilic bioactive compounds, such as drugs, in the pharmaceutical industry, for flavors and antimicrobial agents in the food industry, for solubilizing water-insoluble pesticides in the agrochemical industry, and as a vehicle for skincare and personal products in cosmetics [1–3].

Nanoemulsions have several potential advantages over emulsions for encapsulating functional lipophilic components. The small size of the droplets in nanoemulsions significantly reduced the rate of destabilization mechanisms, such as gravitational separation, flocculation, and coalescence. Another potential advantage of using nanoemulsions is that the small droplet size means they are transparent or only slightly turbid [4].

Ultrasonic emulsification is a high-energy method to produce nanoemulsions and is well documented as a fast and efficient technique for formulating stable nanoemulsions with tiny droplet diameters and low polydispersity. The method applies sound waves with frequencies greater than 20 kHz by using a sonotrode to cause mechanical vibrations followed by the formation of acoustic cavitation. The collapse of these cavities generates powerful shock waves that break the larger droplets. The size of the droplet diameters can be controlled by optimizing the process parameters such as oil concentration, emulsifier concentration, the mixing ratio of oil and surfactant, viscosity of continuous phase, emulsification time, and energy input [2].

Regarding the clinical use of nanoemulsion in the delivery of antimicrobial drugs, nanoemulsion formulations can be at oral and intravenous (IV) administrations. In addition, nanoemulsions can decrease the volatility of the drug, increase the time of the drug in the bloodstream, and improve its absorption by enterocytes [5].

Croton cajucara Benth. (Euphorbiaceae), popularly known as "sacaca", is a plant found in the Amazonian region with a safe history of use in folk medicine. Both the bark and the leaves of *C. cajucara* are popularly used in teas and pills to treat various diseases, including diabetes, diarrhea, stomachaches, fevers, hepatitis, and malaria. In addition, *C. cajucara* also presented anti-genotoxicity, anti-atherogenic, anti-tumor, anti-ulcerogenic, hypoglycemic, hypolipidemic, anti-estrogen, anti-inflammatory, and anti-nociceptive properties [6]. Two morphotypes of *C. cajucara* are known, white "sacaca" and red "sacaca", which are usually identified by the young leaf color and stems. In general, essential oils from the white morphotype are rich in linalool, while those from the red morphotype are rich in 7-hydroxycalamenene [7]. The essential oil of the leaves from the red morphotype and its major constituents were previously described to possess antibacterial, antifungal, and antileishmanial properties [7–10].

Mucormycosis (also known as zygomycosis) is a fungal infection caused by the Mucorales order fungi, which can be present in the soil and decaying organic matter, such as leaves, compost piles, and rotten wood. Mucormycosis is characterized by hyphal invasion of sinus tissue and a time course of less than 4 weeks. Uncontrolled diabetes mellitus and other forms of metabolic acidosis, corticosteroid treatment, organ or bone marrow transplantation, neutropenia, trauma and burns, malignant hematologic disorders, and deferoxamine therapy in hemodialysis patients are all major risk factors for mucormycosis. Therefore, new strategies to prevent and treat mucormycosis are needed, and such strategies can be aided by a thorough understanding of the disease's pathogenesis [11,12].

Candida spp. can cause a wide range of pathologies of varying degrees depending on the pathogen and the host's immune condition. The colonization of the mucous membranes can occur by a change in the microbial population of the microbiota with a preponderant growth of Candida, which can then develop into a disseminated form. The deep infections result from dissemination that leads to a septic state that can evolve to multi-organ failure. Host risk factors associated with candidemia and invasive candidiasis are mainly related to neutropenia, prolonged hospitalization, the use of broad-spectrum antibiotics, chemotherapy, mucosal colonization, vascular catheters, parenteral nutrition, major surgery (mainly the gastrointestinal tract), and renal failure. In addition, some patients have a higher risk of developing candidemia due to their underlying medical conditions before admission as transplant recipients, diabetics, and elderly patients [13].

The aspartic proteases (E.C.3.4.23), also named acid proteases, are a group of endopeptidases with aspartic acid residues at their active site. Aspartic proteases that are excreted are called secreted aspartic proteases (sap's). The main functions of sap's are their use as microbial coagulants in cheese making in substitution of calf rennet, plant invasion of phytopathogens, and fungal invasion in infection of the human host (e.g., zygomycosis and candidemia). The sap's aid in the colonization and penetration of tissues in zygomycosis and candidemia [14].

This study investigated the potential of using the *C. cajucara* essential oil release system for its antifungal activity. Nanoemulsions were developed and evaluated in terms of the emulsification percentage, droplet size, polydispersion index, pH, stability, and morphology by transmission electron microscopy, and their antifungal activity was determined.

2. Materials and Methods

2.1. Plant Material and Essential Oil Extraction

Plant material from *C. cajucara* was obtained from the EMBRAPA Experimental Farm, Amazonas, Brazil. A voucher specimen was deposited at EMBRAPA Amazonia Oriental Herbarium (registry IAN 165013). Leaves of *C. cajucara* were collected between 8 and 9 a.m., dried at room temperature, and coarsely ground into powder just before distillation. The oil was obtained by hydrodistillation in a modified Clevenger apparatus over a 5 h period [7].

2.2. Essential Oil Analysis

C. cajucara essential oil (SO, sacaca oil) was analyzed in an Agilent 6890 N gas chromatograph fitted with a 5%-diphenyl-95%-dimethylpolysiloxane capillary column (HP-5, 25 m × 0.32 mm × 0.25 µm). Mass spectra were obtained with an Agilent 5973 N system, according to Pereira et al. (2011). The results were compared with data from the literature [15,16].

2.3. Oil-in-Water Nanoemulsion Preparation

Different NEs containing SO, as the oily phase, and Pluronic® F-127, as the aqueous phase, were produced. The amount of surfactant in the aqueous phase was prepared in three concentrations: 10%, 12.5%, and 15%. The optimal surfactant concentration was 15%, as it remained in the liquid state, and the amount of essential oil was 5% (Table S1, Supplementary Material). NEs were produced using, first, a Vortex® (KASVI® model K40-1010) for 1 min for homogenization and then, second, an ultrasonic processor (UP100H, Hielscher®) with 100 watts and 30 kHz, in cycle 1. Samples were sonicated under an ice bath at 5 °C. After production, they were tested for storage stability in an incubator at 37 °C, room temperature at 25 °C, and in a refrigerator at 3 °C [17].

2.4. Particle Mean Size and Size Distribution

The mean size of the NEs droplets (diameter in nm) was determined by the dynamic light scattering (DLS) technique using a Zetasizer, Nano® S90 (Malvern Instruments®), with optics of 90° scattering detector angle, at room temperature (25 °C). Transmission electron microscopy was also performed to visualize the structure of the NEs and confirm their size. The NEs were diluted 1:50 in distilled water for these analyses, and the measurements were performed at room temperature (25 °C). DLS was used to screen the preparations, in which the smaller size and lower polydispersity index (PdI) were selected. Analyzes were performed in triplicate, and the results are expressed as the mean ± standard deviation [17].

2.5. Percentage of Essential Oil Emulsification

The percentage of essential oil emulsification was obtained spectrophotometrically (SpectraMax M5/Molecular Devices) by making a standard curve of the *C. cajucara* essential oil and comparing it with ultrasonicated Pluronic® F-127 and the NEs. The percentage of essential oil in nanoemulsion was obtained through logarithmic regression.

2.6. Kinetics Stability

Kinetic stability tests were performed after 7 days of storage of the NEs at room temperature (25 °C) and repeated after 30, 60, 90, 120, and 150 days in storage and evaluated by the percentage of emulsification.

2.7. Hydrogenionic Potential (pH)

The hydrogenionic potential (pH) was measured using the Bante Instrument potentiometer model 922. The readings were performed in fresh and 150-storage-day samples, at room temperature (25 °C) and at the kinetic stability times.

2.8. Antifungal Activity Assay of Nanoemulsion of Croton cajucara (NECC)

The antifungal activity of nanoemulsions containing essential oil of *C. cajucara* red morphotype was evaluated against *Absidia cylindrospora* (URM4476), *Cuninghamella elegans* (URM2084), *Mucor circinelloides* (LIKA0066), *M. mucedo* (LIKA0072), *M. ramosissimus* (URM3087), *Rhizopus microsporus* (LMC123), *R. oryzae* (UCP1506), and *Syncephalastrum racemosum* (UCP1550), as well as *C. albicans* (ATCC 10231), *C. albicans* serotype A (ATCC 36801), and *C. albicans* serotype B (ATCC 36802). Emulsions without the essential oil of *C. cajucara* were also tested as an antifungal activity control. In addition, the purified 7-hydroxycalamenene (7-OH) obtained elsewhere [7] was also tested, and its antifungal minimal inhibitory concentrations (MICs) could be compared with the results obtained for the essential oil of *C. cajucara* nanoemulsions.

The microdilution broth methods were used according to CLSI reference documents M27-A2 [18] for yeasts and M38-A2 [19] for filamentous fungi. Positive and negative growth controls and blanks were made. The antifungal activities of sonicated Pluronic at nanoemulsion concentration were also made and showed no activity to any fungi. All experiments were performed in duplicate and repeated twice. The nanoemulsion was diluted 1:1 in RPMI broth, and an aliquot of 100 µL was placed in the first well of the microplate to initiating serial dilution.

To evaluate the fungicide/fungistatic properties of *C. cajucara* essential oil nanoemulsion, a 10 µL aliquot of serial dilutions was dropped on the surface of potato dextrose agar and incubated at 37 °C for 72 h or Sabouraud agar and incubated at 37 °C for 48 h. If growth is observed, the nanoemulsion activity is fungistatic; if not, it is fungicidal.

2.9. Activity of Extracellular Proteases

In order to evaluate a possible mode of action of NECC, the supernatants of fungi grown in RPMI at MIC conditions were collected and filtered by sterile Millipore (0.22 µm). The supernatants enzymatic activities were determined according to Almeida et al. (2018) [20] with some modifications. First, 20 µL of the supernatant was added to 20 µL BSA (1 mg/mL) and 60 µL buffer (pH 1.0–11.0) onto a 96-well plate. Then, after 1 h of incubation at 37 °C, 100 µL of Bradford solution (0.025% Coomassie Blue G-250, 11.75% ethanol, and 21.25% phosphoric acid) was previously diluted (1:1) and added. Negative control was prepared by adding the substrate immediately after the incubation period. Finally, the plate was read on a spectrophotometer (SpectraMax M5) at 595 nm. One unit of enzyme activity was defined as the total enzyme that causes an increase of 0.001 in absorbance unit under the standard assay conditions.

Alternatively, the supernatants were pre-incubated for 20 min at 37 °C in the presence or absence of pepstatin A (10 mM) and NECC (in the minimum inhibitory concentration). In the latter case, the results are expressed as a relative percentage of activity.

2.10. Hemolytic Activity

Cytotoxicity against erythrocytes was determined by the spectrophotometric assay [21]. Human blood samples (O+) were collected from a healthy volunteer into BD™ Vacutainer™ Citrate tubes. The blood samples were centrifuged (2000 rpm/5 min), washed three times with phosphate buffer saline (PBS, pH 7.2), and a final cellular suspension was prepared (4%, in PBS). Aliquots of 80 µL were distributed into 96-well microplates, where 20 µL of different concentrations (0.03 to 2 mg/mL) of NECC were previously deposited. Emulsions without the essential oil of *C. cajucara* were also tested as a hemolytic activity control. After 1 h at 37 °C, the reaction was slowed down by adding 200 µL of PBS or distilled water (positive control for 100% hemolysis). Next, the microplates were centrifuged, and the supernatant was collected for spectrophotometric analysis at 540 mn (SpectraMax M5, Molecular Devices, CA, USA). Three independent experiments were performed, and the results were expressed as a percentage of hemoglobin released by treated cells relative to the positive control. The blood collection procedures were approved by the Institutional Ethics Board (CAAE 35524814.4.0000.0107). In addition, the informed consent form was duly signed by the volunteer.

3. Results and Discussion

GC-MS of the essential oil from *C. cajucara* showed that it is rich in 7-hydroxycalamenene (Table 1), the expected major constituent of the red morphotype, which has been previously described as responsible for its antimicrobial activities [7–10].

Table 1. Composition of *C. cajucara* essential oil used in the nanoemulsion formulation.

Peak	LRI *	Area %	Identification
1	1459	2.32	aromadendrene<allo>
2	1480	2.43	germacrene D
3	1494	1.14	bicyclogermacrene
4	1498	3.3	α-muurolene
5	1513	6.77	γ-cadinene
6	1522	11.01	δ-cadinene
7	1554	6.1	germacrene B
8	1575	1.08	spathulenol
9	1580	5.48	caryophyllene oxide
10	1626	2.34	dill apiole
11	1640	5.86	τ-cadinol
12	1652	1.47	α-cadinol
13	1803	50.63	7-hydroxycalamenene
Total		99.93	

* Linear retention index.

The nanoemulsion formulations were prepared with Pluronic® F-127 at concentrations of 10%, 12.5%, and 15%. The concentration chosen was the one that remained in the liquid state, which was 15%, the temperature that kept NECC stable was room temperature at 25 °C, and the concentration of 7-hydroxycalamenene in the nanoemulsion obtained was 52.63 mg/mL. The average PdI obtained for the formulation was 0.249 ± 0.014, showing that NECC is monodisperse, indicating size homogeneity. The average size was 45.56 ± 15.76 nm, obtained by the Z-average size parameter of the equipment report.

Using the graph in Figure 1, it was possible to calculate the percentage of essential oil emulsification based on the logarithmic regression equation. The value encountered was 100%.

Figure 2A shows that the size distribution remained within the expected limits of the kinetic stability test. In addition, the evaluation of its shelf-life test showed at least 5 months of size stability.

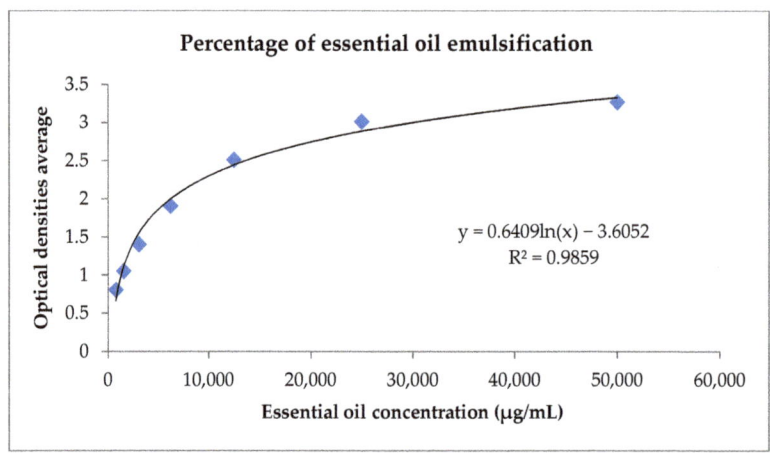

Figure 1. Logarithmic regression to calculate the percentage of emulsification of *C. cajucara* essential oil. Standard curve of the *C. cajucara* essential oil compared with ultrasonicated Pluronic® F-127 and the NEs. The percentage of essential oil in nanoemulsion was based on the equation obtained through logarithmic regression.

Most patients with rhinocerebral zygomycosis have problems with pH due to diabetic ketoacidosis. In systemic acidosis, the iron of proteins is released to the serum, and these two conditions promote the growth of zygomycetes spreading the infection [22]. Therefore, medicines with a neutral or slightly basic pH can help fight infection and help with tissue repair. Thus, the pH of 7.3–8.3 (Figure 2B) obtained by the formulation at the stability study kept at room temperature (25 °C) was considered suitable for human testing.

The NEs were observed by transmission electron microscopy (Figure 3), and a droplet size of about 40 nm measured by DLS was confirmed. The NECCs are spherical, and the shape is regular, as described by de Siqueira et al. 2019 [17]. Arrows indicate small oil drops. Some drops are isolated, and others are agglomerated. This is because TEM requires the removal of the aqueous phase causing agglomeration of the oil droplets of the nanoemulsion. In the clusters of drops, the light parts are oil drops, and the dark parts are the fused surfactant layers. In isolated drops, the light part is the oil drop, and the dark part is the surfactant layer.

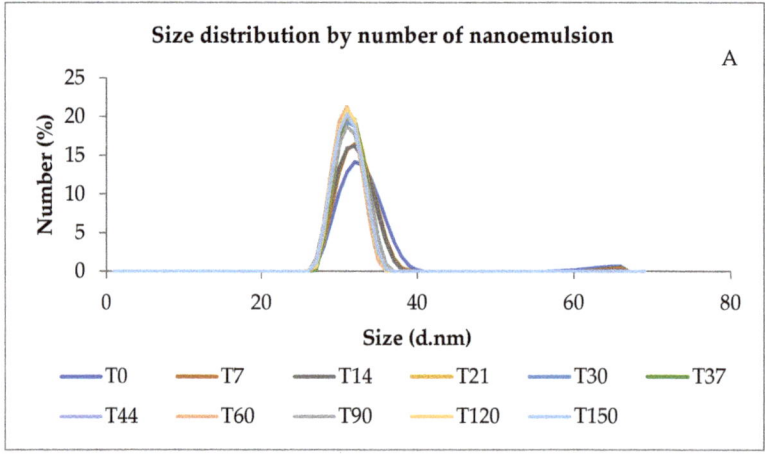

Figure 2. *Cont.*

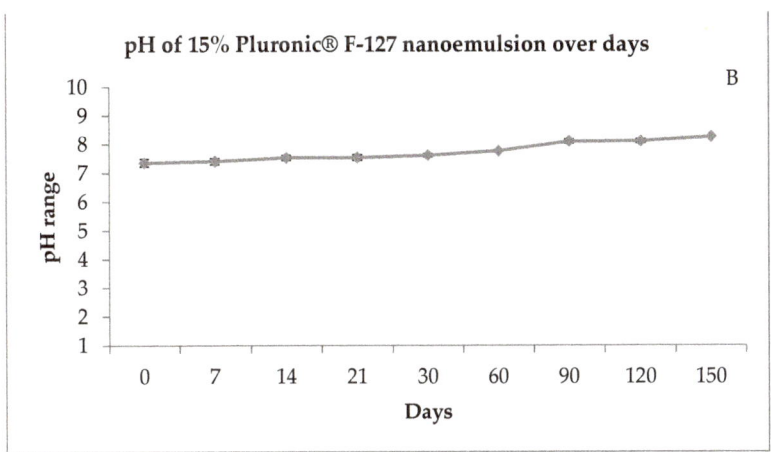

Figure 2. Size distribution of nanoemulsion by number (**A**) and pH of the nanoemulsion prepared with 15% of Pluronic® F-127 over days (**B**). T = time in days.

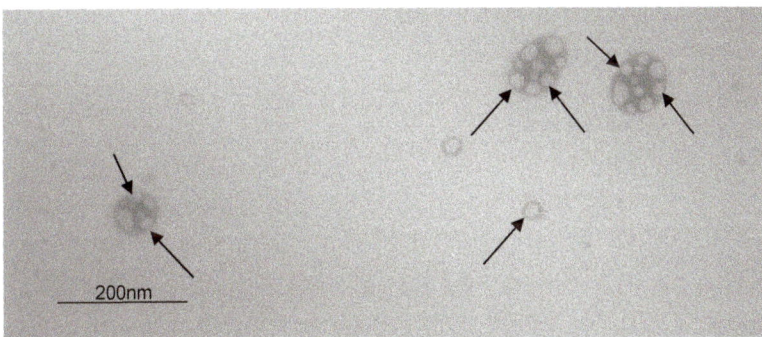

Figure 3. Transmission electron microscopy of NECCs (black arrows) at 71,000× of magnification and 80 kV of accelerating voltage.

The evaluation of NECC activity in inhibiting the microbial growth of microorganisms of medical importance was promising, as can be seen in Table 2. Emulsions without the essential oil of *C. cajucara* were also tested as a control, and no inhibitory activities were detected in all fungi tested.

The Euphorbiaceae family has several species with biological activities as antifungal [23], biolarvicidal and pupicidal [24], antioxidant and anticancer [25], and antibacterial [26]. Our research group has previously described the antifungal [7–9,27], antibacterial [9], antileishmania [10], and antioxidant [9] activities of *Croton cajucara* essential oil.

The MIC assays show that the zygomycetes species tested are very sensitive to NECC and the most promising activities were against *Absidia cylindospora*, *Mucor ramosissimus*, and *Syncephalastrum racemosum*, all common agents of zygomycosis. However, NECC improved the essential oil activity against *M. ramosissimus* and *S. racemosum*, while the non-emulsified essential oil was not effective against these fungi. All *Candida albicans* strains tested were susceptible to NECC. According to Azevedo et al. (2014) [7], zygomycetes were shown to be sensitive to 7-hydroxycalamenene because this substance affected these fungi respiratory chain and spores germination. Azevedo et al. (2016) [27] showed that 7-hydroxycalamenene also demonstrated intense activity against some strains of *C. albicans*, and their proteases were also inhibited. Different authors showed other relevant activities as inhibition of lipidic peroxidation [28], leishmanicidal [10], and therapeutic potential for Alzheimer's disease [29].

Table 2. Minimal inhibitory concentration (MIC) of NECC and 7-hydroxycalamenene (7-OH).

Microorganisms	NECC MIC (µg/mL)	Effect	7-OH MIC (µg/mL)	Effect [1]
Filamentous fungi				
Absidia cylindospora (URM4476)	12.21	Static	19.53	Static
Cuninghamella elegans (URM 2084)	24.41	Static	19.53	Static
Mucor circinelloides (LIKA0066)	48.83	Static	19.53	Cide
M. mucedo (LIKA 0072)	48.83	Static	2500	Static
M. ramosissimus (URM 3087)	12.21	Static	2500	Static
Rhizopus microsporus (LMC123)	195.31	Static	19.53	Static
R. oryzae (UCP 1506)	97.66	Static	39.06	Static
Syncephalastrum racemosum (UCP1550)	12.21	Static	2500	Static
Yeasts				
Candida albicans (ATCC 10231)	25.69	Static	39.06	Static
C. albicans serotype A (ATCC 36801)	25.69	Static	39.06	Static
C. albicans serotype B (ATCC 36802)	51.39	Static	78.12	Static

[1] Cide = fungicide; Static = fungistatic.

Through the growth curve, it is possible to observe the growth over time. Figure 4 shows the interference of NECC on growth.

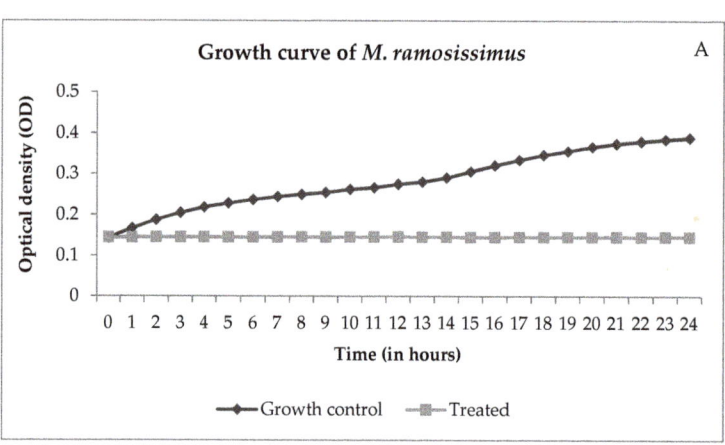

Figure 4. Cont.

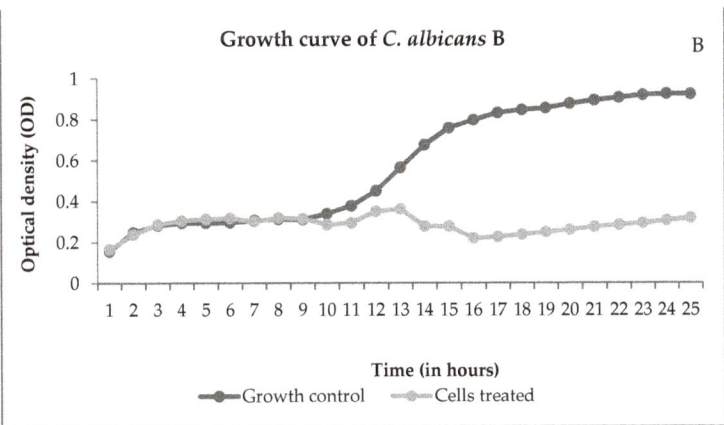

Figure 4. Growth curves of *Mucor ramosissimus* (**A**) and *Candida albicans* B (**B**), controls, and cells treated with NECC at MIC and room temperature (25 °C).

Figure 4A shows that *M. ramosissimus* did not differentiate with treatment with NECC at MIC, and *C. albicans* kept the differentiation until the 9th hour, and then it stopped. In both cases, the microorganisms were not killed, showing that the activity of NECC is fungistatic. Recently, with the COVID-19 pandemic, the incidence of zygomycosis, colloquially called "black fungus", has increased. Spore germination occurs due to various reasons such as low oxygen saturation, high iron levels as evidenced by high ferritin, immunosuppression caused by SARS-CoV-2, decreased phagocytic activity of white blood cells, and hyperglycemia from corticosteroid use [30]. These are all conditions for the development of zygomycosis and candidiasis. Candidiasis is another fungal infection associated with COVID-19. In addition to the factors described, intubation is a risk factor that predisposes the patient to colonization and pulmonary proliferation of *Candida* species [31]. Thus, the development of natural substances with promising antimicrobial activity and low toxicity is of great importance in order to improve patient survival.

The greatest proteases activities for *M. ramosissimus* occurred at pH3 (Figure 5A) and for *C. albicans* at pH4 (Figure 5B). Thus, the following experiment evaluated whether NECC inhibits proteases activities at pH3 (*M. ramosissimus*) and pH4 (*C. albicans*). The aspartic proteases activities of both fungi were completely inhibited when treated with MIC concentrations of NECC (Figure 5C). The inhibition of aspartic proteases activity could be an important way to control these fungi [32]. According to Morace and Borghi (2012) [33], Mucorales of the genus *Mucor* are the second cause of invasive mucormycosis. Challa (2019) [34] stated that aspartic proteases of Mucorales favor host invasion. Azevedo (2014) [7] demonstrated that 7-hydroxycalamenene showed inhibitory activity against rhizopuspepsin (pepsin present in the main genus of zygomycosis, *Rhizopus*). It is also well known that *C. albicans* produces various types of secreted aspartic proteases (Saps), and the production of these Saps varies according to their shape (yeast cells or hyphal form), the pH, and the available substrate. Saps can also hydrolyze various substrates such as keratin, collagen, laminin, fibronectin, salivary lactoferrin, and others [32]. Therefore, the results shown in Figure 5 are promising, as they inhibited 100% of the *Mucor* and *Candida* proteases. These results show that 7-hydroxycalamenene appears to be efficient in inhibiting an important Zygomycetes and Blastomycetes mechanism of action.

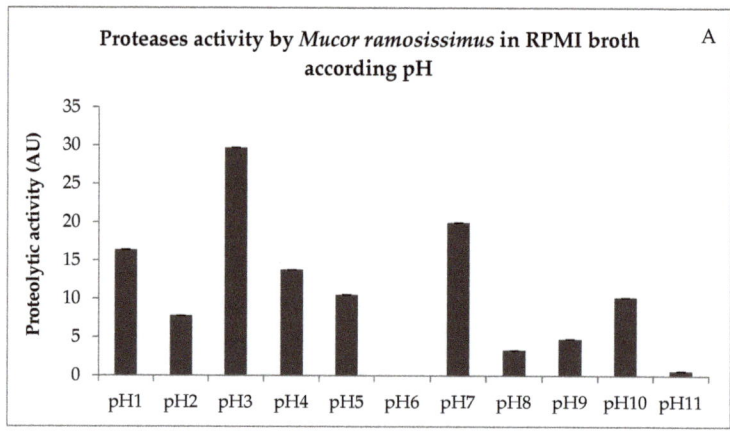
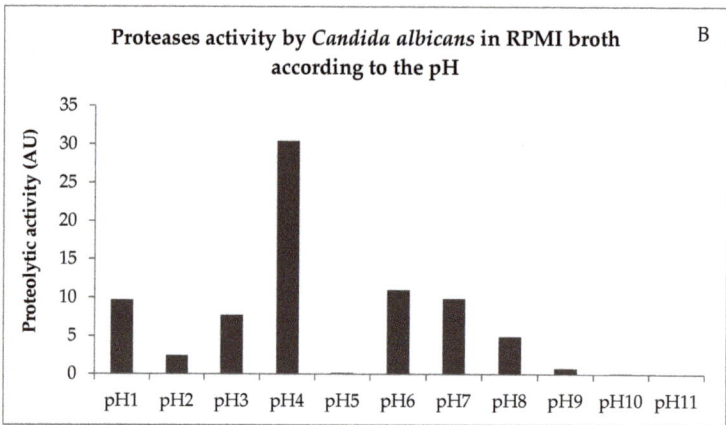
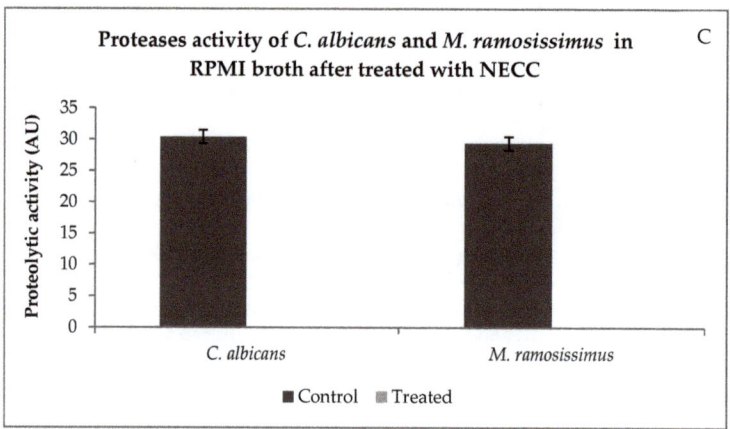

Figure 5. Proteases activity by *M. ramosissimus* (**A**), *C. albicans* (**B**) in RPMI broth according to the pH. Proteases activities by *C. albicans* and *M. ramosissimus* in RPMI broth after treatment with NECC (in arbitrary unit—AU) (**C**).

In addition, NECC demonstrated no hemolytic effect even at the highest concentration tested (2 mg/mL). According to Rodrigues et al. (2013) [10], 7-hydroxycalamenene, which was the main component of the essential oil that they used in their study (>50%), was shown to be non-toxic to peritoneal mouse macrophages at a concentration of 500 µg/mL.

4. Conclusions

In this study, a nanoemulsion was obtained with a 100% emulsification percentage and was stable for more than 150 days at room temperature (25 °C), with a droplet size of around 40 nm. This formulation proved to be effective against zygomycetes, especially against the *Mucor ramosissimus* and *Candida albicans* strains tested. In addition, the nanoemulsion inhibited 100% of their extracellular protease activity. NECC also demonstrated no hemolytic effect at a maximum concentration of 2 mg/mL.

According to the results presented, in vivo experiments should be conducted to confirm the promising activities of the proposed nanoemulsion. However, nanoemulsions containing essential oils can be a way to improve antifungal activities and be widely used as we live in times of resistant microorganisms.

Supplementary Materials: The following are available online at https://www.mdpi.com/article/10.3390/pr9111872/s1, Table S1: NEs formulation optimization. Different NEs were produced containing SO (1 and 5%) as the oily phase and Pluronic® F-127 (10%, 12.5%, and 15%) as the aqueous phase.

Author Contributions: Conceptualization, M.M.B.A.; C.A.A.; C.S.A. and D.S.A., methodology, M.M.B.A.; C.A.A.; F.C.M.C.; E.R.-J.; A.R.G.; and I.A.R.; formal analysis, M.M.B.A.; C.A.A.; E.R.-J.; C.S.A. and D.S.A.; investigation and data curation, M.M.B.A.; C.A.A.; F.C.M.C.; E.R.-J.; A.R.G.; I.A.R.; C.S.A. and D.S.A.; writing—original draft preparation, M.M.B.A.; writing—review and editing, C.A.A.; F.C.M.C.; E.R.-J.; A.R.G.; I.A.R.; C.S.A. and D.S.A.; supervision, C.S.A.; D.S.A.; project administration, C.S.A.; D.S.A.; funding acquisition, C.S.A.; D.S.A. All authors have read and agreed to the published version of the manuscript.

Funding: This study was supported by Fundação Carlos Chagas Filho de Amparo a Pesquisa do Estado do Rio de Janeiro (FAPERJ) grant number E-26/203.035/2017 (233939), Coordenação de Aperfeiçoamento de Pessoal de Nível Superior (CAPES) and Conselho Nacional de Desenvolvimento Científico e Tecnológico (CNPq).

Acknowledgments: The authors thank Maria Barbara Faria Cardoso da Silva for technical assistance and sample preparation. This study was supported by Fundação Carlos Chagas Filho de Amparo a Pesquisa do Estado do Rio de Janeiro (FAPERJ), Coordenação de Aperfeiçoamento de Pessoal de Nível Superior (CAPES) and Conselho Nacional de Desenvolvimento Científico e Tecnológico (CNPq).

Conflicts of Interest: The authors declare no conflict of interest. The funders had no role in the design of the study, in the collection, analyses, or interpretation of data, in the writing of the manuscript, or in the decision to publish the results.

References

1. Sonneville-Aubrun, O.; Simonnet, J.T.; L'alloret, F. Nanoemulsions: A new vehicle for skincare products. *Adv. Colloid Interface Sci.* **2004**, *108*, 145–149. [CrossRef]
2. Ghosh, V.; Mukherjee, A.; Chandrasekaran, N. Ultrasonic emulsification of food-grade nanoemulsion formulation and evaluation of its bactericidal activity. *Ultrason. Sonochem.* **2013**, *20*, 338–344. [CrossRef]
3. Rodrigues, I.A.; Ramos, A.D.S.; Falcão, D.Q.; Ferreira, J.L.P.; Basso, S.L.; Silva, J.R.D.A.; Amaral, A.C.F. Development of nanoemulsions to enhance the antileishmanial activity of *Copaifera paupera* oleoresins. *Biomed Res. Int.* **2018**, *2018*, 9781724. [CrossRef]
4. Chang, Y.; McLandsborough, L.; McClements, D.J. Physical properties and antimicrobial efficacy of thyme oil nanoemulsions: Influence of ripening inhibitors. *J. Agric. Food Chem.* **2012**, *60*, 12056–12063. [CrossRef]
5. Fast, J.P.; Mecozzi, S. Nanoemulsions for intravenous drug delivery. In *Nanotechnology in Drug Delivery*; Springer: New York, NY, USA, 2009; pp. 461–489.
6. Lima, G.S.; Castro-Pinto, D.B.; Machado, G.C.; Maciel, M.A.; Echevarria, A. Antileishmanial activity and trypanothione reductase effects of terpenes from the Amazonian species *Croton cajucara* Benth (Euphorbiaceae). *Phytomedicine* **2015**, *22*, 1133–1137. [CrossRef] [PubMed]

7. Azevedo, M.M.; Almeida, C.A.; Chaves, F.C.; Campos-Takaki, G.M.; Rozental, S.; Bizzo, H.R.; Alviano, C.S.; Alviano, D.S. Effects of 7-Hydroxycalamenene Isolated from *Croton cajucara* Essential Oil on Growth, Lipid Content and Ultrastructural Aspects of *Rhizopus oryzae*. *Planta Med.* **2014**, *80*, 550–556. [CrossRef]
8. Azevedo, M.M.; Pereira, A.Q.; Chaves, F.C.; Bizzo, H.R.; Alviano, C.S.; Alviano, D.S. Antimicrobial activity of the essential oils from the leaves of two morphotypes of *Croton cajucara* Benth. *J. Essent. Oil Res.* **2012**, *24*, 351–357. [CrossRef]
9. Azevedo, M.; Chaves, F.; Almeida, C.A.; Bizzo, H.R.; Duarte, R.S.; Campos-Takaki, G.M.; Alviano, C.S.; Alviano, D.S. Antioxidant and antimicrobial activities of 7-hydroxy-calamenene-rich essential oils from *Croton cajucara* Benth. *Molecules* **2013**, *18*, 1128–1137. [CrossRef] [PubMed]
10. Rodrigues, I.A.; Azevedo, M.M.; Chaves, F.C.; Bizzo, H.R.; Corte-Real, S.; Alviano, D.S.; Alviano, C.S.; Rosa, M.S.S.; Vermelho, A.B. In vitro cytocidal effects of the essential oil from *Croton cajucara* (red sacaca) and its major constituent 7-hydroxycalamenene against *Leishmania chagasi*. *BMC Complement. Altern. Med.* **2013**, *13*, 249. [CrossRef]
11. Tewari, S.; David, J.; Nakhale, S.; David, B. Mucormycosis: Post COVID-19 Fungal Infection. *Int. J. Curr. Microbiol. Appl. Sci.* **2021**, *10*, 64–71.
12. Patil, S.; Sarate, D.; Chopade, S.; Khade, M.; Dhage, S.; Kangate, S. Emerging Challenge of Mucormycosis in post COVID Patients. *IAR J. Med. Case Rep.* **2021**, *2*, 7–10.
13. Di Cosola, M.; Cazzolla, A.P.; Charitos, I.A.; Ballini, A.; Inchingolo, F.; Santacroce, L. *Candida albicans* and Oral Carcinogenesis. A Brief Review. *J. Fungi* **2021**, *7*, 476. [CrossRef]
14. Mandujano-González, V.; Villa-Tanaca, L.; Anducho-Reyes, M.A.; Mercado-Flores, Y. Secreted fungal aspartic proteases: A review. *Rev. Iberoam. Micol.* **2016**, *33*, 76–82. [CrossRef]
15. Adams, R.P. *Identification of Essential oil Components by Gas Chromatography/Mass Spectrometry*, 4th ed.; Allured Publ. Corp.: Carol Stream, IL, USA, 2007; pp. 1–804.
16. Pereira, A.Q.; Chaves, F.C.; Pinto, S.C.; Leitão, S.G.; Bizzo, H.R. Isolation and Identification of cis-7-Hydroxycalamenene from the Essential Oil of *Croton cajucara* Benth. *J. Essent. Oil Res.* **2011**, *23*, 20–23. [CrossRef]
17. De Siqueira, L.B.D.O.; dos Santos Matos, A.P.; da Silva Cardoso, V.; Villanova, J.C.O.; Guimarães, B.D.C.L.R.; Dos Santos, E.P.; Vermelho, A.B.; Santos-Oliveira, R.; Junior, E.R. Clove oil nanoemulsion showed potent inhibitory effect against *Candida* spp. *Nanotechnology* **2019**, *30*, 425101. [CrossRef]
18. Clinical and Laboratory Standards Institute (CLSI). *Reference Method for Broth Dilution Antifungal Susceptibility Testing of Yeasts*; Approved Standard M27-A2; National Committee for Clinical Laboratory Standards: Wayne, NJ, USA, 2002; pp. 1–51.
19. Clinical and Laboratory Standards Institute (CLSI). *Reference Method for Broth Dilution Antifungal Susceptibility Testing of Filamentous Fungi*; Approved Standard M38-A2; National Committee for Clinical Laboratory Standards: Wayne, NJ, USA, 2008; pp. 1–52.
20. Almeida, C.A.; Azevedo, M.; Chaves, F.; Roseo de Oliveira, M.; Rodrigues, I.A.; Bizzo, H.R.; Gama, P.E.; Alviano, D.S.; Alviano, C.S. *Piper* essential oils inhibit *Rhizopus oryzae* growth, biofilm formation, and rhizopuspepsin activity. *Can. J. Infect. Dis. Med. Microbiol.* **2018**, *2018*, 5295619. [CrossRef]
21. Löfgren, S.E.; Miletti, L.C.; Steindel, M.; Bachere, E.; Barracco, M.A. Trypanocidal and leishmanicidal activities of different antimicrobial peptides (AMPs) isolated from aquatic animals. *Exp. Parasitol.* **2008**, *118*, 197–202. [CrossRef]
22. Shinde, Y.B.; Kore, S. A Review on Mucormycosis with recent pharmacological treatment. *J. Drug Deliv. Ther.* **2021**, *11*, 145–149. [CrossRef]
23. Mahmoud, H.; Mohamed, N.T.; Abd-El-Sayed, M.A. Fungicidal Activity of Nanoemulsified Essential Oils Against Botrytis Leaf Blight of Poinsettia (*Euphorbia pulcherrima*) in Egypt. *Egypt. J. Agric. Res.* **2018**, *96*, 1259–1273.
24. Priyadarshini, K.A.; Murugan, K.; Panneerselvam, C.; Ponarulselvam, S.; Hwang, J.S.; Nicoletti, M. Biolarvicidal and pupicidal potential of silver nanoparticles synthesized using *Euphorbia hirta* against *Anopheles stephensi* Liston (Diptera: Culicidae). *Parasitol. Res.* **2012**, *111*, 997–1006. [CrossRef] [PubMed]
25. Javanshir, A.; Karimi, E.; Maragheh, A.D.; Tabrizi, M.H. The antioxidant and anticancer potential of *Ricinus communis* L. essential oil nanoemulsions. *J. Food Meas. Charact.* **2020**, *14*, 1356–1365. [CrossRef]
26. Zhu, Q.; Jiang, M.L.; Shao, F.; Ma, G.Q.; Shi, Q.; Liu, R.H. Chemical Composition and Antimicrobial Activity of the Essential Oil from *Euphorbia helioscopia* L. *Nat. Prod. Commun.* **2020**, *15*, 1934578X20953249. [CrossRef]
27. Azevedo, M.M.; Almeida, C.A.; Chaves, F.C.; Rodrigues, I.A.; Bizzo, H.R.; Alviano, C.S.; Alviano, D.S. 7-hydroxycalamenene effects on secreted aspartic proteases activity and biofilm formation of *Candida* spp. *Pharmacogn. Mag.* **2016**, *12*, 36. [CrossRef] [PubMed]
28. Rodríguez-Chávez, J.L.; Coballase-Urrutia, E.; Nieto-Camacho, A.; Delgado-Lamas, G. Antioxidant capacity of "Mexican arnica" *Heterotheca inuloides* Cass natural products and some derivatives: Their anti-inflammatory evaluation and effect on *C. elegans* life span. *Oxid. Med. Cell. Longev.* **2015**, *2015*, 843237. [CrossRef] [PubMed]
29. Yen, P.L.; Cheng, S.S.; Wei, C.C.; Lin, H.Y.; Liao, V.H.C.; Chang, S.T. Antioxidant Activities and Reduced Amyloid-β Toxicity of 7-Hydroxycalamenene Isolated from the Essential Oil of *Zelkova serrata* Heartwood. *Nat. Prod. Commun.* **2016**, *11*, 1934578X1601100943. [CrossRef]
30. Bhadra, A.; Ahmed, M.S.; Rahman, M.A.; Islam, S. Mucormycosis or black fungus: An emerging threat in COVID-19. *Bangabandhu Sheikh Mujib Med. Univ. J.* **2021**, *14*, 51–56. [CrossRef]
31. Ezeokoli, O.T.; Gcilitshana, O.; Pohl, C.H. Risk factors for fungal co-infections in critically ill COVID-19 patients, with a focus on immunosuppressants. *J. Fungi* **2021**, *7*, 545. [CrossRef]

32. Santos, A.L.S.D. Aspartic proteases of human pathogenic fungi are prospective targets for the generation of novel and effective antifungal inhibitors. *Curr. Enzym. Inhib.* **2011**, *7*, 96–118. [CrossRef]
33. Morace, G.; Borghi, E. Invasive mold infections: Virulence and pathogenesis of *Mucorales*. *Int. J. Microbiol.* **2012**, *2012*, 349278. [CrossRef]
34. Challa, S. Mucormycosis: Pathogenesis and Pathology. *Curr. Fungal Infect. Rep.* **2019**, *13*, 11–20. [CrossRef]

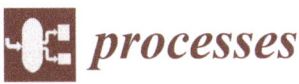

Article

Volatiles from Selected Apiaceae Species Cultivated in Poland—Antimicrobial Activities

Jaroslaw Widelski [1], Konstantia Graikou [2], Christos Ganos [2], Krystyna Skalicka-Wozniak [3] and Ioanna Chinou [2,*]

1. Department of Pharmacognosy, Medical University of Lublin, 1 Chodzki Str., 20-093 Lublin, Poland; jwidelski@pharmacognosy.org
2. Laboratory of Pharmacognosy and Chemistry of Natural Products, Department of Pharmacy, School of Health Science, National and Kapodistrian University of Athens, Panepistimiopolis Zografou, 15771 Athens, Greece; kgraikou@pharm.uoa.gr (K.G.); christos.ganos.19@ucl.ac.uk (C.G.)
3. Independent Laboratory of Natural Products Chemistry, Medical University of Lublin, 1 Chodzki Str., 20-093 Lublin, Poland; kskalicka@pharmacognosy.org
* Correspondence: ichinou@pharm.uoa.gr; Tel.: +30-210-727-4595

Abstract: As part of our ongoing research on phytoconstituents that can act as promising antimicrobial agents, the essential oils of nine selected Apiaceae plants, cultivated in Poland, were studied. The volatiles of the aerial parts with fruits (*herba cum fructi*) of *Silaum silaus*, *Seseli devenyense*, *Seseli libanotis*, *Ferula assa-foetida*, *Glehnia littoralis* and *Heracleum dulce*, in addition to the fruits (*fructi*) of *Torilis japonica* and *Orlaya grandiflora* as well as of the aerial parts (*herba*) of *Peucedanum luxurians* were investigated through Gas Chromatography–Mass Spectrometry to identify more than 60 different metabolites. The essential oils from *S. devenyense*, *H. dulce*, *T. japonica* and *P. luxurians* are reported for the first time. All examined species were also assayed for their antimicrobial activities against several human pathogenic Gram-positive and -negative bacteria and fungi. The species *H. dulce*, *S. devenyense* and *S. libanotis* exerted the strongest antimicrobial activity, mostly against Gram-positive bacteria strains (MIC values 0.90–1.20 mg/mL). To the best of our knowledge, this is the first attempt to determine the antimicrobial activity of the above Apiaceae species.

Keywords: Apiaceae; gas chromatography-mass spectrometry; volatiles; antimicrobial activity; coumarins

1. Introduction

Aromatic plants and their essential oils have been used therapeutically for centuries, while many scientific studies are conducted, describing their remarkable healing properties. Essential oils are complex mixtures of natural volatiles, characterized by a strong odor and formed by aromatic plants as secondary metabolites. They are also proven to exert antimicrobial activity against a large number of bacteria and fungi [1].

Apiaceae is considered as one of the most important plant family, including 3780 species and 434 genera [2]. They are mainly distributed in the Mediterranean basin with high economic importance for the food and cosmetic industry [3]. Plant secondary products typically found in Apiaceae are essential oils, including terpenoids and phenylpropanoids, coumarins and furanocoumarins, sesquiterpenelactones, polyacetylenes (polyines), and further compounds derived from acetate units, such as alkylphthalides and the toxic piperidine alkaloids [4]. Plants of the Apiaceae family are used widely in folk medicine for the treatment of several human ailments [5]. In several scientific studies, they have shown antimicrobial and antioxidant activity, and they are considered as promising sources of bioactive agents [5–8].

In the framework of our ongoing research on umbelliferous plants [1,9–16], we report in this study the chemical analyses of volatiles from nine plants of Apiaceae family, which are cultivated in Poland, which to our knowledge have scarcely been studied phytochemically before.

The incidence of microbial infections has increased dramatically together with emergence of antimicrobial resistant strains [15], thus discovering alternative potentially effective treatments for such infectious diseases is a challenge. Furthermore, phytoconstituents are widely considered as promising agents for antimicrobial therapy [15].

The aim of our study is to evaluate the chemical profile and the antimicrobial activity of nine selected Apiaceae species (Table 1).

Table 1. Apiaceae species analyzed in this study.

Plant Species Studied	Plants Parts Studied	Yield %
Silaum silaus (L.) Schinz & Thell.	aerial parts with fruits (*herba cum fructi*)	0.10
Seseli devenyense Simonkai		0.18
Seseli libanotis (L.) W.D.J.Koch		0.20
Glehnia littoralis F. Schmidt ex Miq.		0.15
Ferula assa-foetida L.		0.32
Heracleum dulce Fisch., C.A.Mey. & Avé-Lall.,		0.18
Torillis japonica (Houtt.) DC.	fruits (*fructi*)	0.25
Orlaya grandiflora (L.) Hoffm		0.22
Peucedanum luxurians Tamamsch.	aerial parts (*herba*)	0.14

The obtained essential oils have been chemically analyzed through GC and GC/MS. Moreover, they have been investigated for their potential antimicrobial activity against Gram-positive and negative bacteria as well as against human pathogenic fungi, as essential oils are known as potential sources of novel compounds with antibacterial properties.

2. Materials and Methods

2.1. Plant Material

The aerial parts and fruits of all studied plant material were collected from three botanical gardens: Botanical Garden of University of Marie Curie-Skłodowska (UMCS), Lublin, Poland; Botanical Garden Adam Mickiewicz University, Poznan, Poland; Pharmacognostic Garden, Dept. of Pharmacognosy, Medical University of Lublin as well as from wild (Lublin region). Species cultivated in Botanical Garden of UMCS were *Seseli libanotis* (voucher specimen: 56_2018) and *Orlaya grandiflora* (voucher specimen: 49_2018). *Peucedanum luxuriansn* was collected in Botanical Garden of Poznań (voucher specimen: 7973_S003). *Torilis japonica* was collected in natural state (190_2019). The rest studied species were cultivated in Pharmacognostic Garden of Lublin: *Silaum silaus* (voucher specimen: 52_2019), *Seseli devenyense* (voucher specimen: 44_2019), *Glehnia littoralis* (voucher specimen: 180_2019), *Ferula asa-foetida* (voucher specimen: 22_2019). Plant material from the Botanical Garden of Poznan was identified by Grażyna Naser while all the rest species (from Lublin) was confirmed by dr Agnieszka Dąbrowska from Botanical Garden of UMCS.

2.2. Experimental

The air dried and powdered plants were submitted to hydrodistillation. About 10 g of the dried whole fruits, crushed leaves and finely chopped stems were subjected to hydro distillation for 2 h in a Clevenger type apparatus containing 200 mL of distilled water. After recording the yield of oil, n-pentane was added to collect the oil, which was stored at $-20\ ^\circ$C until GC/MS and GC analyses. The collected essential oils were dried over anhydrous sodium sulphate.

2.3. GC Analysis

The GC analyses were carried out on a Perkin-Elmer 8500 gas chromatograph with FID, fitted with a Supelcowax-10 fused silica capillary column (30 m × 0.32 mm i.d.,

0.25 µm film thickness). The column temperature was programmed from 60 to 280 °C at a rate of 2.5 °C/min. The injector and detector temperatures were programmed at 230 and 300 °C, respectively. Helium was used as carrier gas, flow rate 1 mL/min.

The GC-MS analyses were performed with an Agilent 7820A Gas Chromatograph System (Shanghai, China) linked to Agilent5977B mass spectrometer system (Santa Clara, CA, USA) equipped with a 30 m length, 0.25 mm id and 0.5 µm film thickness HP5-MS capillary column. The initial column temperature is 60 °C and then increases at a rate of 3 °C/min to a maximum temperature of 280 °C, where it remains for 15 min. Total analysis time was 93 min. Helium was used as a carrier gas at a flow rate of 2.2 mL/min, split ratio 1:10, injector temperature 220 °C, and ionization voltage 70 eV. The compound identification was conducted using the NIST14 library and bibliographic data [17].

2.4. Antimicrobial Activity

In vitro antibacterial study of the studied volatiles was carried out via the agar dilution method in 96-well plates, by measuring the MIC values against two Gram-positive bacteria: *Staphylococcus aureus* (ATCC 25923), *Staphylococcus epidermidis* (ATCC 12228), four Gram-negative bacteria: *Escherichia coli* (ATCC 25922), *Enterobacter cloacae* (ATCC 13047), *Klebsiella pneumoniae* (ATCC 13883) and *Pseudomonas aeruginosa* (ATCC 227853), as well as against three human pathogen fungi: *Candida albicans* (ATCC 10231), *C. tropicalis* (ATCC 13801) and *C. glabrata* (ATCC 28838). Stock solutions of the samples were prepared at 10 and 1 mg/mL, respectively. Serial dilutions of the stock solutions in broth medium (100 µL of Müller–Hinton broth or on Sabouraud broth) were prepared in a microtiter plate (96 wells). All tested organisms have a final cell concentration of 10^7 cell/mL. Then 1 µL of the microbial suspension (the inoculum, in sterile distilled water) was added to each well. For each strain, the growth conditions and the sterility of the medium were checked, and the plates were incubated as referred above. MICs were determined as the lowest concentrations preventing visible growth. Standard antibiotic netilmicin and amoxicillin (at concentrations 4–88 µg/mL) were used in order to control the sensitivity of the tested bacteria, while 5-fluocytosine and amphotericin B (at concentrations 0.5–25 µg/mL) were used as controls against the tested fungi. The experiments were repeated three times, and the results were expressed as average values [18].

3. Results and Discussion

3.1. Chemical Analysis

Silaum silaus (L.) Schinz & Thell., or pepper saxifrage, occurs from Europe to West Siberia and North Caucasus. Plants flowers in summer and fruits are developed by autumn. Whole plant has been used to treat bladder diseases, and leaves are edible as potherbs [19]. The analysis of the essential oil from the aerial parts of *S. silaus* (Table 2) showed the presence of 14 metabolites (87.18% of the total) among which α-pinene (22.48%), myristicin (20.01%), methyl eugenol (9.80%), methyl isoeugenol (7.60%), o-cymene (6.47%), E-β-ocimene (5.97%) and γ-terpinene (4.41%) were the most abundant ones. These results are in agreement with previous bibliographic data for *S. silaus* samples from different areas in Austria. In that study, myristicin was the main compound of the essential oil from the fruits (approx. 60%), followed by E-β-ocimene and α-pinene, while of the leaves and stems, α-pinene (30%) predominated, with E-β-ocimene and myristicin as further major compounds [19]. The abundant chemical category of the compounds in this oil is the monoterpene hydrocarbons followed by phenylpropene and alcohols (Table 3).

Table 2. The composition of Apiaceae essential oils.

Compounds	Silaum silaus	Seseli devenyense	Seseli libanotis	Glehnia littoralis	Ferula assa-foetida	Torilis japonica	Orlaya grandiflora	Peucedanum luxurians
α-pinene	22.48	0.84	1.90	0.50	5.24	-	-	-
camphene	-	0.2	0.20	-	-	-	-	-
sabinene	0.65	-	18.37	-	1.28	-	-	-
myrcene	3.02	-	1.25	-	18.74	-	-	1.33
β-pinene	-	0.48	0.57	2.30	-	-	-	-
propyl octanoate	-	-	-	18.80	-	-	-	-
β-elemene	-	-	1.97	-	-	18.12	-	-
γ-elemene	-	-	2.20	5.94	-	-	-	-
δ-elemene	-	-	-	-	-	-	-	5.10
β-caryophyllene	-	3.30	28.70	-	-	11.02	18.83	8.84
limonene	-	0.48	-	-	4.01	-	-	-
β-phellandrene	-	-	13.16	16.26	0.18	-	-	-
δ-3-carene	2.49	0.05	-	1.21	1.45	-	-	-
p-cymene	-	0.17	1.66	0.55	-	-	-	-
o-cymene	6.47	-	-	-	-	-	-	-
tricyclene	-	-	0.41	-	-	-	-	-
geranyl acetate	-	5.31	-	-	-	-	-	-
Z-β-ocimene	-	0.38	-	-	0.16	-	-	-
E-β-ocimene	5.97	0.08	-	-	0.38	-	-	-
α-amorphene	-	7.97	0.60	-	-	-	8.56	-
eugenol	0.10	-	-	-	8.05	-	-	-
methyl eugenol	9.80	-	-	-	20.75	-	-	-
Z-methyl isoeugenol	0.95	-	-	-	-	-	-	-
γ-terpinene	4.41	0.11	0.36	-	2.83	-	-	-
meta-tolualdeyde	-	0.35	-	-	0.21	-	-	-
terpinolene	0.34	0.06	-	-	1.93	-	-	-
anethole	-	-	-	1.81	0.11	-	-	-
β-cubebene	-	-	-	-	0.35	-	-	-
α-humulene	-	-	-	-	-	0.97	-	-
trans-β-farnesene	-	-	1.36	1.73	-	-	-	16.35
germacrene D	2.80	4.70	1.96	0.65	5.75	9.33	7.27	13.76
bicyclo-germacrene	-	-	1.67	-	-	-	-	-
α-germacrene	-	-	-	-	-	8.29	-	-
α-muurolene	-	3.57	-	-	-	-	-	-

Table 2. Cont.

Compounds	Silaum silaus	Seseli devenyense	Seseli libanotis	Glehnia littoralis	Ferula assa-foetida	Torilis japonica	Orlaya grandiflora	Peucedanum luxurians
γ-muurolene	-	3.67	-	-	-	-	-	-
E-methyl isoeugenol	7.60	-	-	-	25.46	-	-	-
α-zingiberene	-	-	-	-	-	-	-	10.58
β-sesquiphellandrene	-	17.79	-	-	-	-	-	3.72
δ-cadinene	-	-	-	0.79	0.70	1.12	10.83	-
α-cadinene	-	-	-	-	-	-	2.48	-
myristicin	20.01	-	-	-	-	-	-	-
palmitic acid	-	-	-	16.45	-	-	-	-
spathulenol	0.09	5.70	12.80	0.59	0.31	-	–	-
germacrene B	-	-	-	4.06	-	-	0.33	-
calamenene	-	-	-	0.42	-	-	-	-
t-cadinol	-	-	-	-	0.71	-	5.33	-
1,6-germacradien-5-ol	-	-	-	-	-	38.46	-	-
4,5-dehydro-isolongifolene	-	-	-	2.48	-	-	-	-
linoleic acid	-	-	-	9.70	-	-	-	-
oleic acid	-	-	-	3.17	-	-	-	-
unknown compounds	-	29.09	-	-	-	-	28.64	26.50
Total (%)	87.18	84.30	89.14	87.41	98.6	87.31	82.27	86.18

-: not detected.

Table 3. Chemical categories (% area) in the studied Apiaceae essential oils.

Chemical Categories	S. silaus	S. devenyense	S. libanotis	G. littoralis	F. assa-foetida	H. dulce	T. japonica	O. grandiflora	P. luxurians
Monoterpene hydrocarbons	45.83	2.85	37.88	20.82	36.2	-	-	-	1.33
Sesquiterpene hydrocarbons	2.80	41.0	38.46	16.07	6.8	2.01	48.85	48.3	58.35
Phenylpropene	20.01	-	-	1.81	0.11	-	-	-	-
Aldehydes	-	0.35	-	-	0.21	-	-	-	-
Alcohols	18.54	5.70	12.80	0.59	55.28	-	38.46	5.33	-
Esters	-	5.31	-	18.80	-	-	-	-	-
Fatty acids	-	-	-	29.32	-	27.84	-	-	-
Coumarins	-	-	-	-	-	58.38	-	-	-
Unknown	-	29.09	-	-	-	-	-	28.64	26.50

Seseli devenyense Simonkai (*Seseli elatum* subsp. *osseum* (Crantz) P.W.Ball.) was studied exhaustively previously, by our scientific team [12,13] as a source of several coumarins, which have been isolated and structurally determined, while its essential oil has never been studied before. In the present work, *S devenyense* yielded 0.18% of essential oil, consisting of 19 components (Table 2) with β-sesquiphellandrene (17.8%), amorphene (8%), spathulenol (5.7%) and geranyl acetate (5.30%) as main ones. Sesquiterpene hydrocarbons is the abundant chemical category with percentage 41% of the total (Table 3).

Seseli libanotis (L.) W.D.J. Koch is an aromatic plant widely distributed from Central Europe to West Siberia. In Turkish folk medicine, the aerial parts of the plant were popularly used against inflammations as well as antinociceptive agent probably due to its coumarins' content. The leaves of *S. libanotis* are consumed as a vegetable in Turkey [1]. The essential oil composition from different geographic areas in Austria has been studied, and monoterpenes such as α-pinene, sabinene and β-myrcene and the sesquiterpene germacrene D were present in all essential oils from its aerial parts [20]. Root's volatiles have been also studied and were dominated by α-pinene [20], while in a study on the fruits of the plant [1] sabinene and β-phellandrene appeared as the most abundant metabolites. Volatiles obtained from the aerial parts of the plant from Iran has shown trans-caryophyllene (20%) as the main constituent, followed by limonene, α-pinene and caryophyllene oxide [21]. The essential oil from *S. libanotis*, in the present study (yield 0.20%), appeared a rich chemical profile (Table 2) with 17 identified metabolites (89.14%), dominated by β-carryophyllene (28.70%), sabinene (18.37%), together with β-phellandrene (13.16%) and spathulenol (12.80%) as major ones. In this oil the percentage of monoterpene and sesquiterpene hydrocarbons is equally high (~38%).

Glehnia littoralis F. Schmidt ex Miq. essential oils from aerial and root parts have been investigated previously only in Japan, and the main constituents of the essential oils were found to be α-pinene, limonene, β-phellandrene, germacrene B, spathulenol, β-oplopenone, panaxynol, propyl octanoate, hexadecanoic acid and linoleic acid [22]. Moreover, oral administration of certain extracts of *Glehnia* root prolonged pentobarbital-induced sleeping time due to inhibition of liver metabolizing enzymes and have caused analgesic effects in vivo in mice [23]. In this study, the composition of the essential oil (yield 0.15%) of the aerial parts together with fruits (Table 2) is comparable to previously investigated essential oil from aerial and root parts [22] as propyl octanoate (18.80%), palmitic acid (16.45%), β-phellandrene (16.26%), γ-elemene (5.94%) and germacrene B (4.06%) were the most abundant compounds. It is noteworthy that this is the only essential oil with high percentage of fatty acids (29.32%), followed by monoterpene and sesquiterpene hydrocarbons as well as by esters.

Ferula assa-foetida L. is a perennial herb distributed throughout the Mediterranean area and central Asia. It is reputed in Iranian and Indian traditional medicine for its therapeutic applications against a number of different disorders [24,25] and in food industry, due to the occurrence of essential oils and/or mainly oleoresin possessing strong aromatic scent [26]. It contains mainly sesquiterpene coumarins, phenolics and volatile compounds (especially sulfur compounds) [26,27]. The most frequent compounds that occurred among the main constituents of *Ferula* oils were α-pinene, β-pinene, myrcene and limonene (among monoterpene hydrocarbons); linalool, α-terpineol and neryl acetate (among oxygenated monoterpenes); β-caryophyllene, germacrene B, germacrene D and δ-cadinene (among sesquiterpene hydrocarbons); caryophyllene oxide, α-cadinol, guaiol and spathulenol (among oxygenated sesquiterpenes) and sec-butyl-(Z)-propenyl disulfide and sec-butyl-(E)-propenyl disulfide (among sulfur-containing compounds) [24]. In our study, the essential oil (yield 0.32%) exerted a rich chemical profile of 20 constituents (Table 2) belonging to monoterpene and sesquiterpene hydrocarbons. Methyl isoeugenol (25.46%), methyl eugenol (20.75%), myrcene (18.74%), germacrene D (5.75%), α-pinene (5.24%), and limonene (4.01%) have been detected in *F. assa-foetida*, while it is characteristic the absence of sulfur-containing compounds (butyl-propenyl disulfides) which have been referred in other chemical studies and the fact that alcohols is the abundant category (more than 50%).

Furthermore, the aerial parts of *Heracleum dulce* Fisch., C.A.Mey. & Avé-Lall., not having been previously studied phytochemically, showed a unique chemical profile (Table 4) as it contained mainly coumarins (58.38%), several of which have been identified and a high percentage of fatty acids.

Table 4. The composition of the essential oil from *Heracleum dulce*.

Compounds	H. dulce
Psoralene	0.73
palmitic acid	0.77
psoralene-8-hydroxy (xanthotoxol)	4.87
xanthotoxin	2.88
bergapten	1.04
germacrene D	2.01
linoleic acid	7.10
oleic acid	19.46
8-heptadecenoic acid	0.51
coumarin	0.84
coumarin	18.04
coumarin	5.58
coumarin	5.39
coumarin	13.33
coumarin	0.61
coumarin	0.47
allo-imperatorin	0.75
coumarin	3.85
Hexadecyl oleate	0.67
Total (%)	88.90

Torilis japonica D.C. (Japanese name "Jabujirami") is widespread in East Asia (China, Korea, Mongolia and Russia), also naturalized in the warmer areas of Europe. Its fruits were used as a substitute medicament of the She-Chuang-Zi (*Cnidium monnieri* fructi, snowparsley), known for promoting healthy libido and fertility levels. They have been studied phytochemically twice before and had afforded to new hemiterpenoid pentol and monoterpenoid glycosides [28] as well as guaiane-type sesquiterpenoid glycosides [29]. The essential oil of the plant, to the best of our knowledge, has never been investigated before. In the present study, through the chemical investigation of its volatiles (yield 0.25%), the metabolites 1,6-germacradien-5-ol (38.46%), β-elemene (18.12%), β-caryophyllene (11.02%), germacrene D (9.33%) and α-germacrene (8.29%) appeared as the main compounds (Table 2). In this essential oil, only sesquiterpenes and alcohols are present.

The essential oil of the aerial parts of *Orlaya grandiflora* (L.) Hoffm., the white laceflower, growing wild in Central Balkan area, has been reported once before [30], where sabinene, a-pinene followed by γ-terpinene, β-caryophyllene and germacrene D have been identified as abundant compounds. The volatiles from the fruits essential oil of *O. grandiflora* (yield 0.22%) have been examined in this study, where β-caryophyllene (18.83%), δ-cadinene (10.83%), α-amorhene (8.56%) and germacrene D (7.27%) appeared as the major constituents and all of them belong to sesqiterpenes (Table 2). It is obvious that out of the identification of germacrene D in both oils, their chemical profiles did not show any other similarities.

Finally, herba of *Peucedanum luxurians* was studied phytochemically before, as a source of rare bioactive furanocourmarins with unique structures by our scientific team [3,6–8], while its volatiles have never been studied until now. *P luxurians* is an endemic plant from Armenia, growing in the area around Mount Ararat [31]. In the present study, the analysis revealed the presence of *trans*-β-farnesene (16.35%), germacrene D (13.76%) α-zingiberene (10.58%) and β-caryophyllene (8.84%), as the most abundant constituents (Table 2). Among its constituents, one (26.50%) remained unidentified, which unfortunately due to the low yield of the oil (0.14%) was not possible to be further isolated and structurally determined, while the majority of the identified compounds belong to the sesquiterpenes (Table 3).

3.2. Antimicrobial Activity Evaluation

All essential oils assayed against a panel of nine human pathogenic microbia, two Gram-positive (*Staphylococcus aureus, S. epidermidis*), four Gram-negative (*Escherichia coli, Pseudomonas aeruginosa, Klebsiella pneumoniae* and *Enterobacte cloacae*) as well as against three fungi strains (*Candida albicans, C. tropicalis* and *C. glabrata*). According to the results presented in Table 5, the essential oils of *G. littoralis* and *T. japonica* appeared completely inactive against all assayed microbial strains. *S. silaus* showed a moderate activity against Gram-positive bacteria *S. aureus* and *S. epidermidis* (MIC values 1.25, 1.48 mg/mL, respectively) and a very weak activity against Gram-negative bacteria (MIC values 7.38–13.45 mg/mL), while being inactive against all *Candidas'* strains. *O. grandiflora* compared to *S. silaus* exerted a stronger activity specifically against both Gram-positive strains (1.52 and 1.60 mg/mL). *S. libanotis* aerial parts' volatiles exerted moderate activity against Gram-positive bacteria (MIC 1.35, 1.47 mg/mL, respectively) and weak activities against all the Gram-negative bacteria and the fungi. Corresponding results to that of *S. libanotis* were revealed from *S. devenyense* (MIC 1.35, 1.20 mg/mL). These results are in agreement with previously published data, where Gram-negative bacteria are less sensitive to essential oils obtained from plants belonging to the Apiaceae family [1]. The essential oil from *F. assa-foetida* showed a weak activity against all tested microorganisms, while *P. luxurians* appeared together with *H. dulce* as the most active among all assayed essential oils exerting activity against all assayed microorganisms. More specifically *H. dulce* showed strong activity against Gram-positive bacteria (MIC values 0.90 and 0.87 mg/mL) and a moderate one against the rest Gram-negative ones (MIC values 3.30–4.05 mg/mL), while it was the only one, which exhibited activity (weak) against the three assayed fungi (MIC values 4.0–4.9 mg/mL). *P. luxurians* expressed also strong activity against Gram-positive bacteria (MIC values 1.0–1.20 mg/mL) and weaker against Gram-negative one (MIC values 2.80–5.76 mg/mL) and the tested fungi (MIC values 4.87–6.89 mg/mL).

Table 5. Antimicrobial activity of the tested essential oils compared to common antimicrobial agents (mg/mL).

	S. aureus	S. epidermidis	P. aeruginosa	E. cloacae	K. pnaumioniae	E. coli	C. albicans	C. tropicalis	C. glabrata
S. silaus	1.80	1.25	8.70	13.45	10.27	7.38	>20	>20	>20
S. devenyense	1.35	1.20	12.80	12.00	11.62	13.41	10.70	9.65	9.00
S. libanotis	1.35	1.47	5.68	6.00	6.32	6.70	12.35	11.45	10.80
G. littoralis	>20	>20	>20	>20	>20	>20	>20	>20	>20
F. assa-foetida	7.23	6.80	5.70	4.65	5.23	4.35	7.65	5.43	4.30
H. dulce	0.90	0.87	3.30	3.84	4.05	3.92	4.90	4.78	4.00
T. japonica	>20	>20	>20	>20	>20	>20	>20	>20	>20
O. grandiflora	1.60	1.52	8.70	9.60	12.32	15.70	16.30	12.27	11.90
P. luxurians	1.20	1.00	2.80	>20	5.76	3.43	6.89	5.94	4.87
itraconazol	nt	nt	nt	nt	nt	nt	1.0×10^{-3}	0.1×10^{-3}	1×10^{-3}
5-flucytocine	nt	nt	nt	nt	nt	nt	0.1×10^{-3}	1.0×10^{-3}	9.7×10^{-3}
amphotericin B	nt	nt	nt	nt	nt	nt	1.0×10^{-3}	0.5×10^{-3}	0.4×10^{-3}
amoxicillin	1.8×10^{-3}	1.5×10^{-3}	2.5×10^{-3}	2.7×10^{-3}	3.1×10^{-3}	2.1×10^{-3}	nt	nt	nt
netilmicin	3.0×10^{-3}	2.9×10^{-3}	7.0×10^{-3}	7.8×10^{-3}	6.8×10^{-3}	3.1×10^{-3}	nt	nt	nt

nt: not tested.

4. Conclusions

The analyses of the essential oils of nine selected Apiaceae plants, all of them cultivated in Poland, resulted to some new data for *Seseli devenyense*, *Heracleum dulce*, *Torillis japonica* and *Peucedanum luxurians* as they have never been studied before for their volatiles. Moreover, the essential oils from *Silaum silaus* and *Orlaya grandiflora* have been analyzed for the second time, showing differences in their chemical profile probably due to different cultivation, climate and geographic conditions [32–34]. *Glehnia littoralis* essential oil, cultivated in Europe, was analyzed for the first time, while *Seseli libanotis* was studied for the second time in Europe showing differences in comparison with published data. *Ferula assa-foetida* was also analyzed in this study due to its wide use and in order to compare its chemical profile with previously reported data.

In general, the identified compounds showed a great variability among investigated Apiaceae species. Among approx. 60 different metabolites, which were identified, sesquiterpene germacrene D was the only metabolite common in all nine essential oils. It is noteworthy that the chemical profile of *Heracleum dulce* was completely different from all the other studied species, as it contains mainly coumarins. Moreover, it is also of interest that the high proportion content of myristicin in the *S. silaus* essential oil, which together with α-pinene, and α-caryophyllene were also present in many other plants of the Apiaceae family.

The essential oils or some of their constituents are very effective against a large variety of organisms including bacteria and fungi. As typical lipophiles, they disrupt the structure of the cytoplasmic membrane and permeabilize them. In bacteria, the permeabilization of the membranes is associated with loss of ions and reduction of membrane potential [1,15].

Throughout the antimicrobial tests, *Peucedanum luxurians* together with *Heracleum dulce* appeared as the most active among all assayed essential oils, exerting activity against all assayed microorganisms. These results are in agreement with bibliographic data, as selected *Peucedanum* plants (*P. paniculatum*, *P. alsaticum*, *P. cervaria*, *P. graveolens*, *P. ruthenicum*, *P. zenkeri* and *P. ostruthium*) have been used for centuries as antibacterial agents, and for some of them, the activity was confirmed by biological and pharmacological studies, showing moderate or high activity against different human pathogens [15].

Additionally, *Heracleum dulce* essential oil was full of coumarins, and its exerted bioactivity could be contributed mainly to these compounds. Coumarins, naturally plant-derived metabolites, possess a wide variety of known bioactivities. Series of coumarin analogues naturally-isolated coumarins, as well as their chemically modified analogs, are being extensively studied due to their broad spectrum, low toxicity, and lower drug resistance properties [9,11,13–15]. Moreover, isolated furanocoumarins, from different Apiaceae species (like imperatorin, bergapten, ostruthin, and isoimperatorin) were found to be very active antimicrobial agents [35–37]. The above data suggest that several among the studied essential oils may be an alternative promising way to treat various infections with further extension towards cosmetic and pharmaceutical applications.

Author Contributions: Conceptualization, I.C., J.W., K.G.; methodology, K.G.; investigation, I.C., K.G., J.W., C.G., K.S.-W.; data curation, K.G., J.W.; writing—original draft preparation, K.G., C.G., I.C.; writing—review and editing, K.G., I.C.; supervision, I.C. All authors have read and agreed to the published version of the manuscript.

Funding: This research was founded by DS 28, Medical University of Lublin.

Acknowledgments: Authors would like to thank Justyna Wiland-Szymańska and Grażyna Naser (Botanical Garden of Adam Mickiewicz University in Poznań) and Grażyna Szymczak and Agnieszka Dąbrowska (Botanical Garden of UMCS) for plant material of excellent quality and great assistance in obtaining it and identifying the numerous species used in the study.

Conflicts of Interest: The authors declare no conflict of interest.

References

1. Skalicka-Wozniak, K.; Los, R.; Glowniak, K.; Malm, A. Comparison of Hydrodistillation and Headspace Solid-Phase Micro-extraction Techniques for Antibacterial Volatile Compounds from the Fruits of *Seseli libanotis*. *Nat. Prod. Commun.* **2010**, *5*, 1427–1430. [PubMed]
2. Sayed-Ahmad, B.; Talou, T.; Saad, Z.; Hijazi, A.; Merah, O. The Apiaceae: Ethnomedicinal family as source for industrial uses. *Ind. Crop. Prod.* **2017**, *109*, 661–671. [CrossRef]
3. Kamte, S.L.N.; Ranjbarian, F.; Cianfaglione, K.; Sut, S.; Dall'Acqua, S.; Bruno, M.; Afshar, F.H.; Iannarelli, R.; Benelli, G.; Cappellacci, L.; et al. Identification of highly effective antitrypanosomal compounds in essential oils from the Apiaceae family. *Ecotoxicol. Environ. Saf.* **2018**, *156*, 154–165. [CrossRef]
4. Chizzola, R. Essential Oil Composition of Wild Growing Apiaceae from Europe and the Mediterranean. *Nat. Prod. Commun.* **2010**, *5*, 1477–1492. [CrossRef] [PubMed]
5. Zengin, G.; Sinan, K.I.; Ak, G.; Mahomoodally, M.F.; Paksoy, M.Y.; Picot-Allain, C.; Glamocilja, J.; Sokovic, M.; Jekő, J.; Cziá-ky, Z.; et al. Chemical profile, antioxidant, antimicrobial, enzyme inhibitory, and cyto-toxicity of seven Apiaceae species from Turkey: A comparative study. *Ind. Crops Prod.* **2020**, *153*, 112572. [CrossRef]
6. Hasheminya, S.-M.; Dehghannya, J. Chemical composition, antioxidant, antibacterial, and antifungal properties of essential oil from wild *Heracleum rawianum*. *Biocatal. Agric. Biotechnol.* **2021**, *31*, 101913. [CrossRef]
7. Pateiro, M.; Munekata, P.E.; Sant'Ana, A.S.; Domínguez, R.; Rodríguez-Lázaro, D.; Lorenzo, J.M. Application of essential oils as antimicrobial agents against spoilage and pathogenic microorganisms in meat products. *Int. J. Food Microbiol.* **2021**, *337*, 108966. [CrossRef]
8. Süzgeç-Selçuk, S.; Dikpınar, T. Phytochemical evaluation of the Ferulago genus and the pharmacological activities of its coumarin constituents. *J. Herb. Med.* **2021**, *25*, 100415. [CrossRef]
9. Melliou, E.; Magiatis, P.; Mitaku, S.; Skaltsounis, A.-L.; Chinou, E.; Chinou, I. Natural and Synthetic 2,2-Dimethylpyranocoumarins with Antibacterial Activity. *J. Nat. Prod.* **2005**, *68*, 78–82. [CrossRef]
10. Chinou, I.; Widelski, J.; Fokialakis, N.; Magiatis, P.; Glowniak, K. Coumarins from *Peucedanum luxurians*. *Fitoterapia* **2007**, *78*, 448–449. [CrossRef]
11. Widelski, J.; Popova, M.; Graikou, K.; Glowniak, K.; Chinou, I. Coumarins from *Angelica lucida* L.-Antibacterial Activities. *Molecules* **2009**, *14*, 2729–2734. [CrossRef] [PubMed]
12. Widelski, J.; Melliou, E.; Fokialakis, N.; Magiatis, P.; Glowniak, K.; Chinou, I. Coumarins from the Fruits of *Seseli devenyense*. *J. Nat. Prod.* **2005**, *68*, 1637–1641. [CrossRef]
13. Widelski, J.; Grzegorczyk, A.; Malm, A.; Chinou, I.; Główniak, K. Antimicrobial activity of petroleum ether and methanolic extracts from fruits of Seseli devenyense Simonk. and the herb of *Peucedanum luxurians* Tamam. *Curr. Issues Pharm. Med. Sci.* **2015**, *28*, 257–259. [CrossRef]
14. Widelski, J.; Kukula-Koch, W.; Baj, T.; Kedzierski, B.; Fokialakis, N.; Magiatis, P.; Pozarowski, P.; Rolinski, J.; Graikou, K.; Chinou, I.; et al. Rare Coumarins Induce Apoptosis, G1 Cell Block and Reduce RNA Content in HL60 Cells. *Open Chem.* **2017**, *15*, 1–6. [CrossRef]

15. Widelski, J.; Vlad Luca, S.; Skiba, A.; Chinou, I.; Marcourt, L.; Wolfender, J.L.; Skalicka-Woźniak, K. Isolation and antimicrobi-al activity of coumarin derivatives from fruits of *Peucedanum luxurians* Tamamsh. *Molecules* **2018**, *23*, 1222. [CrossRef] [PubMed]
16. Kontaratou, V.; Widelski, J.; Wojtowicz, I.; Glowniak, K.; Chinou, I. Volatiles from three Apiaceae species. In Proceedings of the 5th International Symposium on Chromatography of Natural Products, Lublin, Poland, 19–22 June 2006.
17. Adams, R.P. *Identification of Essential Oil Components by Gas Chromatography/Mass Spectrometry*; Allured Publishing Corporation: Carol Stream, IL, USA, 2007; Volume 456.
18. Atsalakis, E.; Chinou, I.; Makropoulou, M.; Karabournioti, S.; Graikou, K. Evaluation of Phenolic Compounds in Cistus cre-ticus Bee Pollen from Greece. Antioxidant and Antimicrobial Properties. *Nat. Prod. Commun.* **2017**, *12*, 1813–1816.
19. Chizzola, R. Variability of the Volatile Oil Composition in a Population of *Silaum silaus* from Eastern Austria. *Nat. Prod. Commun.* **2008**, *3*, 1141–1144. [CrossRef]
20. Chizzola, R. Chemodiversity of Essential Oils in Seseli libanotis (L.) W.D.J. Koch (*Apiaceae*) in Central Europe. *Chem. Biodivers.* **2019**, *16*. [CrossRef]
21. Masoudi, S.; Esmaeili, A.; Ali khalilzadeh, M.; Rustaiyan, A.; Moazami, N.; Akhgar, M.R.; Varavipoor, M. Volatile Constitu-ents of *Dorema aucheri* Boiss., *Seseli libanotis* (L.) WD Koch *var. armeniacum* Bordz. and *Conium maculatum* L. Three Umbel-liferae Herbs Growing Wild in Iran. *Flavour Fragr. J.* **2006**, *21*, 801–804. [CrossRef]
22. Miyazawa, M.; Kurose, K.; Itoh, A.; Hiraoka, N. Comparison of the Essential Oils of Glehnia littoralis from Northern and Southern Japan. *J. Agric. Food Chem.* **2001**, *49*, 5433–5436. [CrossRef] [PubMed]
23. Okuyama, E.; Hasegawa, T.; Matsushita, T.; Fujimoto, H.; Ishibashi, M.; Yamazaki, M.; Hosokawa, M.; Hiraoka, N.; Anetal, M.; Masuda, T. Analgesic Components of Glehnia Root (*Glehnia littoralis*). *J. Nat. Med.* **1998**, *52*, 491–501.
24. Sahebkar, A.; Iranshahi, M. Volatile Constituents of the Genus Ferula (*Apiaceae*): A Review. *J. Essent. Oil Bear. Plants* **2011**, *14*, 504–531. [CrossRef]
25. Mohammad, N.S.; Dehpour, A.A.; Ebrahimzadeh, M.A.; Fazel, N.S. Antioxidant activity of the methanol extract of Ferula assafoetida and its essential oil composition. *Grasas Aceites* **2009**, *60*, 405–412. [CrossRef]
26. Farhadi, F.; Iranshahi, M.; Taghizadeh, S.F.; Asili, J. Volatile sulfur compounds: The possible metabolite pattern to identify the sources and types of asafoetida by headspace GC/MS analysis. *Ind. Crop. Prod.* **2020**, *155*. [CrossRef]
27. Kavoosi, G.; Tafsiry, A.; Ebdam, A.A.; Rowshan, V. Evaluation of Antioxidant and Antimicrobial Activities of Essential Oils from *Carum copticum* Seed and *Ferula asafoetida* Latex. *J. Food Sci.* **2013**, *78*, T356–T361. [CrossRef] [PubMed]
28. Kitajima, J.; Suzuki, N.; Tanaka, Y. ChemInform Abstract: New Guaiane-Type Sesquiterpenoid Glycosides from Torilis japonica Fruit. *Chem. Pharm. Bull.* **1998**, *46*, 1743–1747. [CrossRef]
29. Kitajima, J.; Suzuki, N.; Ishikawa, T.; Tanaka, Y. New Hemiterpenoid Pentol and Monoterpenoid Glycoside of Torilis japonica Fruit, and Consideration of the Origin of Apiose. *Chem. Pharm. Bull.* **1998**, *46*, 1583–1586. [CrossRef]
30. Kapetanos, C.; Karioti, A.; Bojović, S.; Marin, P.; Veljić, M.; Skaltsa, H. Chemical and Principal-Component Analyses of the Essential Oils of Apioideae Taxa (*Apiaceae*) from Central Balkan. *Chem. Biodivers.* **2008**, *5*, 101–119. [CrossRef]
31. Sarkhail, P. Traditional uses, phytochemistry and pharmacological properties of the genus *Peucedanum*: A review. *J. Ethnopharmacol.* **2014**, *156*, 235–270. [CrossRef]
32. Şanli, A.; Karadoğan, T. Geographical Impact On Essential Oil Composition Of Endemic Kundmannia Anatolica Hub.-Mor. (*Apiaceae*). *Afr. J. Tradit. Complement. Altern. Med.* **2017**, *14*, 131–137. [CrossRef]
33. Mekinić, I.G.; Šimat, V.; Ljubenkov, I.; Burčul, F.; Grga, M.; Mihajlovski, M.; Lončar, R.; Katalinić, V.; Skroza, D. Influence of the vegetation period on sea fennel, *Crithmum maritimum* L. (*Apiaceae*), phenolic composition, antioxidant and anticholinesterase activities. *Ind. Crop. Prod.* **2018**, *124*, 947–953. [CrossRef]
34. Msaada, K.; Hosni, K.; Ben Taarit, M.; Chahed, T.; Kchouk, M.E.; Marzouk, B. Changes on essential oil composition of coriander (*Coriandrum sativum* L.) fruits during three stages of maturity. *Food Chem.* **2007**, *102*, 1131–1134. [CrossRef]
35. Schinkovitz, A.; Gibbons, S.; Stavri, M.; Cocksedge, M.J.; Bucar, F. Ostruthin: An Antimycobacterial Coumarin from the Roots of *Peucedanum ostruthium*. *Planta Medica* **2003**, *69*, 369–371. [CrossRef] [PubMed]
36. Gökay, O.; Kühner, D.; Los, M.; Götz, F.; Bertsche, U.; Albert, K. An efficient approach for the isolation, identification and evaluation of antimicrobial plant components on an analytical scale, demonstrated by the example of *Radix imperatoriae*. *Anal. Bioanal. Chem.* **2010**, *398*, 2039–2047. [CrossRef] [PubMed]
37. Ngwendson, J.N.; Bedir, E.; Efange, S.M.N.; Okunji, C.O.; Iwu, M.M.; Schuster, B.G.; Khan, I.A. Constituents of *Peucedanum zenkeri* seeds and their antimicrobial effects. *Pharm.-Int. J. Pharm. Sci.* **2003**, *58*, 587–589.

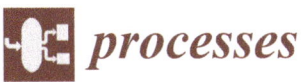

Article

Chemical Profiling of *Pistacia lentiscus* var. *Chia* Resin and Essential Oil: Ageing Markers and Antimicrobial Activity

Vasiliki K. Pachi [1], Eleni V. Mikropoulou [1], Sofia Dimou [2], Mariangela Dionysopoulou [2], Aikaterini Argyropoulou [3], George Diallinas [2,4] and Maria Halabalaki [1,*]

[1] Division of Pharmacognosy and Natural Products Chemistry, Department of Pharmacy, National and Kapodistrian University of Athens, Panepistimiopolis Zografou, 15771 Athens, Greece; vpachi@pharm.uoa.gr (V.K.P.); elenamik@pharm.uoa.gr (E.V.M.)
[2] Department of Biology, National and Kapodistrian University of Athens, Panepistimiopolis Zografou, 15784 Athens, Greece; sofiadimou123@gmail.com (S.D.); mariangeladiony@gmail.com (M.D.); diallina@biol.uoa.gr (G.D.)
[3] PharmaGnose S.A., 57th km Athens—Lamia National Road, 32011 Oinofyta, Greece; kargyropoulou@pharmagnose.com
[4] Institute of Molecular Biology and Biotechnology, Foundation for Research and Technology, 70013 Heraklion, Greece
* Correspondence: mariahal@pharm.uoa.gr; Tel.: +30-2107-2747-81

Abstract: Chios Mastic Gum (CMG) and Chios Mastic Oil (CMO) are two unique products of the tree *Pistacia lentiscus* var. *Chia*, cultivated exclusively on the Greek island of Chios. In the present study, the method proposed by the European Pharmacopoeia for mastic identification was employed using HPTLC together with an in-house method. A GC-MS methodology was also developed for the chemical characterization of CMOs. α-Pinene and β-myrcene were found in abundance in the fresh oils; however, in the oil of the aged collection, oxygenated monoterpenes and benzenoids such as verbenone, pinocarveol, and α-campholenal were found at the highest rates. Additionally, the antimicrobial activity of Chios Mastic Gums (CMGs) with their respective Chios Mastic Oils (CMOs) was evaluated, with growth tests against the fungi *Aspergillus nidulans*, *Aspergillus fumigatus*, *Candida albicans*, *Mucor circinelloides*, and *Rhizopus oryzae*, and the bacteria *Escherichia coli*, *Pseudomonas aeruginosa* and *Bacillus subtilis*, with the samples exhibiting a moderate activity. To our knowledge, this is the first time that an HPTLC method is proposed for the analysis of mastic and its essential oil and that a standardized methodology is followed for the distillation of CMO with a parallel assessment of the ageing effect on the oil's composition.

Keywords: *Pistacia lentiscus* var. *Chia*; Chios mastic; ageing; chemical profile; antibacterial; antifungal; α-pinene; β-myrcene; GC-MS; HPTLC

Citation: Pachi, V.K.; Mikropoulou, E.V.; Dimou, S.; Dionysopoulou, M.; Argyropoulou, A.; Diallinas, G.; Halabalaki, M. Chemical Profiling of *Pistacia lentiscus* var. *Chia* Resin and Essential Oil: Ageing Markers and Antimicrobial Activity. *Processes* **2021**, *9*, 418. https://doi.org/10.3390/pr9030418

Academic Editors: Adriana Trifan, Elwira Sieniawska and Greige-Gerges Helene

Received: 29 January 2021
Accepted: 21 February 2021
Published: 25 February 2021

Publisher's Note: MDPI stays neutral with regard to jurisdictional claims in published maps and institutional affiliations.

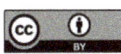

Copyright: © 2021 by the authors. Licensee MDPI, Basel, Switzerland. This article is an open access article distributed under the terms and conditions of the Creative Commons Attribution (CC BY) license (https://creativecommons.org/licenses/by/4.0/).

1. Introduction

Pistacia lentiscus var. *chia* (Anacardiaceae) is an evergreen shrub cultivated exclusively in the southern part of the Greek island of Chios [1]. The most characteristic products are the resin or Chios Mastic Gum (CMG), produced from the wounds of the bark and branches, and the essential oil, Chios Mastic oil (CMO), which is obtained by hydrodistillation from the resin. Even though the *Pistacia* species are widely distributed in the Mediterranean basin and in circum-Mediterranean areas, CMG is a unique resin of the mastic trees grown only in the southern part of the island of Chios. Attempts to cultivate it in different areas, even at the north part of the island, were not successful, failing to produce resin with specific physicochemical and organoleptic characteristics. In that view, CMG and CMO are both Protected Designation of Origin (PDO) products [2] while the know-how of cultivating mastic on the island of Chios was included by UNESCO in the Representative List of the Intangible Cultural Heritage of Humanity [3]. In 2015, *Pistacia lentiscus* L. resin (mastix or mastic), was recognized by the European Medicines Agency (EMA) as a traditional herbal medicinal product with two indications, i.e., for the treatment of mild dyspeptic disorders, skin inflammations, and as an aid in the healing of minor wounds [4].

For over 2500 years, the resin has been used in the ethnopharmacology of the Mediterranean populations. In the 1st century AD, Dioscorides, reported in his work "De Materia Medica" that CMG and CMO were effective against minor gastrointestinal disorders and proposed their use for the skin's and the oral cavity's care [5]. In the 2nd century AD, Galen also reported the beneficial effects of CMG against stomachache and dysentery [6]. Later on, several references can be found containing mastic as an ingredient of multiple medicinal preparations, with probably the most noteworthy being the "Jerusalem balsam", which was served as a "panacea" and was included in numerous European Pharmacopoeias until the 20th century [7].

In contemporary times, CMG and CMO have been studied for their composition as well as their biological and pharmacological properties. However, the number of available studies remains relatively small. CMG and CMO have been reported as potent antioxidant [8,9], anti-inflammatory [10,11], cardioprotective [12–14], and chemopreventive agents [15–19]. Over the recent years, the increasing number of clinical or intervention trials examining the effect of mastic administration on different disease models further validates the Mediterranean populations' inherent knowledge regarding mastic's therapeutic potential. Interestingly, CMG's anti-inflammatory activity has been demonstrated in pilot studies involving patients with active Crohn's disease and inflammatory bowel syndrome (IBS) [10,20], and CMG has been suggested as a possible cardioprotective and hepatoprotective agent in a pilot study describing a long term mastic administration in a human cohort [21]. Moreover, in a prospective, randomized, placebo-controlled clinical study, daily mastic consumption by healthy volunteers led to a significant decrease of their total cholesterol and glucose levels [22], while in a recently published research, mastic administration led to the regulation on peripheral and aortic blood pressure hemodynamics in hypertensive patients [23].

It is worth mentioning that one of the first pharmacological properties of CMG and CMO that were examined by modern day science was their antimicrobial activity, and especially their efficacy against *Helicobacter pylori* and oral and periodontal pathogens [24–30]. In fact, according to the study of Miyamoto et al., CMO exhibits a notable anti-*H. pylori* activity against four different strains, established from patients with gastritis, gastric ulcer, and gastric cancer [26]. In addition, CMO was found potent against several food-borne microorganisms such as *Staphylococcus aureus, Escherichia coli,* and *Salmonella* sp. [24,25,27,29,31]. Furthermore, both CMG and CMO are used in numerous products and have a wide spectrum of applications. CMO is used due to its distinguishing aroma in alcoholic drinks [32] and as a perfume and a perfume stabilizer [33] as well as in cosmetic products for the mouth and skin care [34]. CMG is incorporated in many traditional bakery products, confections, and desserts [32,35]. Moreover, the resin is widely found in food supplements and phytotherapeutic products due to its long-term documented ethnobotanical medicinal use as well as recent studies [34].

From a chemical point of view, CMG constitutes an entity of more than 120 compounds reported thus far, primarily terpenes. Triterpenes, mainly tetracyclic and pentacyclic, constitute the major chemical group of CMG, comprising approximately 65–70% of the total resin weight. Its composition is complemented by the fraction of volatile components which constitute the essential oil of mastic (CMO) [1]. All these compounds coexist with the natural polymer, poly-β-myrcene (25–30% of the dry weight), forming the resin structure. CMO is typically produced by steam and/or water distillation [36], while Supercritical Fluid Extraction (SFE) has been recently developed as an alternative method to the existing ones [37]. CMO constitutes approximately 3% of the resin weight when harvested by the traditional way and about 13% when harvested in a fluid form [38]. The chemical composition of the essential oil has been studied mainly by the GC-MS and GC-FID techniques [38–40].

CMG is often extensively adulterated because of the resin's uniqueness and high commercial value [41]. Adulteration is mainly achieved by mixing mastic with similar resins of lower economic value such as Iranian mastic (*Pistacia atlantica*), *Boswellia* resin (frankincense), or *Pinus* resin, together with packing falsification [42]. However, special attention should be paid to the fact that the *Pistacia lentiscus* var. *Chia* tree, as well as its resin, can be found in the literature with various different names such as "schinos" or "lentisk" without the authors specifying the geographical origin or variety. Additionally, very often, the source of the resin and/or the essential oil under investigation is vague or not defined, a fact which further complicates the identification of *Pistacia lentiscus* originating from Chios island (var *Chia*), which is distinguished for its unique aroma characteristics [43]. CMG is often found in the market as simply mastic or mastic gum, Chios masticha, mastiha, mastihi, and mastix. Moreover, another misperception is often encountered regarding mastic oil or "mastichelaion" (as described by Dioscorides), which is the essential oil of the resin and is often confused with *Pistacia lentiscus* oil or "schinelaion", the essential oil obtained possibly from the plant's berries. Despite the obvious confusion in the literature regarding both the provenance of the resin and its essential oil but also the terminology employed, CMO is used to this day to define and differentiate CMG from other resins in the respective monograph of the European Pharmacopoeia (Ph. Eur.) [44]. For the identification of the resin according to the Ph. Eur. method, only the analysis of its essential oil is used, including a specific distillation yield (10 mL of essential oil/kg of dry resin) and a TLC method for a visual evaluation [44]. Thus far, there is no other suitable and efficient analytical method available for authentication and quality control of CMG and, therefore, adulteration detection [1].

In the present study, different *P. lentiscus* var. *Chia* resin (CMG) samples together with their produced essential oils (CMO) after hydrodistillation were investigated. Two analytical methods, namely High Performance Thin Layer Chromatography (HPTLC) and GC-MS, were employed for sample profiling, and the Ph. Eur. proposedTLC method was also used for comparison purposes. Special emphasis was given to the exploration of the ageing effect on the CMG and CMO composition, which is a critical parameter of quality and authentication. Finally, both types of samples were evaluated for their antifungal and antibacterial properties against different fungi and bacteria strains, with the *Aspergillus nidulans*, *Aspergillus fumigatus*, *Mucor circinelloides*, and *Rhizopus oryzae* being tested for the first time. Moreover, to our knowledge, it is the first time that a high number of original CMG and CMO samples are analyzed, and the ageing parameter is investigated so extensively in the essential oil, employing two analytical methods and in comparison to the official monograph of the Ph. Eur.

2. Materials and Methods

2.1. Chemicals and Standards

Toluene [Ph. Eur., ≥99.7% (GC)] and sulfuric acid (puriss. meets analytical specification of Ph. Eur., BP, 95–97%) were obtained from Sigma-Aldrich (St. Louis, MO, USA). Dimethyl sulfoxide (for analysis) was purchased from Merck (Kenilworth, NJ, USA). Methanol [≥99.8% (HPLC)] and ethanol absolute (99.8% HPLC grade) were purchased from Fischer Chemical (Pittsburg, PA, USA). Petroleum ether (RPE, for analysis) and ethanol 96° were provided by Carlo Erba Reagents (Milan, Italy). Dichloromethane (reagent grade) (Scharlau, Barcelona, Spain) was used after distillation for the dilution of the resins and their essential oils for all HPTLC and GCMS analyses. Vanillin used (Acros Organics, Fair Lawn, NJ, USA) was 99% pure. The alkane C10–C40 analytical standard mixture and the standards borneol (97% purity) and eugenol (99% purity) were obtained from Sigma-Aldrich (St. Louis, MO, USA).

2.2. Starting Material and Production of Essential Oil

Eleven CMG samples were kindly provided by the Chios Mastiha Growers Association (CMGA). Eight samples (CMG_1–8) were analyzed fresh (2 and 6 months after collection) or slightly aged (2 years), whilst three (CMG_9–11) were aged for a longer time period (over 10 years). The distillation process of the resins was conducted according to the Ph.

Eur. monograph of Mastic (01/2008:1876), within a period of two weeks for all samples. In brief, 20 g of resin was reduced to a coarse powder and then distilled for 2 h in a 500 mL round-bottomed flask, using 200 mL of distilled water and a Clevenger apparatus [44]. The produced oils (CMO_1–9) were collected and stored at 4 °C. Two of the aged resins (CMG_10–11) did not produce essential oil and, therefore, were not analyzed further.

2.3. Profiling of the Resin and Essential Oil by HPTLC

Eleven resin samples (CMG_1–11) and their respective essential oils (CMO_1–9) were analyzed by HPTLC. Two methods were applied, the 1st according to the Ph. Eur. monograph and the 2nd developed in-house. According to the monograph's instructions, 1 g of resin was diluted in 10 mL of dichloromethane, filtered after 1–2 min, and used as the test solution. Moreover, the preparation of a reference solution involving the dilution of 25 mg of eugenol and 25 mg of borneol in 3 mL of dichloromethane was carried out as indicated in the monograph. For the in-house method, 10 mg of the tested resins were diluted in 1 mL of dichloromethane with the aid of an ultrasonic bath for 1–2 min. In both methodologies, CMOs were dissolved in dichloromethane at a concentration of 2 mg/mL.

HPTLC analyses were conducted using a CAMAG system (CAMAG®, Muttenz, Switzerland) consisting of an automatic TLC sampler (ATS4), an automatic development chamber (ADC2), a Visualizer 2 Documentation System, and a Derivatizer, under the control of the software platform VisionCats 2.5 (CAMAG®, Muttenz, Switzerland). The samples were applied onto 20 × 10 cm HPTLC Silica gel 60 F_{254} glass plates (Merck, Kenilworth, NJ, USA). Standard and sample solutions were applied band wise with the autosampler ATS4 using a syringe of 25 µL (Hamilton, Reno, NV, USA) and a nitrogen aspirator with the following standard settings: Tracks with 8.0 mm bands, 8 mm distance from the lower edge, 20 mm from the left and right edges, and 11.4 mm between the different tracks, 200 nL/s delivery speed. For the Ph. Eur. method, application volume was set to 1 µL, and the mobile phase consisted of light petroleum of reagent grade (R), toluene R (5:95 v/v). For the in-house methodology, the mobile phase consisted of dichloromethane, methanol (98:2 v/v), and the application volume was set to 10 µL. In both methodologies, the application volume of the essential oils was 20 µL. The standard settings used in ADC2 were the following: 20 min chamber saturation, 10 min of plate activation (conditioning) at 33% relative humidity using $MgCl_2$ as a desiccant, and 5 min of plate drying. The solvent front was set to 8.5 cm. Plate images at 254 nm and 366 nm before spraying and at white light after spraying were recorded. For visualization of the spots, the plates were sprayed with vanillin reagent R [i.e., 2 mL of sulfuric acid added to 100 mL of a 10 g/L solution of vanillin in ethanol (96°)] and heated at 100–105 °C for 5 min in the oven. An optical evaluation of the color and shape of the spots was performed according to the monograph's instructions.

2.4. Determination of Essential Oil Constituents by GC-MS

All CMO samples were diluted in dichloromethane at a concentration of 2 mg/mL. Analyses were performed on a Finnigan Trace GC Ultra 2000 apparatus (Thermo Electron Corporation, Waltham, MA, USA) with an AI 3000 autosampler. The system was coupled with a Finnigan Trace DSQ mass selective detector at Electron Impact (EI) mode. The separation was achieved on a Trace TR-5MS capillary column (30 m × 0.25 mm; film thickness 0.25 m) (Thermo Scientific, Waltham, MA, USA). Helium (1 mL/min) was used as a carrier gas. 1 µL of essential oil was directly injected at splitless mode. The initial oven temperature was set to 40 °C, reaching 240 °C with a gradient of 3 °C/min. When the temperature reached 240 °C, it was kept steady for 10 min. The injector and source temperatures were set to 220 °C and 250 °C, respectively. The mass range was set to 40–400 Da and electron energy to 70 eV. Spectra acquisition and analysis were performed using the XCalibur 2.2 software platform (Thermo, Waltham, MA, USA). Compound identification was conducted by mass spectra comparison to Willey/NIST 0.5 and in-house libraries [45,46]. For the compounds of C14 and above, the method of retention indices (RI) as defined by IUPAC for temperature-programmed GC was additionally used in terms of a better structural verification [47]. A relative quantification of detected compounds was performed by employing the Area % feature and the auto integration using the ICIS algorithm.

2.5. Media and Growth Conditions

Standard minimal media (MM) for *A. nidulans* was used for the growth of *A. nidulans*, *A. fumigatus*, *M. circinelloides*, and *R. oryzae*. Media and supplemented auxotrophies were used at the concentrations given in Fungal Genetics Stock Center (FGSC) [48]. Glucose 1% (w/v) and 5 mM urea were used as the carbon and nitrogen sources, respectively. Growth tests were performed at 37 °C, at pH 6.8, and scored after 3–6 days. The *C. albicans* strain was incubated at 30 °C in YPD broth pH 6.8 (2% Bacto peptone, 1% yeast extract, 2% dextrose) at 200 rpm. Liquid bacterial cultures were incubated in Luria-Bertani (LB) medium pH 6.8 (BactoTryptone 10 g, NaCl 10 g, BactoYeast Extract 5 g for 1 L) at 250 rpm. Media and chemical reagents were obtained from Sigma-Aldrich or AppliChem. Mastic resins (CMG_1–8) were diluted in 100% DMSO or ethanol and added to the media in a final concentration of 0.2 mg/mL and 0.4 mg/mL, respectively (final 1% DMSO or 1% ethanol). Mastic essential oils (CMO_1–8) were diluted in 100% DMSO and added to the media in a final concentration of 0.2 mg/mL (1% DMSO). Controls were treated with the same concentration of solvent (final 1% DMSO or ethanol).

2.6. Epifluorescence Microscopy

For wide-field epifluorescence microscopy, conidiospores were incubated overnight in glass bottom 35 mm l-dishes (ibidi) in liquid minimal media, for 16–22 h at 25 °C, supplemented with glucose 1% (w/v) and urea at 5 mM. Mastic resins (CMG_1–8) were diluted in ethanol and added to the media in a final concentration of 0.4 mg/mL (1% ethanol). Images were obtained using an inverted Zeiss Axio Observer Z1 (Zeiss, White Plains, NY, USA) equipped with a Hamamatsu ORCA Flash 4.0 CMOS camera using the Zen lite 2012 software (Hamamatsu Photonics Deutschland GmbH, Herrsching am Ammersee, Germany). Images were processed and annotated in Adobe Photoshop CS4 Extended version 11.0.2 (Adobe, San Jose, CA, USA).

3. Results and Discussion

3.1. Hydrodistillation Yield

The yield of hydrodistillation plays a key role in CMG identification, since according to the Ph. Eur. monograph for mastic, a minimum of 10 mL of essential oil/kg of anhydrous resin is required as a quality marker [44]. In the current study, only the fresh and slightly aged samples (CMG_1–8) produced essential oil, whilst the three aged samples (CMG_9–11) produced CMO either in traces (CMG_9) or none (CMG_10–11). As shown in Table 1, the distillation yields differed significantly among the analyzed resins, providing an average of 14.7 mL/kg of essential oil.

Moreover, in the case of CMG_6, the yield was found below the limit set by the monograph, with CMG_1 and 2 barely surpassing it. Since these samples were collected at the same period as two of the highest CMO-producing resins (CMG_3,5), it seems that other parameters such as the age of the tree or climatic conditions might play a significant role in essential oil content. Nonetheless, it was verified that ageing decreases CMO yield, leading to almost none or traces production after a long period of storage. Interestingly, according to Papanicolaou et al., the loss of essential oil during storage was attributed mainly to the transformation of volatiles to non-volatiles and, to a lesser degree, to evaporation [49]. Consequently, distillation yield in itself does not constitute an adequate marker of quality, and the proposed levels might need to be reconsidered. However, given that our results on the loss of volatiles during ageing and the average calculated yield corroborated with those reported elsewhere [50,51], we consider that essential oil yield might provide meaningful information that should be examined in conjunction with findings from other techniques.

To our knowledge, in previous studies investigating this aspect, the number of analyzed samples was significantly low and, therefore, a direct comparison is infeasible [38].

Table 1. Hydrodistillation yields, performed according to the Ph. Eur. instructions.

Collection Time (month/year)	Resin	Essential Oil	Yield (mL/kg)
01/2020	CMG_1	CMO_1	11.9
01/2020	CMG_2	CMO_2	10.3
02/2020	CMG_3	CMO_3	23.4
02/2020	CMG_4	CMO_4	19.5
02/2020	CMG_5	CMO_5	24.8
06/2020	CMG_6	CMO_6	9.9
06/2020	CMG_7	CMO_7	14.3
11/2018	CMG_8	CMO_8	3.5
	Minimum		3.5
	Maximum		24.8
	Average ± SD [1]		14.7 ± 7.3
2010	CMG_9	CMO_9	traces
2010	CMG_10	CMO_10	-
2010	CMG_11	CMO_11	-

[1] SD = Standard Deviation.

3.2. HPTLC Profiling

Apart from distillation yields, a TLC method was also described in the Ph. Eur. monograph for the identification of CMG, accompanied by a visual inspection of substances considering the color and the shape of certain zones. Eugenol and borneol were used as reference compounds. In the current study, the Ph. Eur. method was used for the analysis of all 11 CMG samples, together with the respective CMOs, utilizing an HPTLC approach [44]. Additionally, an in-house elution method was developed for the profiling of both sample types (Figure 1).

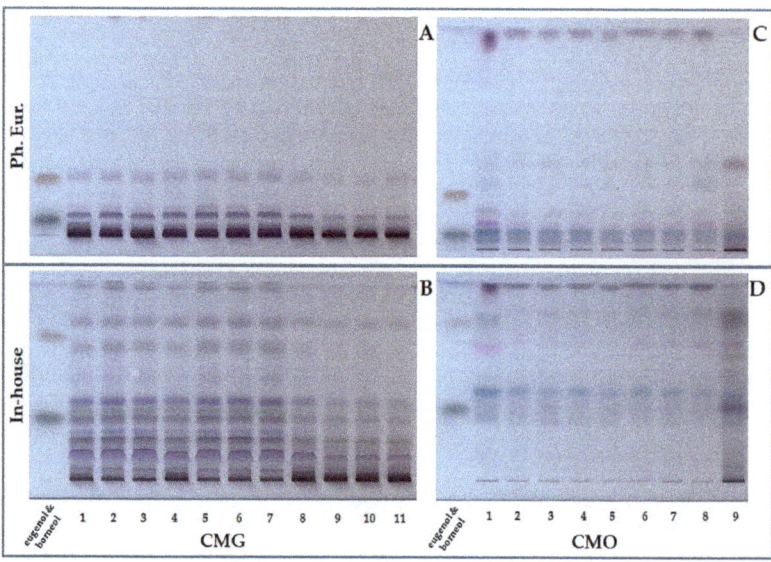

Figure 1. HPTLC chromatograms of Chios Mastic Gum (CMG) (**A,B**) and Chios Mastic Oil (CMO) (**C,D**) samples developed with the Ph. Eur. (**A,C**) and in-house (**B,D**) methods. Detection at visible light after spraying with vanillin reagent.

According to the Ph. Eur. monograph, six zones of different coloring after spraying were evaluated and compared with the reference standards indicating the resin's identity. As shown in Figure 1A, the solvent system proposed by the Ph. Eur. was not suitable for profiling and compound monitoring, since most of the constituents were concentrated on the baseline together with the poly-β-myrcene polymer (dark brown). The same remark could be made for the CMO samples (Figure 1C). In order to resolve this issue, the development of an in-house method was deemed necessary. To that end, different solvent systems (e.g., toluene/ethyl acetate/heptane/formic acid 80:20:10:3, cyclohexane/diisopropyl ether/acetic acid 60:40:10, dichloromethane/methanol 98:2) and methanol for resin dilution were tested for the development of a suitable HPTLC method (data not shown). Moreover, the dilution of the resin in different solvents, i.e., dichloromethane, methanol, acetone, and acetonitrile, were also tested. Finally, dichloromethane/methanol 98:2 as an elution system was selected as the most suitable, and dichloromethane for resin dilution was found to be the most appropriate solvent. Furthermore, the initial concentration of the samples was reduced to 10 mg/mL for crude mastic powder (compared to 100 mg/mL proposed by Ph. Eur.) in order to achieve an improved sample dilution and, therefore, an enhanced separation and a more rigid and uniform elution of constituents. Lastly, filtration of samples prior to application was omitted, ensuring a greater metabolite coverage. As observed in Figure 1B,D, with the elution system employed, the separation of the compounds was more efficient, the resolution was greatly improved, and even minor qualitative and/or quantitative alterations could be detected.

Based on the HPTLC data, a comparison between the fresh and aged samples could be made regardless of the method used, even if, with the in-house method, the assessment was considerably more straightforward. Figures S1–S4, present the different chemical profiles between the fresh and aged collections in 254 and 366 nm. The effect of ageing could be observed in both CMG and CMO samples. In the aged resin samples in particular (CMG_9–11), the absence of zones and/or quantitative decrease was clearly evident, possibly indicating the instability of the resin over time and the decomposition of numerous constituents. Moreover, it seems that the formation of β-myrcene polymer was favored over time as it was manifested by the obvious relative intensification of the dark brown zone at the baseline. Poly-β-myrcene, which is derived from myrcene polymerization present in CMO, undergoes further oxidation reactions affording diverse oxidation products [52]. In general, according to Behr et al., the storage of myrcene is a difficult task since it polymerizes spontaneously at room temperature. One-third is lost by polymerization in a 3-month period leading to a higher viscosity index and the formation of peroxides [53]. The addition of vitamin E has been suggested as a means of impeding polymerization and oxidation phenomena [49], while other agents have also been proposed, such as 0.1% *p-tert*-butylcatechol and a mixture of 0.05% *p-tert*-butylcatechol and 0.05% butylhydroxyanisol [53]. This observation was also evident in the profiles of the CMO samples, where polymer formation along with the appearance of several new zones of increased polarity, clearly sets the oil produced from the 10-year-old resin (CMO_9) apart from the rest. In fact, CMO could be suggested as an even better substrate for ageing detection, given that its profile presents many more differences with fresh and slightly aged samples compared to its respective crude resin.

Finally, it is worth mentioning that despite the importance of CMO's chemical composition for the quality control of the resin, a fact recognized even by the Ph. Eur., the number of studies aiming to assess the effect of ageing on the essential oil's yield and profile is quite limited and outdated, while the investigated storage period is usually restricted to a few months [38,49]. In addition, to our knowledge, there is no HPTLC methodology in the literature for CMG and/or CMO profiling, an alternative to the Ph. Eur. monograph. It is important to state that given that the technique is the advanced form of Thin-Layer Chromatography (TLC), automation, low operating cost, improved application of the samples, higher separation, resolution, data acquisition and processing, faster analysis time, and lower volumes of mobile phase are ensured [54]. Moreover, HPTLC is characterized as a state-of-the-art method and a useful analytical tool in the case of complex mixtures, e.g., plant extracts [55].

3.3. GC-MS Analysis

Amongst analytical techniques, GC-MS has been almost exclusively used for the chemical characterization of CMO as well as CMG [50,56,57]. More precisely, GC-MS constitutes the method of choice as it is often employed for the detection of adulteration phenomena in the oil and, generally, for its quality assessment [51]. In the current study, 8 samples of essential oils produced from fresh and slightly aged resins (CMO_1–8) were analyzed. Due to the minimal production of essential oils from resins aged 10 years and more, only one sample, namely CMG_9, provided oil in an adequate quantity (CMO_9) and was, therefore, forwarded for analysis. In Figure 2, superimposed total ion chromatograms (TIC) of representative samples (CMO_1, CMO_8, and CMO_9) are presented, clearly demonstrating the chemical transformations taking place over time.

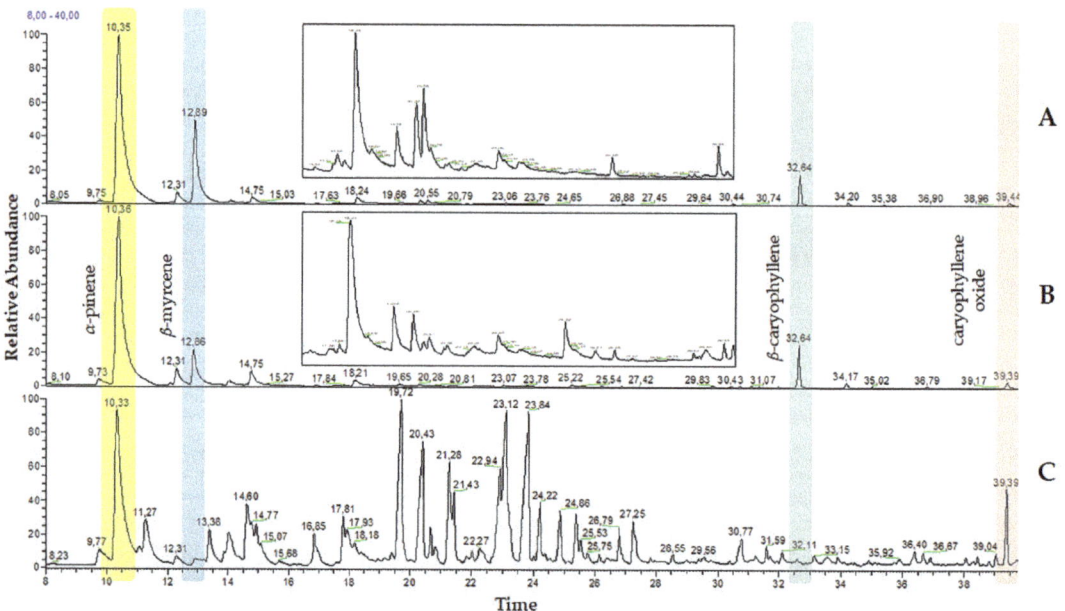

Figure 2. GC-MS chromatograms of Chios Mastic Oils (CMOs) obtained from (**A**) a fresh (CMO_1), (**B**) a 2-year-old (CMO_8) and (**C**) a 10-year-old resin (CMO_9).

Based on the GC-MS data explained in detail in Table 2, 33 compounds were identified in fresh CMO samples (CMO_1–7) (97.69%) together with 7 non-identified (1.10%).

The main categories of metabolites found in fresh samples (CMO_1–7) were monoterpene hydrocarbons (86.01%), oxygenated monoterpenes and benzenoids (4.60%), sesquiterpene hydrocarbons (4.99%), oxygenated sesquiterpenes (0.63%), and diterpene hydrocarbons (1.47%). The oil produced from a 10-year-old resin (CMO_9) demonstrated a significantly different profile verifying the HPTLC observations and 25 compounds were identified in total (70.85%). A more comprehensive annotation of a fresh and aged sample is presented in Figure S5. Even from a preliminary inspection of the available chromatograms, it is obvious that ageing has a profound effect on the composition of CMO, and hence it shall be discussed in greater detail in the following Section 3.4.

Table 2. GC-MS analysis of the essential oil composition of fresh CMO samples (CMO_1–7).

A/A	Rt (min) [1]	Compound	Molecular Formula	MW (g/mol) [2]	Main Fragments (Descending Intensity)	RI [3]	IM [4]
1	9.75	N/I_C01	$C_{10}H_{16}$	136.23	93, 67, 49, 41, 84, 79, 108, 121, 136	-	MS
2	10.36	α-Pinene	$C_{10}H_{16}$	136.23	93, 77, 105, 121, 67, 41, 53, 136	-	MS
3	12.10	Sabinene	$C_{10}H_{16}$	136.23	93, 77, 41, 136, 121, 105	-	MS
4	12.31	β-Pinene	$C_{10}H_{16}$	136.23	93, 69, 41, 79, 121, 136	-	MS
5	12.88	β-Myrcene	$C_{10}H_{16}$	136.23	69, 93, 41, 79, 53, 121, 107, 136	-	MS
6	14.06	o-Methyl-anisole	$C_8H_{10}O$	122.16	122, 107, 77, 91, 51, 69, 41, 83	-	MS
7	14.76	D-Limonene	$C_{10}H_{16}$	136.23	68, 93, 79, 107, 53, 121, 41, 136	-	MS
8	16.22	N/I_C02	$C_{10}H_{18}O$	154.25	49, 84, 93, 41, 69, 77, 121, 107, 136	-	MS
9	16.88	N/I_C03	$C_{10}H_{18}O$	154.25	49, 84, 93, 69, 41, 79, 107, 122, 137, 152	-	MS
10	17.64	Terpinolene	$C_{10}H_{16}$	136.23	93, 121, 136, 69, 79, 41, 105, 152	-	MS
11	17.86	Camphenol	$C_{10}H_{16}O$	152.23	93, 108, 67, 41, 79, 121, 137, 152	-	MS
12 & 13	18.25	Perillene & α-Linalool	$C_{10}H_{14}O$ & $C_{10}H_{18}O$	150.22 & 154.25	69, 71, 41, 93, 55, 81, 150, 121, 107, 135	-	MS
14	18.81	N/I_C04	$C_{10}H_{18}O$	154.25	69, 71, 93, 41, 55, 84, 121, 150, 107, 136, 154	-	MS
15	19.67	α-Campholenal	$C_{10}H_{16}O$	152.23	108, 93, 67, 41, 81, 150, 119, 136	-	MS
16	20.30	Pinocarveol	$C_{10}H_{16}O$	152.23	55, 92, 69, 41, 83, 109, 119, 134, 150	-	MS
17	20.57	Cis-Verbenol	$C_{10}H_{16}O$	152.23	109, 41, 81, 91, 69, 119, 150, 137	-	MS
18	21.40	N/I_C05	$C_{11}H_{18}$	150.26	49, 84, 69, 41, 108, 93, 135, 122, 150	-	MS
19	22.33	Verbenol	$C_{10}H_{16}O$	152.23	59, 94, 79, 69, 83, 41, 109, 119, 136, 150	-	MS
20	23.07	Myrtenal	$C_{10}H_{14}O$	150.22	79, 107, 91, 41, 67, 119, 135, 150	1203.0	RI, MS
21	23.81	Verbenone	$C_{10}H_{14}O$	150.22	107, 91, 79, 135, 67, 41, 150, 122	1220.5	RI, MS
22	26.27	N/I_C06	$C_{10}H_{16}O$	152.23	93, 69, 49, 41, 84, 79, 136, 164, 121, 109, 150	-	MS
23	26.89	Bornyl acetate	$C_{12}H_{20}O_2$	196.29	95, 43, 121, 136, 108, 67, 55, 80, 154, 196	1291.6	RI, MS
24	29.46	N/I_C07	$C_{15}H_{26}O$	222.37	105, 161, 119, 49, 91, 69, 41, 84, 58, 204, 148, 133	-	MS
25	29.64	α-Longipinene	$C_{15}H_{24}$	204.35	119, 105, 93, 133, 69, 41, 55, 79, 204, 161, 152, 189	1354.4	RI, MS
26	30.46	α-Ylangene	$C_{15}H_{24}$	204.35	105, 119, 93, 161, 41, 69, 79, 55, 133, 204, 189, 148	1373.0	RI, MS
27	30.76	α-Copaene	$C_{15}H_{24}$	204.35	105, 119, 161, 93, 69, 81, 41, 148, 133, 204, 189	1379.6	RI, MS
28	31.10	β-Bourbonene	$C_{15}H_{24}$	204.35	81, 123, 91, 105, 41, 69, 161, 148, 133, 204	1387.3	RI, MS

Table 2. Cont.

A/A	Rt (min) [1]	Compound	Molecular Formula	MW (g/mol) [2]	Main Fragments (Descending Intensity)	RI [3]	IM [4]
29	31.33	β-Elemene	$C_{15}H_{24}$	204.35	93, 81, 69, 148, 41, 105, 121, 133, 161, 189, 176, 204	1392.7	RI, MS
30	31.98	Isocaryophyllene	$C_{15}H_{24}$	204.35	93, 69, 133, 105, 41, 79, 55, 148, 119, 161, 189, 175, 204	1407.6	RI, MS
31	32.65	β-Caryophyllene	$C_{15}H_{24}$	204.35	93, 133, 105, 69, 79, 41, 55, 120, 147, 161, 189, 175, 204	1423.9	RI, MS
32	34.21	α-Humulene	$C_{15}H_{24}$	204.35	93, 121, 80, 107, 147, 67, 41, 53, 204, 136, 189, 161, 175	1461.1	RI, MS
33	35.11	α-Muurolene	$C_{15}H_{24}$	204.35	105, 161, 91, 119, 79, 133, 69, 41, 204, 55, 148, 189, 178	1482.3	RI, MS
34	35.39	D-Germacrene	$C_{15}H_{24}$	204.35	161, 105, 91, 79, 119, 41, 148, 133, 69, 204, 178	1489.0	RI, MS
35	39.46	Caryophyllene oxide	$C_{15}H_{24}O$	220.35	79, 93, 41, 69, 107, 55, 121, 135, 147, 161, 178, 187, 205, 220	1591.2	RI, MS
36	40.68	α-Humulene epoxide II	$C_{15}H_{24}O$	220.35	109, 67, 96, 138, 43, 55, 81, 123, 178, 148, 164, 205, 191, 220	-	MS
37	50.40	p-Camphorene/Dimyrcene	$C_{20}H_{32}$	272.47	69, 41, 93, 105, 55, 119, 79, 133, 229, 147, 187, 161, 272, 175, 202, 216, 243, 257	-	MS
38	51.15	Dimyrcene	$C_{20}H_{32}$	272.47	69, 93, 41, 105, 55, 79, 121, 187, 147, 229, 133, 159, 203, 272, 175, 257, 215, 243	-	MS
39	52.26	m-Camphorene/Dimyrcene	$C_{20}H_{32}$	272.47	69, 41, 91, 105, 119, 79, 133, 55, 147, 229, 203, 161, 187, 272, 257, 173, 216, 243	-	MS
40	53.58	Dimyrcene	$C_{20}H_{32}$	272.47	69, 93, 41, 105, 79, 133, 119, 55, 229, 147, 203, 161, 187, 272, 257, 175	-	MS

[1] Rt = Retention time; [2] MW = Molecular Weight; [3] RI = Retention Indices calculated against n-alkanes; [4] IM = Identification Method.

Regarding the fresh samples' chemical composition (CMO_1–7), the dominant compounds are α-pinene (Rt 10.3 min) ranging from 56.4 to 73.0% (avg. 64.8%) and β-myrcene (Rt 12.8 min) ranging from 12.6 to 19.9% (avg. 16.4%), verifying available information [15,51]. Other compounds detected in significant levels included β-pinene (2.47–3.08%), limonene (1.24–1.98%), perillene coeluting with α-linalool (0.84–2.53%), and β-caryophyllene (2.21–6.38%). Interestingly, perillene has only been reported in two studies thus far [11,51] while the compounds camphor, 1-ethenyl-2,4-dimethylbenzene or 1-methyl-4-(2-propenyl)-benzene, β-methyl-cinnamaldehyde, trimethyl-hydroquinone, 3,8,8-trimethyl-1,2,3,4,5,6,7,8-octahydro-2-naphthalenyl methyl acetate, and 4-acetyl-1-methylcyclohexene are reported for the first time in the 10-year old CMO.

The major compounds found in mastic's essential oil, α-pinene and β-myrcene have been proposed in the past as quality markers for CMO [51], however, most available studies did not follow a standardized methodology for the resin's distillation and/or the storage period was not mentioned. Therefore, a direct comparison of the calculated metabolites' content was not possible, especially when the geographical origin of the starting material was not clear [26] or market samples of CMO were analyzed [51]. As a consequence, the reported levels of those two major compounds varied considerably in the existing literature, i.e., for α-pinene between 30–90% and for β-myrcene between 1–60% [50,58,59]. In fact, it appears that sample origin is so crucial to the essential oil's composition that in some cases of essential oil acquired from a different *Pistacia lentiscus* variety, β-myrcene was reported at very low levels (<4%) or it was completely absent [26,60,61]. Impressively, in one case, α-copaene is mentioned as one of the major compounds, while according to our findings it constitutes one of the minor constituents [62].

We hereby have to note that despite the existence of a limited number of studies assessing CMO's chemical composition, to our knowledge, there is only one previous research work by Paraschos and colleagues where a considerable number of authentic mastic oil samples have been analyzed similar to the current study [51]. Nevertheless, even in this comprehensive effort, the samples were not acquired through a controlled laboratory process, instead, they were commercial specimens provided by the official producers. In that scope, the present work attempts to narrow down the proposed limits of marker compounds in CMO, following a standardized methodology for its distillation, as proposed by an official authority (Ph. Eur.).

3.4. Essential Oil Ageing

Ageing together with storage are critical for quality assessment; hence monitoring of marker compounds during the ageing process is deemed essential. In the current study, the ageing effect on the resin and the produced essential oils was assessed in samples collected 2 and 10 years prior to analysis with the view to provide further insight on the chemical transformations taking place in mastic samples overtime. Table 3 summarizes the qualitative and/or quantitative differences in specific constituents between fresh and aged samples.

Table 3. CMO chemical composition in fresh (CMO_1-7), aged for 2 years (CMO_8) and aged for 10 years (CMO_9) samples analyzed.

Compounds	(Min–Max) % in Fresh Samples (*n* = 7)	Average % ± SD in Fresh Samples (*n* = 7)	% in the 2-Year-Old Sample (*n* = 1)	% in the 10-Year-Old Sample (*n* = 1)
Monoterpene hydrocarbons	79.40–91.15	86.01 ± 4.37	81.96	13.2
Oxygenated monoterpenes [1] & Benzenoids [2]	3.75–6.25	4.60 ± 0.78	4.35	52.51
Sesquiterpene hydrocarbons	2.84–7.94	4.99 ± 1.96	5.91	0.08
Oxygenated sesquiterpenes	0.29–0.96	0.63 ± 0.26	0.90	1.91
Diterpene hydrocarbons	0.29–2.62	1.47 ± 0.89	3.23	-
Ketones	-	-	-	3.23
Total identified	96.12–98.43	97.69 ± 0.79	96.35	70.85
Total non-identified	0.76–1.66	1.10 ± 0.31	1.98	29.00
Compounds	(Min–Max) % in Fresh Samples (*n* = 7)	Average % ± SD in Fresh Samples (*n* = 7)	% in the 2-Year-Old Sample (*n* = 1)	% in the 10-Year-Old Sample (*n* = 1)
Monoterpene Hydrocarbons				
α-Pinene	56.42–72.99	64.83 ± 5.78	65.65	12.00
β-Pinene	2.47–3.08	2.75 ± 0.25	3.81	0.45
β-Myrcene	12.6–19.94	16.40 ± 3.17	8.90	-
Sabinene	0.18–0.3	0.23 ± 0.04	0.28	-
D-Limonene	1.24–1.98	1.66 ± 0.32	3.24	-
Terpinolene	0.11–0.2	0.15 ± 0.04	0.08	-
Camphene	-	-	-	0.75
Oxygenated Monoterpenes [1] & Benzenoids [2]				
Perillene [1] & α-Linalool [1]	0.84–2.53	1.68 ± 0.64	1.73	-
Camphenol [1]	0.06–0.09	0.08 ± 0.01	0.07	-
α-Campholenal [1]	0.33–0.47	0.39 ± 0.05	0.42	6.32
Pinocarveol [1]	0.31–0.72	0.50 ± 0.14	0.29	5.16
cis-Verbenol [1]	0.3–1.05	0.61 ± 0.25	0.2	-
Verbenol [1]	0.15–0.31	0.21 ± 0.057	0.17	-
Verbenone [1]	0.07–0.22	0.13 ± 0.059	0.07	7.21
Bornyl acetate [1]	0.07–0.2	0.11 ± 0.046	0.06	0.98
Campholene group [1]	-	-	-	4.62

Table 3. Cont.

Compounds	(Min–Max) % in Fresh Samples ($n = 7$)	Average % ± SD in Fresh Samples ($n = 7$)	% in the 2-Year-Old Sample ($n = 1$)	% in the 10-Year-Old Sample ($n = 1$)
Oxygenated Monoterpenes [1] & Benzenoids [2]				
Camphor [1]	-	-	-	0.78
3,6,6-Trimethyl norpinan-2-one [1] & Pinocarvone [1]	-	-	-	4.99
cis-3-Pinanone [1]	-	-	-	0.27
cis-Carveol [1]	-	-	-	1.47
1-Ethenyl-2,4-dimethylbenzene or 1-Methyl-4-(2-propenyl)-benzene [2] & o-Methyl-anisole [2]	0.36–0.84	0.60 ± 0.16	1.14	1.93
o-, p- & m-Cymene [2]	-	-	-	5.30
β-Methyl-cinnamaldehyde [2]	-	-	-	0.15
Myrtenal [1] & p-Cymen-8-ol [2]	0.22–0.39	0.28 ± 0.058	0.2	11.11
Carvone [1] & Trimethyl-hydroquinone [2]	-	-	-	2.22
Sesquiterpene Hydrocarbons				
β-Caryophyllene	2.21–6.38	4.13 ± 1.53	4.74	-
α-Humulene	0.28–0.91	0.54 ± 0.22	0.69	-
α-Longipinene	0.01–0.07	0.03 ± 0.02	0.02	-
α-Ylangene	0.04–0.16	0.10 ± 0.04	0.08	0.08
α-Copaene	0.02–0.08	0.05 ± 0.02	0.06	-
β-Bourbonene	0.01–0.07	0.04 ± 0.02	0.07	-
β-Elemene	0.01–0.09	0.04 ± 0.03	0.07	-
Isocaryophyllene	0.02–0.11	0.06 ± 0.03	0.07	-
a-Muurolene	0.03–0.09	0.05 ± 0.02	0.08	-
D-Germacrene	0.05–0.1	0.06 ± 0.02	0.03	-
Oxygenated Sesquiterpenes				
Caryophyllene oxide	0.27–0.89	0.58 ± 0.24	0.82	1.63
α-Humulene epoxide II	0.02–0.07	0.05 ± 0.02	0.08	-
3,8,8-Trimethyl-1,2,3,4,5,6,7,8-octahydro-2-naphthalenyl methyl acetate	-	-	-	0.28
Ketones				
4-Acetyl-1-methylcyclohexene	-	-	-	1.53
2-Undecanone	-	-	-	1.70

[1] Oxygenated monoterpenes; [2] Benzenoids.

Even from a preliminary analysis of the results, it is obvious that CMG undergoes severe alterations to its chemical composition. In more detail, it seems that monoterpene hydrocarbons decrease slightly in the 2-year storage (81.96%) and significantly in the 10 years one (13.2%). Oxygenated monoterpenes and benzenoids have similar rates over the 2-year period, but in the 10-year-old sample, they constitute more than half of the oil's composition (52.5%); thus, chemical processes such as oxidation are implied. Sesquiterpene hydrocarbons appeared to be almost absent in the 10-year aged sample, whilst their oxygenated counterparts were higher compared to the fresh samples. In the only study investigating the ageing in a 3-year storage period, there was only a slight decline in the monoterpene hydrocarbons, while all the other categories exhibited similar rates [38].

Investigating individual compounds, it is obvious that the fresh collections contain α-pinene and β-myrcene at the highest rates. It has been reported that under thermal oxidation conditions, α-pinene and β-pinene can be transformed to oxygenated monoterpenes [63,64]. α-Pinene seems to be unaffected in the collection aged for 2 years (65.7%), verifying an existing study reporting a 3-year storage [38]. However, its content was found significantly lower (12.0%) in the sample aged over a 10-year period. Evidently, as time goes by, both compounds suffer from a definitive loss in content, however, β-myrcene, clearly stands out as the one most affected by long storage periods. As a matter of fact, in the collection of 2018, i.e., CMG_8, which produced little oil (CMO_8), β-myrcene was found at a lower rate in contrast to the other fresh collections, while in the oil produced from the 10-year aged collection, β-myrcene was completely absent. Therefore, β-myrcene could be suggested as a marker for ageing as it clearly demonstrates a gradual decrease over time [38]. Indeed, the ratios of β-myrcene/α-pinene and β-pinene/β-myrcene have been previously proposed as quality markers for CMO [38,51]. According to our findings presented in detail in Table S1, the ratio of β-myrcene/α-pinene was more suitable for the qualitative evaluation of CMO's ageing process, as it displayed a more evident decrease in oils procured from aged resins and a low SD amongst samples of fresh collection. In fact, when this rate equals zero, as in the case of the 10-year old collection, it can be safely assumed that the oil is entirely aged. The ratios calculated herein coincide with those previously reported [11,38,51], with β-myrcene/α-pinene ranging from 0.14–0.35 and β-pinene/β-myrcene from 0.13–0.43.

Apart from the gradual degradation of marker-compounds such as α-pinene and β-myrcene, other compounds were also decreased over time, with the most characteristic being β-caryophyllene (Rt 32.6 min), giving its place to its oxidized product, caryophyllene oxide (Rt 39.4 min). In the same context, oxidized products of monoterpenes such as pinocarveol (Rt 20.4 min) and verbenone (Rt 23.8 min) dominated the profile of the 10-year aged sample. Based on our data, these compounds, along with α-campholenal (Rt 19.7 min) were detected <1% in fresh samples, whereas pinocarvone (Rt 21.3 min) and *cis*-carveol (Rt 24.2 min) were only detected in the aged sample (Figure 3).

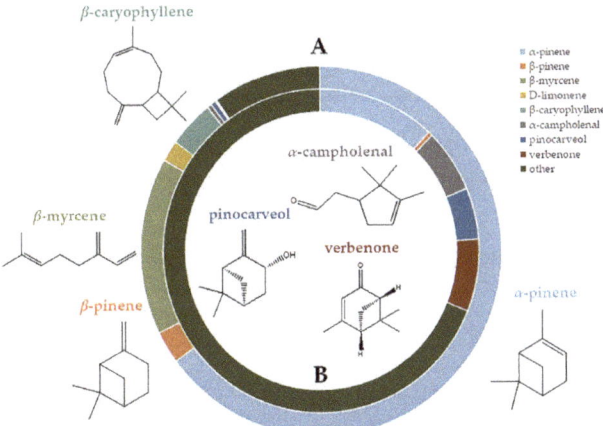

Figure 3. % Content of different volatiles in CMOs obtained from (**A**) fresh and (**B**) 10-year-old resin.

Pinocarvone, however, has been mentioned thus far only in one study of samples from a fresh collection [11]. Moreover, camphene (Rt 11.0 min), eluting close to α-pinene, appears only in the aged sample, implying a possible isomerization of the latter [38]. Other transformations taking place include the conversion of D-limonene (Rt 14.7 min) to benzenoid cymene derivatives (Rt 14.6 min) and that of perillene and α-linalool (Rt 18.2 min) to the oxygenated campholene ones (Rt 17.8 min). Benzenoid cymene derivatives have also been found to increase in samples of aged wine [65], and as for D-limonene, Karlberg et al. suggested its possible transformation into carvone under air exposure [66].

Similar observations could be made for benzenoid compounds and cymene derivatives such as *p*-cymen-8-ol, carvone (Rt 25.3 min), as well as *o*-, *p*- and *m*-cymene, which constitute characteristic examples. The presence of *p*-cymene has been reported in three studies of fresh collections (<0.4%) [11,30,60]. Moreover, in the aged collection sample, myrtenal (Rt 23.1 min) seemed to co-elute with *p*-cymen-8-ol (Rt 22.9 min), a compound referenced only in one study of a fresh collection of mastic [11]. *o*-Methyl-anisole is a compound found both in fresh and aged oils; however, in the 10-year old oil, it seemed to co-elute with 1-ethenyl-2,4-dimethylbenzene or 1-methyl-4-(2-propenyl)-benzene (Rt 14.0 min). In accordance with our findings, in the only work studying the ageing of CMG during a 3-year storage period, camphene, limonene, β-pinene, *p*-cymene, myrtenal, and *trans*-carveol were augmented [38]. An interesting and somewhat contradictory observation, though, was that β-pinene and D-limonene seem to be increased in the 2-year storage verifying the previous reference whilst the first decreases significantly (<1%) and the second disappears in the 10-year-old sample.

Finally, regarding the presence of dimyrcenes, their content was found higher in the 2-year collection sample compared to the fresh ones, but they were absent from the 10-year collection. A plausible explanation could be the gradual polymerization of myrcene first to its dimer (after a short storage period) and then to its polymer over a longer ageing time. Dimyrcenes have only been detected in fresh collections in the Seville's and Izmir's essential oils of *Pistacia lentiscus* resin at levels similar to those presented herein [11,60]. Finally, two ketones, namely 4-acetyl-1-methylcycloxene (Rt 13.3 min) and 2-undecanone (Rt 27.2 min), have been detected only in the 10-year-old sample. The existence of 2-undecanone at a low rate (<0.2%) has been reported in only two studies analyzing samples of fresh collections [30,60].

To summarize, according to our findings, the oil produced from the resin aged for 2 years presented few differences with the fresh ones, with the only evident exception being β-myrcene, the compound, which seems to be the most affected by ageing. On the other hand, in the oil produced from the resin stored for a period longer than 10 years, the chemical composition was completely altered with oxidized products such as verbenone, pinocarveol, and α-campholenal dominating the oil's profile. α-Pinene is still one of the major constituents of the aged oil, and β-myrcene is completely absent, probably due to extensive polymerization phenomena.

3.5. Antifungal and Antibacterial Effects of Resins and Essential Oils

All resins (CMG_1–7) and essential oils (CMO_1–7) from fresh collections together with the resin stored for 2 years (CMG_8) and the respective oil (CMO_8) were tested for their antifungal and antibacterial activity. In vivo growth tests were performed against the following microorganisms: Fungi: *Aspergillus nidulans, Aspergillus fumigatus, Candida albicans, Mucor circinelloides,* and *Rhizopus oryzae*. Bacteria: *Escherichia coli, Pseudomonas aeruginosa,* and *Bacillus subtilis*. The rationale for the choice of fungi to be tested is the following. *A. nidulans* is a non-pathogenic well-studied model system that permits unique genetic, molecular, and cellular approaches [67] that would have enabled us to address the mechanism of any potential action of the mastic compounds tested. *A. fumigatus* and *C. albicans* are two of the most prominent major fungal (ascomycete) human pathogens in immunocompromised people [68,69]. *M. circinelloides* and *R. oryzae* are clinical isolates of Mucorales, a genus of emerging pathogens that often includes strains resistant to antifungal pharmacological therapy [70–72]; provided by Dr. George Chamillos, IMMB]. The bacteria tested are standard strains that represent Gram− (*E. coli*) or Gram+ (*B. subtilis*) model eubacteria, whereas *P. aeruginosa* is a common Gram− bacterium that can cause disease in plants and animals, including humans.

Figure 4 and Figure S6 summarize results obtained with fungi and bacteria, respectively.

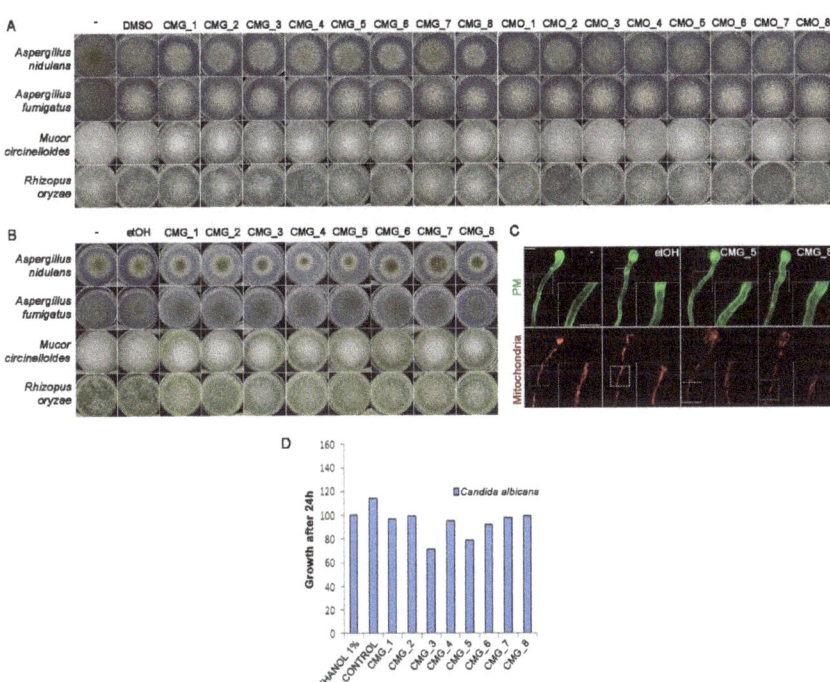

Figure 4. Effect of resins and essential oils against fungi. (**A,B**) Comparative growth test of *A. nidulans*, *A. fumigatus*, *M. circinelloides*, and *R. oryzae* on Minimal Media (MM) after 3 days at 37 °C in the presence or absence (control/solvent) of samples. In (**A**) Mastic resins (CMG_1–8) and essential oils (CMO_1–8) were diluted in DMSO and added to MM in a final concentration of 0.2 mg/mL (1% DMSO). In (**B**), mastic resins were diluted in ethanol and added to the minimal media in a final concentration of 0.4 mg/mL (1% ethanol). (**C**) Epifluorescence microscopy of an *A. nidulans* strain co-expressing a plasma membrane (PM) purine transporter tagged with GFP (AzgA-GFP) and a mitochondrial marker tagged with DsRed (CitA-DsRed) in the presence or absence of resins (CMG_1–8). CMG_5 and CMG_8 depict representative results of the effect of all mastic resins tested. Scale bar: 5 µm (**D**) The bar graph depicts growth rate of *Candida albicans* in the presence of mastic resins (CMG_1–8) after 24 h of incubation. The standard deviation in all cases was <1%.

Figure 4A shows that all samples tested, when dissolved in DMSO, had minor or no effect on fungal growth. More specifically, in the case of *A. nidulans*, all led to a moderate reduction in colony diameter and no effect on apparent conidiospore production. Among those, CMG_8 (2.2 cm), followed by CMG_6 and CMG_1 (2.5 cm), had the most prominent effect, compared to the control (3.2 cm). It is important to note that the most potent was the most aged between the analyzed samples. The respective oils (CMO_1–8) had practically no effect on *A. nidulans* colonies. CMG_8 also had the strongest effect on *A. fumigatus* (2.5 cm versus 3.2 cm in control), while other CMGs had minor effects on growth. Nearly all CMGs had an effect on hyphal density in *M. circinelloides*, not evident in *R. oryzae*, but did not affect the rate of colony growth in any of the two Mucorales. CMOs had no effect on *M. circinelloides*, but CMO_2 and CMO_7 led to a significant reduction of hyphal density in *R. oryzae*.

Based on these results, we retested all CMGs at 2-fold increased concentration, this time diluted in ethanol. Results shown in Figure 4B demonstrate that CMG_4, CMG_5, and CMG_8 had a negative effect on *A. nidulans* colony diameter, reducing it from 2.2 cm to 1.4–1.7 cm, while again CMG_8 also led to a significant reduction of growth in *A. fumigatus*

(1.9 cm compared to 2.6 cm in the control). Overall, CMG_8 showed the most consistent negative effect on the growth of both Aspergilli (22–37% reduction of colony diameter).

As far as it concerns Mucorales, again, most CMGs led to a significant reduction in hyphal density in *M. circinelloides*, but not in *R. oryzae*. Based on the result for growth tests, it became apparent that the CMG_8 had a promising antifungal effect mostly against Aspergilli, but possibly also against *M. circinelloides*. To investigate possible cellular defects underlying its action, but also of other CMG and CMO samples, we took advantage of available genetic strains expressing specific fluorescent molecular markers in *A. nidulans*, and in particular a strain stably expressing a plasma membrane (PM) protein (purine transporter AzgA) and a mitochondrial protein (citrate synthase CitA), tagged with GFP or DsRed, respectively [73,74]. Several known antifungal agents have a targeting effect on the cell wall or PM biosynthesis or in mitochondrial functioning and morphology [72,75]. In previous reports, oils have been shown to have minimal and variable activity against some fungi (e.g., *Saccharomyces cerevisiae*, *Zygosaccharomyces bailii*, *Aspergillus flavus*, *Penicillium roquefortii*, *Eurotium amstelodami*; [76]), but to our knowledge, there were practically no reports on mastic resins against fungi, except a report related to the phytopathogenic fungus *Rhizoctonia solani* [61]. Figure 4C shows representative results with CMG_8 and CMG_5. None of the samples tested had any detectable effect on the general morphology of *A. nidulans* hyphal cells, or in the localization, stability, and turnover of PM or mitochondrial proteins.

As shown in Figure 4D, we did not detect any significant effect against *C. albicans*. Moreover, all tested samples did not seem to have any significant effect on the growth of the bacterial strains tested. Figure S6 shows optical densities of bacterial strains after 24 h of growth in the presence of samples compared to the control culture. No effect was also observed at earlier incubation times (8 and 16 h, data not shown).

From the aforementioned results, specific CMGs do have a moderate antifungal activity, which apparently is not directly related to the integrity of the cell wall, the PM of the functioning of mitochondria. It is interesting to note that the most potent resin was the one after 2 years' storage, while the respective oil did not present any activity. A reasonable assumption is that degradation and/or oxidized forms of terpenes were most probably responsible for the observed effects, while a possible role of the relatively increased levels of poly-β-myrcene cannot also be ignored.

4. Conclusions

In the present study, 11 different authentic mastic resins (CMG) from different collection times were investigated together with their respective essential oils (CMO). All samples were analyzed by HPTLC using the elution system proposed by the Ph.Eur. monograph and a new one developed in-house with the new system providing an improved separation and a higher resolution for the detected constituents. HPTLC could be used as a fast screening method for CMG and CMO samples and is even suitable for the detection of the ageing effect on both sample types. Based on our results, the two criteria set by the Pharmacopoeia, namely distillation yield, and the TLC method, were found to be insufficient and inaccurate for the successful identification of the resin and adulteration detection and, therefore, they should be reconsidered.

CMOs were also analyzed by GC-MS, and more than 30 compounds were identified in the fresh oils, and specific content ranges were proposed for the major components of CMOs originating exclusively from *P. lentiscus* var *Chia*. Major differences were observed in CMO's major compound classes during the ageing process. Monoterpene hydrocarbons were found to gradually decrease over time, followed by a simultaneous increase in oxygenated monoterpenes and benzenoids. A similar pattern is observed between sesquiterpene hydrocarbons and oxygenated sesquiterpenes. α-Pinene and β-myrcene, which are quality markers for CMO, were found in high levels in fresh samples, also showing a continuing decline over time. However, β-myrcene seems to be a more suitable marker of ageing since, due to extensive polymerization after 10 years, it is not detectable. Similarly, camphene appears only in aged samples as an isomerization product of α-pinene. Amongst these lines, other compounds such as α-campholenal, pinocarveol, verbenone, and pinocarvone could also be proposed as ageing markers.

Regarding the antimicrobial properties of the samples, overall, the resins were found to be more potent compared to oils and specifically against *A. nidulans, A. fumigatus,* and *M. circinelloides* as judged on their effect on colony diameter and growth in general. Here, we also obtained direct cellular evidence that the moderate effect of the most potent mastic compounds does not seem to be associated with major morphological defects of the PM, nuclei organization, or the mitochondria of *A. nidulans*. Interestingly also, the most active was compound CMG_8 was a resin sample stored for 2 years, while the relative fresh sample showed moderate activity.

Supplementary Materials: The following are available online at https://www.mdpi.com/2227-9717/9/3/418/s1, Figure S1: HPTLC chromatogram of CMG with the Ph. Eur. Method. Detection at (A) 254 nm and (B) 366 nm. Figure S2: HPTLC chromatogram of CMO with the Ph. Eur. Method. Detection at (A) 254 nm and (B) 366 nm. Figure S3: HPTLC chromatogram of CMG developed with the in-house method. Detection at A) 254 nm and B) 366 nm. Figure S4: HPTLC chromatogram of CMO developed with the in-house method. Detection at (A) 254 nm and (B) 366 nm. Figure S5: Zoomed superimposed total ion chromatograms (TIC) of a fresh (CMO_1) and an aged sample (CMO_9). Figure S6: Effect of resins and essential oils against bacteria. Comparison of bacterial growth (E. coli, P. aeruginosa and B. subtilis), as expressed by measuring optical density values (550 nm), in the presence of resins (CMG_1–8) or essential oils (CMO_1–8), after 24 h of incubation at 37 °C. Values in graphs represent % of growth in the presence of mastic extracts relative to control (no mastic extract added) taken as 100%. In the left panel mastic resins and essential oils diluted in DMSO were added at a final concentration of 0.2 mg/mL (1% DMSO), whilst in the right penal mastic resins diluted in ethanol were added at final concentration of 0.4 mg/mL (1% ethanol). Standard deviation in all cases was <1%. Table S1: Minimum, maximum, and average values for the ratios of major compounds in CMO samples (CMO_1–8, CMO_9).

Author Contributions: Conceptualization, V.K.P., G.D., and M.H.; methodology, V.K.P., E.V.M., S.D., M.D., and A.A.; resources, G.D. and M.H.; writing—original draft preparation, V.K.P., S.D., M.D., and E.V.M.; writing—review and editing, A.A., G.D., and M.H.; visualization, V.K.P., S.D., M.D., and E.V.M.; supervision, G.D. and M.H.; project administration, V.K.P. and M.H.; funding acquisition, G.D. and M.H. All authors have read and agreed to the published version of the manuscript.

Funding: Vasiliki K. Pachi is co-financed by Greece and the European Union (European Social Fund-ESF) through the Operational Programme «Human Resources Development, Education and Lifelong Learning» in the context of the project "Strengthening Human Resources Research Potential via Doctorate Research" (MIS-5000432), implemented by the State Scholarships Foundation (IKY). Eleni V. Mikropoulou is financed through a Stavros Niarchos Foundation (SNF) grant to the National and Kapodistrian University of Athens. The present work was co-funded by the European Union (ERDF) and Greek national funds through the Operational Program "Competitiveness, Entrepreneurship and Innovation", under the call "STRENGTHENING RESEARCH AND INNOVATION INFRASTRUCTURES" (project code: 5002803–PlantUP).

Institutional Review Board Statement: Not applicable.

Informed Consent Statement: Not applicable.

Data Availability Statement: The data presented in this study are available on request from the corresponding author.

Acknowledgments: The authors would like to thank Chios Mastiha Growers Association and especially Smyrnioudis Ilias for kindly providing the CMG samples. The authors are also thankful to Iasis Pharma Hellas S.A. for the valuable information and assistance.

Conflicts of Interest: The authors declare no conflict of interest.

References

1. Pachi, V.K.; Mikropoulou, E.V.; Gkiouvetidis, P.; Siafakas, K.; Argyropoulou, A.; Angelis, A.; Mitakou, S.; Halabalaki, M. Traditional Uses, Phytochemistry and Pharmacology of Chios Mastic Gum (*Pistacia lentiscus* Var. *Chia*, Anacardiaceae): A Review. *J. Ethnopharmacol.* **2020**, *254*. [CrossRef]
2. European Commission. Commission Regulation (EC) No 123/97 of 23 January 1997 Supplementing the Annex to Commission Regulation (EC) No 1107/96 on the Registration of Geographical Indications and Designations of Origin. *Off. J.* **1997**, *L 22*, 19–20.
3. United Nations Educational, Scientific and Cultural Organization. Decision of the Intergovernmental Committee: 9.COM 10.18, Inscribing the Know-How of Cultivating Mastic on the Island of Chios on the Representative List of the Intangible Cultural Heritage of Humanity. 2014. Available online: https://ich.unesco.org/en/Decisions/9.COM/10.18 (accessed on 1 November 2020).
4. European Medicines Agency. Assessment Report on Pistacia lentiscus, L., Resin (Mastix). 2015. Available online: https://www.ema.europa.eu/en/documents/herbal-report/draft-assessment-report-pistacia-lentiscus-l-resin-mastic_en.pdf (accessed on 1 November 2020).
5. Dioscorides, P. *De Materia Medica*, 1st ed.; Militos: Alimos, Greece, 1999.
6. Galen. *Pharmacy*, 2nd ed.; Lindsay and Blakiston: Philadelphia, PA, UAS, 1846.
7. Moussaieff, A.; Fride, E.; Amar, Z.; Lev, E.; Steinberg, D.; Gallily, R.; Mechoulam, R. The Jerusalem Balsam: From the Franciscan Monastery in the Old City of Jerusalem to Martindale 33. *J. Ethnopharmacol.* **2005**, *101*, 16–26. [CrossRef] [PubMed]
8. Assimopoulou, A.N.; Zlatanos, S.N.; Papageorgiou, V.P. Antioxidant Activity of Natural Resins and Bioactive Triterpenes in Oil Substrates. *Food Chem.* **2005**, *92*, 721–727. [CrossRef]
9. Dedoussis, G.V.Z.; Kaliora, A.C.; Psarras, S.; Chiou, A.; Mylona, A.; Papadopoulos, N.G.; Andrikopoulos, N.K. Antiatherogenic Effect of *Pistacia lentiscus* via GSH Restoration and Downregulation of CD36 MRNA Expression. *Atherosclerosis* **2004**, *174*, 293–303. [CrossRef] [PubMed]
10. Kaliora, A.C.; Stathopoulou, M.G.; Triantafillidis, J.K.; Dedoussis, G.V.Z.; Andrikopoulos, N.K. Chios Mastic Treatment of Patients with Active Crohn's Disease. *World J. Gastroenterol.* **2007**, *13*, 748–753. [CrossRef] [PubMed]
11. Tabanca, N.; Nalbantsoy, A.; Kendra, P.E.; Demirci, F.; Demirci, B. Chemical Characterization and Biological Activity of the Mastic Gum Essential Oils of *Pistacia lentiscus* Var. *Chia* from Turkey. *Molecules* **2020**, *25*, 2136. [CrossRef] [PubMed]
12. Vallianou, I.; Peroulis, N.; Pantazis, P.; Hadzopoulou-Cladaras, M. Camphene, a Plant-Derived Monoterpene, Reduces Plasma Cholesterol and Triglycerides in Hyperlipidemic Rats Independently of HMG-CoA Reductase Activity. *PLoS ONE* **2011**, *6*, e20516. [CrossRef] [PubMed]
13. Andreadou, I.; Mitakou, S.; Paraschos, S.; Efentakis, P.; Magiatis, P.; Kaklamanis, L.; Halabalaki, M.; Skaltsounis, L.; Iliodromitis, E.K. "*Pistacia lentiscus*", L. Reduces the Infarct Size in Normal Fed Anesthetized Rabbits and Possess Antiatheromatic and Hypolipidemic Activity in Cholesterol Fed Rabbits. *Phytomedicine* **2016**, *23*, 1220–1226. [CrossRef] [PubMed]
14. Tzani, A.I.; Doulamis, I.P.; Konstantopoulos, P.S.; Pasiou, E.D.; Daskalopoulou, A.; Iliopoulos, D.C.; Georgiadis, I.V.; Kavantzas, N.; Kourkoulis, S.K.; Perrea, D.N. Chios Mastic Gum Decreases Renin Levels and Ameliorates Vascular Remodeling in Renovascular Hypertensive Rats. *Biomed. Pharmacother.* **2018**, *105*, 899–906. [CrossRef]
15. Spyridopoulou, K.; Tiptiri-Kourpeti, A.; Lampri, E.; Fitsiou, E.; Vasileiadis, S.; Vamvakias, M.; Bardouki, H.; Goussia, A.; Malamou-Mitsi, V.; Panayiotidis, M.I.; et al. Dietary Mastic Oil Extracted from *Pistacia lentiscus* Var. *Chia* Suppresses Tumor Growth in Experimental Colon Cancer Models. *Sci. Rep.* **2017**, *7*, 3782–3796. [CrossRef] [PubMed]
16. Magkouta, S.; Stathopoulos, G.T.; Psallidas, I.; Papapetropoulos, A.; Kolisis, F.N.; Roussos, C.; Loutrari, H. Protective Effects of Mastic Oil from *Pistacia lentiscus* Variation *Chia* against Experimental Growth of Lewis Lung Carcinoma. *Nutri. Cancer* **2009**, *61*, 640–648. [CrossRef] [PubMed]
17. Loutrari, H.; Magkouta, S.; Pyriochou, A.; Koika, V.; Kolisis, F.N.; Papapetropoulos, A.; Roussos, C. Mastic Oil from *Pistacia lentiscus* Var. *Chia* Inhibits Growth and Survival of Human K562 Leukemia Cells and Attenuates Angiogenesis. *Nutr. Cancer* **2006**, *55*, 86–93. [CrossRef] [PubMed]
18. Loutrari, H.; Magkouta, S.; Papapetropoulos, A.; Roussos, C. Mastic Oil Inhibits the Metastatic Phenotype of Mouse Lung Adenocarcinoma Cells. *Cancers* **2011**, *3*, 789–801. [CrossRef] [PubMed]
19. Buriani, A.; Fortinguerra, S.; Sorrenti, V.; Dall'Acqua, S.; Innocenti, G.; Montopoli, M.; Gabbia, D.; Carrara, M. Human Adenocarcinoma Cell Line Sensitivity to Essential Oil Phytocomplexes from *Pistacia* Species: A Multivariate Approach. *Molecules* **2017**, *22*, 1336. [CrossRef] [PubMed]
20. Papada, E.; Amerikanou, C.; Torović, L.; Kalogeropoulos, N.; Tzavara, C.; Forbes, A.; Kaliora, A.C. Plasma Free Amino Acid Profile in Quiescent Inflammatory Bowel Disease Patients Orally Administered with Mastiha (*Pistacia lentiscus*); a Randomised Clinical Trial. *Phytomedicine* **2019**, *56*, 40–47. [CrossRef] [PubMed]
21. Triantafyllou, A.; Chaviaras, N.; Sergentanis, T.N.; Protopapa, E.; Tsaknis, J. Chios Mastic Gum Modulates Serum Biochemical Parameters in a Human Population. *J. Ethnopharmacol.* **2007**, *111*, 43–49. [CrossRef]
22. Kartalis, A.; Didagelos, M.; Georgiadis, I.; Benetos, G.; Smyrnioudis, N.; Marmaras, H.; Voutas, P.; Zotika, C.; Garoufalis, S.; Andrikopoulos, G. Effects of Chios Mastic Gum on Cholesterol and Glucose Levels of Healthy Volunteers: A Prospective, Randomized, Placebo-Controlled, Pilot Study (CHIOS-MASTIHA). *Eur. J. Prev. Cardiol.* **2015**, *23*, 722–729. [CrossRef] [PubMed]

23. Kontogiannis, C.; Georgiopoulos, G.; Loukas, K.; Papanagnou, E.-D.; Pachi, V.K.; Bakogianni, I.; Laina, A.; Kouzoupis, A.; Karatzi, K.; Trougakos, I.P.; et al. Chios Mastic Improves Blood Pressure Haemodynamics in Patients with Arterial Hypertension: Implications for Regulation of Proteostatic Pathways. *Eur. J. Prev. Cardiol.* **2019**, *26*, 328–331. [CrossRef]
24. Sterer, N. Antimicrobial Effect of Mastic Gum Methanolic Extract Against *Porphyromonas gingivalis*. *J. Med. Food* **2006**, *9*, 290–292. [CrossRef]
25. Koychev, S.; Dommisch, H.; Chen, H.; Pischon, N. Antimicrobial Effects of Mastic Extract Against Oral and Periodontal Pathogens. *J. Periodontol.* **2017**, *88*, 511–517. [CrossRef]
26. Miyamoto, T.; Okimoto, T.; Kuwano, M. Chemical Composition of the Essential Oil of Mastic Gum and Their Antibacterial Activity Against Drug-Resistant *Helicobacter pylori*. *Nat. Prod. Bioprospecting* **2014**, *4*, 227–231. [CrossRef]
27. Karygianni, L.; Cecere, M.; Skaltsounis, A.L.; Argyropoulou, A.; Hellwig, E.; Aligiannis, N.; Wittmer, A.; Al-Ahmad, A. High-Level Antimicrobial Efficacy of Representative Mediterranean Natural Plant Extracts against Oral Microorganisms. *BioMed Res. Int.* **2014**, *2014*, 839019. [CrossRef] [PubMed]
28. Tassou, C.C.; Nychas, G.J.E. Antimicrobial Activity of the Essential Oil of Mastic Gum (*Pistacia lentiscus* Var. *Chia*) on Gram Positive and Gram Negative Bacteria in Broth and in Model Food System. *Int. Biodeterior. Biodegrad.* **1995**, *36*, 411–420. [CrossRef]
29. Vrouvaki, I.; Koutra, E.; Kornaros, M.; Avgoustakis, K.; Lamari, F.N.; Hatziantoniou, S. Polymeric Nanoparticles of *Pistacia lentiscus* Var. *Chia* Essential Oil for Cutaneous Applications. *Pharmaceutics* **2020**, *12*, 353. [CrossRef] [PubMed]
30. Magiatis, P.; Melliou, E.; Skaltsounis, A.L.; Chinou, I.B.; Mitaku, S. Chemical Composition and Antimicrobial Activity of the Essential Oils of *Pistacia lentiscus* Var. *Chia*. *Planta Med.* **1999**, *65*, 749–752. [CrossRef]
31. Sharifi, M.S.; Hazell, S.L. Fractionation of Mastic Gum in Relation to Antimicrobial Activity. *Pharmaceuticals* **2009**, *2*, 2–10. [CrossRef]
32. Paraskevopoulou, A.; Kiosseoglou, V. Chios Mastic Gum and Its Food Applications. In *Functional Properties of Traditional Foods*; Springer: Berlin/Heidelberg, Germany, 2016; pp. 271–287.
33. Fazeli-Nasab, B.; Fooladvand, Z. Classification and Evaluation of Medicinal Plant and Medicinal Properties of Mastic. *Int. J. Adv. Biol. Biomed. Res.* **2014**, *2*, 2155–2161.
34. CMGA. Available online: https://www.gummastic.gr/en (accessed on 5 November 2020).
35. Mavrakis, C.; Kiosseoglou, V. The Structural Characteristics and Mechanical Properties of Biopolymer/Mastic Gum Microsized Particles Composites. *Food Hydrocoll.* **2008**, *22*, 854–861. [CrossRef]
36. Paraschos, S. *Phytochemical and Pharmacological Study of Chios Mastic Gum*; National and Kapodistrian University of Athens: Athens, Greece, 2010. [CrossRef]
37. Xynos, N.; Termentzi, A.; Fokialakis, N.; Skaltsounis, L.A.; Aligiannis, N. Supercritical CO_2 extraction of Mastic Gum and Chemical Characterization of Bioactive Fractions Using LC-HRMS/MS and GC–MS. *J. Supercrit. Fluids* **2018**, *133*, 349–356. [CrossRef]
38. Papanicolaou, D.; Melanitou, M.; Katsaboxakis, K. Changes in Chemical Composition of the Essential Oil of Chios "Mastic Resin" from *Pistacia lentiscus* Var. *Chia* Tree during Solidification and Storage. *Dev. Food Sci.* **1995**, *37*, 303–310. [CrossRef]
39. Daferera, D.; Pappas, C.; Tarantilis, P.A.; Polissiou, M. Quantitative Analysis of α-Pinene and β-Myrcene in Mastic Gum Oil Using FT-Raman Spectroscopy. *Food Chem.* **2002**, *77*, 511–515. [CrossRef]
40. Koutsoudaki, C.; Krsek, M.; Rodger, A. Chemical Composition and Antibacterial Activity of the Essential Oil and the Gum of *Pistacia lentiscus* Var. *Chia*. *J. Agric. Food Chem.* **2005**, *53*, 7681–7685. [CrossRef]
41. Hellenic Republic, Ministry of Rural Development and Food. Available online: www.minagric.gr (accessed on 25 November 2020).
42. Ierapetritis, D.; Fotaki, M. Συνεταιριστική Κοινωνική Επιχειρηματικότητα: Η ανάπτυξη δικτύου καταστημάτων λιανικής πώλησης τησ Ένωσης Μαστιχοπαραγωγών Χίου και οι επιπτώσεις της (text in Greek). In *Kainotomo-Epicheiro*; Lioukas, S., Ed.; Athens University of Economics and Business: Athens, Greece, 2013.
43. Rigling, M.; Fraatz, M.A.; Trögel, S.; Sun, J.; Zorn, H.; Zhang, Y. Aroma Investigation of Chios Mastic Gum (*Pistacia lentiscus* Variety *Chia*) Using Headspace Gas Chromatography Combined with Olfactory Detection and Chiral Analysis. *J. Agric. Food Chem.* **2019**, *67*, 13420–13429. [CrossRef]
44. *European Pharmacopoeia 9.0*; 2011; Volume 1, pp. 2277–2278. Available online: https://www.tsoshop.co.uk/?DI=647707 (accessed on 28 January 2021).
45. Adams, R.P. *Identification of Essential Oil Components by Gas Chromatography/Mass Spectrometry*, 4th ed.; Allured Publishing Corporation: Carol Stream, IL, USA, 2007.
46. NIST. Available online: https://webbook.nist.gov/chemistry/ (accessed on 20 October 2020).
47. Maryutina, T.A.; Savonina, E.Y.; Fedotov, P.S.; Smith, R.M.; Siren, H.; Hibbert, D.B. Terminology of Separation Methods (IUPAC Recommendations 2017). *Pure Appl. Chem.* **2018**, *90*, 181–213. [CrossRef]
48. FGSC. Available online: http://www.fgsc.net (accessed on 2 November 2020).
49. Papanicolaou, D.; Melanitou, M.; Katsaboxakis, K. Effect of α-Tocopherol (Vitamin E) on the Retention of Essential Oil, Color and Texture of Chios Mastic Resin during Storage. *Dev. Food Sci.* **1998**, *40*, 689–694. [CrossRef]
50. Papageorgiou, V.P.; Mellidis, A.S.; Argyriadou, N. The Chemical Composition of the Essential Oil of Mastic Gum. *J. Essent. Oil Res.* **1991**, *3*, 107–110. [CrossRef]

51. Paraschos, S.; Magiatis, P.; Gikas, E.; Smyrnioudis, I.; Skaltsounis, A.-L. Quality Profile Determination of Chios Mastic Gum Essential Oil and Detection of Adulteration in Mastic Oil Products with the Application of Chiral and Non-Chiral GC–MS Analysis. *Fitoterapia* **2016**, *114*, 12–17. [CrossRef] [PubMed]
52. Van Den Berg, K.J.; Van Der Horst, J.; Boon, J.J.; Sudmeijer, O.O. Cis-1,4-Poly-β-Myrcene: The Structure of the Polymeric Fraction of Mastic Resin (*Pistacia lentiscus*, L.) Elucidated. *Tetrahedron Lett.* **1998**, *39*, 2645–2648. [CrossRef]
53. Behr, A.; Johnen, L. Myrcene as a Natural Base Chemical in Sustainable Chemistry: A Critical Review. *ChemSusChem* **2009**, *2*, 1072–1095. [CrossRef] [PubMed]
54. Mikropoulou, E.V.; Petrakis, E.A.; Argyropoulou, A.; Halabalaki, M.; Skaltsounis, L.A. Quantification of Bioactive Lignans in Sesame Seeds Using HPTLC Densitometry: Comparative Evaluation by HPLC-PDA. *Food Chem.* **2019**, *288*, 1–7. [CrossRef] [PubMed]
55. Meier, B.; Spriano, D. Modern HPTLC-A Perfect Tool for Quality Control of Herbals and Their Preparations. *J. AOAC Int.* **2010**, *93*, 1399–1409. [CrossRef] [PubMed]
56. Assimopoulou, A.N.; Papageorgiou, V.P. GC-MS Analysis of Penta- and Tetra-Cyclic Triterpenes from Resins of Pistacia Species. Part, I. *Pistacia lentiscus* Var. *Chia. Biomed. Chromatogr.* **2005**, *19*, 285–311. [CrossRef]
57. Papageorgiou, V.P.; Bakola-Christianopoulou, M.N.; Apazidou, K.K.; Psarros, E.E. Gas Chromatographic-Mass Spectroscopic Analysis of the Acidic Triterpenic Fraction of Mastic Gum. *J. Chromatography A* **1997**, *769*, 263–273. [CrossRef]
58. Serifi, I.; Tzima, E.; Bardouki, H.; Lampri, E.; Papamarcaki, T. Effects of the Essential Oil from *Pistacia lentiscus* Var. *Chia* on the Lateral Line System and the Gene Expression Profile of Zebrafish (*Danio rerio*). *Molecules* **2019**, *24*, 3919. [CrossRef]
59. Papageorgiou, V.P.; Sagredos, A.N.; Mose, R. GLC-MS Computer Analysis of the Essential Oil of Mastic Gum. *Chim. Chronica New Ser.* **1981**, *10*, 119–124.
60. Boelens, M.H.; Jimenez, R. Chemical Composition of the Essential Oils from the Gum and from Various Parts of *Pistacia lentiscus* L. (Mastic Gum Tree). *Flavour Fragr. J.* **1991**, *6*, 271–275. [CrossRef]
61. Duru, M.E.; Cakir, A.; Kordali, S.; Zengin, H.; Harmandar, M.; Izumi, S.; Hirata, T. Chemical Composition and Antifungal Properties of Essential Oils of Three Pistacia Species. *Fitoterapia* **2003**, *74*, 170–176. [CrossRef]
62. Burham, B.O.; EL-Kamali, H.H.; EL-Egami, A.A. Volatile Components of the Resin of *Pistacia lentiscus* "Mistica" Used in Sudanese Traditional Medicine. *J. Chem. Pharm. Res.* **2011**, *3*, 478–482.
63. Neuenschwander, U.; Guignard, F.; Hermans, I. Mechanism of the Aerobic Oxidation of α-Pinene. *ChemSusChem* **2010**, *3*, 75–84. [CrossRef]
64. Neuenschwander, U.; Meier, E.; Hermans, I. Peculiarities of β-Pinene Autoxidation. *ChemSusChem* **2011**, *4*, 1613–1621. [CrossRef] [PubMed]
65. Slaghenaufi, D.; Ugliano, M. Norisoprenoids, Sesquiterpenes and Terpenoids Content of Valpolicella Wines during Aging: Investigating Aroma Potential in Relationship to Evolution of Tobacco and Balsamic Aroma in Aged Wine. *Front. Chem.* **2018**, *6*, 1–13. [CrossRef] [PubMed]
66. Karlberg, A.; Magnusson, K.; Nilsson, U. Air Oxidation of D-limonene (the Citrus Solvent) Creates Potent Allergens. *Contact Dermat.* **1992**, *26*, 332–340. [CrossRef] [PubMed]
67. Scazzocchio, C. Aspergillus: A Multifaceted Genus. In *Encyclopedia of Microbiology*; Academic Press: Cambridge, MA, USA, 2009; ISBN 9780123739445.
68. Jerez Puebla, L.E. Fungal Infections in Immunosuppressed Patients. In *Immunodeficiency*; InTech: Rijeka, Croatia, 2012.
69. Latgé, J.P.; Chamilos, G. Aspergillus Fumigatus and Aspergillosis in 2019. *Clin. Microbiol. Rev.* **2020**, *33*. [CrossRef]
70. Ghuman, H.; Voelz, K. Innate and Adaptive Immunity to Mucorales. *J. Fungi* **2017**, *3*, 48. [CrossRef]
71. Chamilos, G.; Lewis, R.E.; Kontoyiannis, D.P. Lovastatin Has Significant Activity against Zygomycetes and Interacts Synergistically with Voriconazole. *Antimicrob. Agents Chemother.* **2006**, *50*, 96–103. [CrossRef]
72. Wiederhold, N.P. Antifungal Resistance: Current Trends and Future Strategies to Combat. *Infect. Drug Resist.* **2017**, *10*, 249–259. [CrossRef] [PubMed]
73. Pantazopoulou, A.; Lemuh, N.D.; Hatzinikolaou, D.G.; Drevet, C.; Cecchetto, G.; Scazzocchio, C.; Diallinas, G. Differential Physiological and Developmental Expression of the UapA and AzgA Purine Transporters in *Aspergillus nidulans*. *Fungal Genet. Biol.* **2007**, *44*, 627–640. [CrossRef] [PubMed]
74. Toews, M.W.; Warmbold, J.; Konzack, S.; Rischitor, P.; Veith, D.; Vienken, K.; Vinuesa, C.; Wei, H.; Fischer, R. Establishment of MRPF1 as a Fluorescent Marker in *Aspergillus nidulans* and Construction of Expression Vectors for High-Throughput Protein Tagging Using Recombination in Vitro (GATEWAY). *Curr. Genet.* **2004**, *45*, 383–389. [CrossRef] [PubMed]
75. Sant, D.G.; Tupe, S.G.; Ramana, C.V.; Deshpande, M.V. Fungal Cell Membrane—Promising Drug Target for Antifungal Therapy. *J. Appl. Microbiol.* **2016**, *121*, 1498–1510. [CrossRef] [PubMed]
76. Gkogka, E.; Hazeleger, W.C.; Posthumus, M.A.; Beumer, R.R. The Antimicrobial Activity of the Essential Oil of *Pistacia lentiscus* Var. *Chia. J. Essent. Oil Bear. Plants* **2013**, *16*, 714–729. [CrossRef]

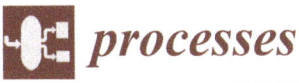

Article

Biofilm Degradation of Nontuberculous Mycobacteria Formed on Stainless Steel Following Treatment with Immortelle (*Helichrysum italicum*) and Common Juniper (*Juniperus communis*) Essential Oils

Dolores Peruč [1,*], Dalibor Broznić [2], Željka Maglica [3], Zvonimir Marijanović [4], Ljerka Karleuša [5] and Ivana Gobin [1]

1. Department of Microbiology and Parasitology, Faculty of Medicine, University of Rijeka, 51000 Rijeka, Croatia; ivana.gobin@uniri.hr
2. Department of Medical Chemistry, Biochemistry and Clinical Chemistry, Faculty of Medicine, University of Rijeka, 51000 Rijeka, Croatia; dalibor.broznic@medri.uniri.hr
3. Department of Biotechnology, University of Rijeka, 51000 Rijeka, Croatia; zeljka.maglica@uniri.hr
4. Department of Food Technology and Biotechnology, Faculty of Chemistry and Technology, University of Split, 21000 Split, Croatia; zvonimir.marijanovic@ktf-split.hr
5. Department of Physiology and Immunology, Faculty of Medicine, University of Rijeka, 51000 Rijeka, Croatia; ljerka.karleusa@medri.uniri.hr
* Correspondence: dolores.peruc@uniri.hr; Tel.: +385-(0)51-651-145; Fax: +385-(0)51-651-177

Abstract: Nontuberculous mycobacteria, like other opportunistic premise plumbing pathogens, produce resistant biofilms on various surfaces in the plumbing system including pipes, tanks, and fittings. Since standard methods of water disinfection are ineffective in eradicating biofilms, research into new agents is necessary. Essential oils (EOs) have great potential as anti-biofilm agents. Therefore, the purpose of this research was to investigate the potential anti-biofilm effect of common juniper (*Juniperus communis*) and immortelle (*Helichrysum italicum*) EOs. Minimum inhibitory concentrations (MIC), minimum bactericidal concentrations (MBC), and minimum effective concentrations of EOs on *Mycobacterium avium*, *M. intracellulare*, and *M. gordonae* were tested. Additionally, biofilms on the surface of a stainless steel disc were treated with single or mixed concentration of EOs, in order to investigate their degeneration via the bacterial count and confocal laser scanning microscopy (CLSM). *H. italicum* EO showed the strongest biofilm degradation ability against all Mycobacteria strains that were tested. The strongest effect in the biofilm degradation after the single or mixed applications of EOs was observed against *M. gordonae*, followed by *M. avium*. The most resistant was the *M. intracellulare* biofilm. Synergistic combinations of *J. communis* and *H. italicum* EOs therefore seem to be an effective substance in biofilm degradation for use in small water systems such as baths or hot tubs.

Keywords: biofilm; common juniper; immortelle; nontuberculous mycobacteria; stainless steel

1. Introduction

Mycobacteria originated 150 million years ago [1]. The *genus Mycobacterium* is the only member of the family *Mycobacteriaceae* from the *order Actinomycetales* and the class *Actinomycetes*. Today, more than 200 species belong to the genus *Mycobacterium*, which include obligate and opportunistic pathogens and saprophytes [2]. Nontuberculous mycobacteria (NTM) are a heterogeneous group of environmental bacteria mainly isolated from water, soil, dust, various animals, milk, and dairy products [3]. Although mostly apathogenic, nowadays, they increasingly represent important environmental opportunistic pathogens [4]. *Mycobacterium avium* and *M. intracellulare* are members of the *Mycobacterium avium* complex (MAC). These are slow-growing unpigmented mycobacteria that form smooth, flat, transparent colonies. MACs are the most frequently isolated pathogenic NTM species from respiratory samples [5]. *M. gordonae* is a mycobacterium that forms smooth orange colonies and is a mostly apathogenic, saprophytic species of NTM [5,6]. In Croatia, it is one of the most common isolates from the respiratory tract, but is extremely rarely associated with clinically proven infection [7]. Inhalation of infectious aerosol is a major transmission route for pulmonary infections caused by NTM [8]. The source of infection can be drinking tap water, well water, taps in residential, hospital and laboratory areas, hot tub water, house dust, potted soil, forest soil, domestic animals, or sea water [8–10]. The presence of NTM in these sources is mainly a result of their ability to form biofilms and to survive in free-living amoebae [9]. Due to a high content of complex lipids and mycolates, the cell wall of mycobacteria is extremely hydrophobic, which greatly facilitates their binding to various surfaces and biofilm formation and contributes to their resistance to phagocytosis, disinfectants, and antimicrobial drugs [2]. The research revealed that tap water is often a source of NTM colonization and/or infection [11]. In the aquatic environment, *M. avium* has an exceptional ability to form biofilm [4]. As a result, this mycobacterium, along with *Legionella pneumophila, Pseudomonas aeruginosa,* and *Acinetobacter baumannii,* is classified as an opportunistic premise plumbing pathogen (OPPP) [12]. Twice as many *Mycobacterium* spp. were found in biofilm samples from showerheads than were found in drinking water samples. *M. gordonae, M. avium, M. intracellulare,* and *M. xenopi* were the species most frequently isolated from these biofilms, while drinking water contained significant amounts of *M. gordonae, M. chelonae, M. fortuitum,* and *M. terrae* [13,14].

Most studies comparing the formation of biofilms of slow-growing NTMs in the aquatic environment have identified three key determinants: First, NTMs can, independently, without the presence of other microorganisms, create a suitable substrate and begin biofilm formation. Second, plastic and siliconized substrates widely used in medicine and in the water supply system can be very quickly colonized with mycobacteria. Third, NTMs can produce biofilms under the conditions of low nutrient levels such as in the water supply system, without significantly impairing their growth potential [15].

The Mediterranean area is known as the natural habitat of a large number of medicinal plants that have long been utilized in traditional medicine. According to the available data, the Croatian flora consists of over 4000 species [16]. Research on the antimicrobial effect of certain plant species and natural substances, the effective concentration of which has no harmful effects on the human body, represents an important contribution to the improvement of therapeutic and preventive protocols. The biochemical and physiological properties of each plant species directly depend on its chemical composition. This primarily refers to the fact that each individual species inhabiting a particular geographical area will have a genome encoding specific enzyme system, which in turn produces a specific range of certain chemical compounds [17]. Essential oils (EO) are extracts characterized as a complex mixture of volatile constituents having a strong scent. They are formed by the secondary metabolism of plants [18]. There is substantial data in the literature on the antibacterial, antifungal, and antiviral effects of different EOs [19–21], but few studies have been made on the effects of EOs on mycobacteria [22,23].

Common juniper (*Juniperus communis*) is an evergreen coniferous shrub that grows in the hilly regions of the Northern Hemisphere. Its needles and dried fruit are used in traditional medicine as diuretic, uroantiseptic, carminative, digestive, and antioxidant agents [24]. The main bioactive substances in *J. communis* EO are: α- and β-pinene, β-myrcene, sabinene, limonene, terpinene-4-ol and β-caryophyllene [25–27]. Immortelle (*Helichrysum italicum*), a perennial flowering plant belonging to the genus *Helichrysum*, from the family *Asteraceae*, is widely distributed along the Adriatic coast and islands and is used in traditional medicine for its anti-inflammatory, antimicrobial, and antioxidant properties [28]. *H. italicum* EO, produced from the flowering plant, is most commonly reported to contain: α-pinene, neryl acetate, β-curcumene, γ-curcumene, β-caryophyllene, limonene, α-cadrene, and geranyl acetate [17,29,30].

The first aim of this study was to determine the chemical compositions of *J. communis* and *H. italicum* EOs as well as to examine the antimicrobial effects of these EOs on *M. avium, M. intracellulare,* and *M.gordonae* and to determine their minimum inhibitory concentration (MIC) and minimum bactericidal concentration (MBC). The second aim was to examine the interaction of *J. communis* and *H. italicum* EOs on selected NTMs and their effect on the degradation of mycobacterial biofilms formed on stainless steel.

2. Material and Methods

2.1. Essential Oils

The natural EOs of common juniper (*Juniperus communis*) and immortelle (*Helichrysum italicum*) used in this research were purchased from IREX AROMA d.o.o., Zagreb, Croatia. The EOs were produced in 2018. Gas chromatography and mass spectrometry (GC/MS) analyses of EOs were done [31]. EOs have been shown to have chemical composition characteristic for the said essential oils. Each EO was dissolved in dimethylsulfoxide (DMSO; Kemika, Zagreb, Croatia) to obtain a stock suspension, which was stored in sterile glass vials in the dark at 4 °C prior to use.

2.2. Strains and Growth Media

American Type Culture Collection (ATCC) strains were used in these experiments: *Mycobacterium avium* ssp. *avium* (serotype 2) ATCC 25291, *Mycobacterium intracellulare* ATCC 13950, and *Mycobacterium gordonae* ATCC 14470, and were cultured as described previously [27,32,33]. Briefly, bacterial strains were subcultured twice in Middlebrook 7H9 broth (7H9S, Difco, Detroit, Michigan, USA) containing 10% albumin-dextrose-catalase enrichment (ADC, Biolife Italiana, Milano, Italy) and 0.05% Tween 80 (Biolife Italiana, Milano, Italy) at 30 °C (*M. gordonae*) or 37 °C (*M. avium* and *M. intracellulare*) for at least 14 days to obtain 10^8 CFU mL^{-1}. The bacteria were kept frozen at −80 °C in 7H9S with 10% glycerol (Kemika, Zagreb, Croatia). For each experiment, an aliquot was thawed and subcultured in 7H9S for at least 14 days and then on Middlebrook 7H10 agar (7H10S, Difco, Detroit, Michigan, USA) with 10% oleic acid-albumin-dextrose-catalase enrichment (OADC, Biolife Italiana, Milan, Italy) and 0.05% Tween 80 at 30 °C (*M. gordonae*) or 37 °C (*M. avium* and *M. intracellulare*) for another 14 days. The number of bacteria in the initial inocula were verified by diluting and plating the culture onto 7H10S and incubating at 30 °C (*M. gordonae*) or 37 °C (*M. avium* and *M. intracellulare*) for four to six weeks, after which colonies were counted.

2.3. Sterile Tap Water Sample

In all experiments, tap water from the public water supply system of the city of Rijeka was used. Physicochemical parameters of tap water in Rijeka are regularly monitored by authorized Croatian testing laboratories certified to provide chemical analysis of drinking water and show values that rarely deviate. The water is colorless and odorless, with a normal temperature parameter depending on seasonal variations. It has low turbidity, neutral to slightly alkaline pH (from 7.5 to 8.0), low conductivity (0.211–0.250 mS cm^{-1} at 20 °C), and moderate total hardness (135 mg L^{-1}). According to these parameters, it is considered as medium hard. The tap water sample in a glass bottle was left at room temperature for two days to allow for dechlorination. The water sample was then autoclaved at 121 °C for 15 min and cooled to room temperature and stored at 4 °C until use.

2.4. Checkerboard Synergy Method

To determine the potential interaction effect of *J. communis* and *H. italicum* EOs on NTM, the checkerboard synergy method was used, as described previously [33–35]. Briefly, stock solutions and serial two-fold dilutions of each EO were prepared in 7H9S. These dilutions were arrayed in a grid pattern, with the *J. communis* EO dilution series running perpendicular to that of the *H. italicum* EO. The combinations of concentrations of each EO tested are shown in the results section (Figure 1). An inoculum of each *Mycobacterium* isolate (10^6 CFU mL^{-1}) was prepared in 7H9S and added along with 0.015% resazurin solution (Sigma-Aldrich, Darmstadt, Germany) to wells containing diluted EOs. Positive (bacterial inoculum in 7H9S) and negative (7H9S) growth controls were prepared. Additionally, the antibiotic amikacin (Sigma-Aldrich, Darmstadt, Germany) was also tested against all three mycobacteria. The final concentration of DMSO as a solvent was approximately 10% and its effect was tested against the selected mycobacteria. The plates were incubated for four days under aerobic conditions at 30 °C (*M. gordonae*) or 37 °C (*M. avium* and *M. intracellulare*), and then dilutions from each well were inoculated on 7H10S in duplicate and incubated for a further four weeks. Fractional inhibitory concentration or fractional bactericidal concentration [36] and fractional inhibitory concentration index (FIC_i) or fractional bactericidal concentration index (FBCi) were determined as previously described by Bassole et al. and White et al. [20,37]. Baes on the FIC_i or FBC_i values, a combination of EOs was considered synergistic if FIC_i/FBC_i was ≤ 0.5, additive if FIC_i/FBC_i was >0.5 and ≤ 1.0, indifferent when FIC_i/FBC_i was >1.0 and ≤ 4, and antagonistic if FBC_i was >4 [38].

2.5. Effect of Juniperus communis and Helichrysum italicum Essential Oils on Mycobacterial Biofilm on Stainless Steel Discs in Sterilized Tap Water

The effect of different concentrations of *J. communis* and *H. italicum* EOs as well as synergistic or additive combinations of these EOs on the degradation of the biofilm of *M. avium*, *M. intracellulare*, and *M. gordonae* was tested on stainless steel discs (diameter, 5 mm; American Iron and Steel Institute (AISA) type 316) in sterilized tap water (STW). The discs were left overnight in 70% ethanol (Kemika, Zagreb, Croatia), rinsed with distilled water, air dried, dry heat sterilized at 160 °C, and then aseptically transferred to the wells of microtiter plates (24-well microtiter plates, Falcon, Becton Dickinson, Franklin Lakes, New Jersey, USA). Then, a suspension of 10^6 CFU mL^{-1} of mycobacterial cells was prepared in STW and added to wells containing discs to form a biofilm. The plates were incubated for 72 h at 30 °C (*M. gordonae*) or 37 °C (*M. avium* and *M. intracellulare*), then carefully washed with STW to remove planktonic cells and transferred to new microtiter plates. *J. communis* EO or *H. italicum* EO in MIC, 2 × MIC and their synergistic (for *M. avium* and *M. gordonae*) or additive (for *M. intracellulare*) combinations were added to the biofilm and were then incubated for an additional 24 h at 30 °C (*M. gordonae*) or 37 °C (*M. avium* and *M. intracellulare*). Untreated mycobacterial cells served as controls. Discs were then washed three times with STW and sonicated in a water bath (Bactosonic, Bandelin, Berlin, Germany) at 40 kHz for 1 min. Mycobacteria were quantified by culturing on 7H10S at 37 °C for 14 days, until colonies were observed. The percentage of degradation in the biofilm on the stainless steel discs that resulted from this was determined as described previously by Teanpaisan et al. [39]:

$$\text{Percentage of degradation } (\%) = 1 - \frac{\text{CFU of sample treated with EO}}{\text{CFU of negative control}} \times 100$$

2.6. Determination of Cell Viability in Biofilms Growing on Stainless Steel Coupons, after Treatment with Juniperus communis and Helichrysum italicum Essential Oils

Cell viability assays were performed (Live/Dead BacLight Bacterial Viability Kit; Invitrogen, Carlsbad, California, USA) according to the manufacturer's protocol. Briefly, a biofilm of *M. avium* and *M. intracellulare* was grown for three days on round stainless steel discs. These were exposed to the individual effect of *J. communis* or *H. italicum* EOs, in synergistic or additive combinations, for 22 h at 37 °C. The stainless steel discs were carefully washed with STW to remove planktonic cells. Fluorescent-stain working solution was prepared by adding 3 μL of the SYTO® 9 stain and 3 μL of the propidium iodide (PI) stain to 1 mL of filter-sterilized water. This staining solution was then applied to the surface of the disc and incubated in the dark for 15 min. The samples were then washed with sterile saline to remove excess dye. Fluorescence from the stained cells was observed using an Olympus confocal microscope FV300 (Olympus Optical Company, Tokyo, Japan) with a 40x LCPlanF objective. The excitation/emission maxima for these dyes are around 480/500 nm for the SYTO® 9 stain and 490/635 nm for PI. Simultaneous dual-channel imaging was used to display green and red fluorescence. The obtained images were saved in TIFF format, and further processed using ImageJ 1.47. A minimum of three images per term were analyzed.

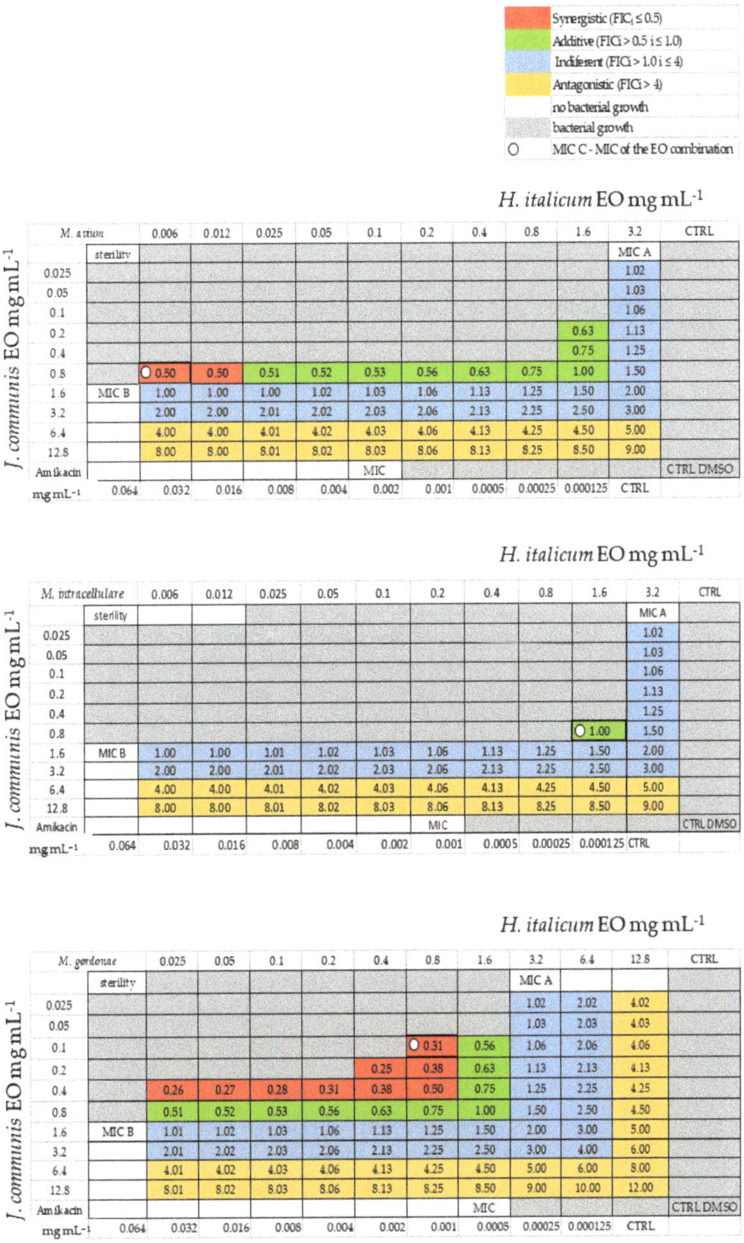

Figure 1. Checkerboard synergy method for the potential interaction of *J. communis* and *H. italicum* EOs on nontuberculous mycobacteria (NTM). MIC—minimal inhibitory concentration; FIC—fractional inhibitory concentration; FIC$_i$—fractional inhibitory concentration index; CTRL—control; EO—essential oil.

2.7. Statistical Analysis

All assays were repeated three times. Experimental data were expressed as means with standard deviations and analyzed using STATISTICA commercial software, 12.0

(StatSoft, Tulsa, OK, USA). Differences between groups of samples were analyzed using the Kruskal–Wallis ANOVA on ranks test, while the effects of EOs on mycobacterium were tested using the Mann–Whitney U test. Differences with $p < 0.05$ were considered to be statistically significant.

3. Results

3.1. Checkerboard Synergy Method

The MIC and MBC values obtained for *J. communis* and *H. italicum* EOs against *M. avium*, *M. intracellulare*, and *M. gordonae* were 1.6 mg mL^{-1} and 3.2 mg mL^{-1}, respectively (Figures 1 and 2). For the control antibiotic, amikacin, MIC was 0.002 mg mL^{-1} for *M. avium*, 0.001 mg mL^{-1} for *M. intracellulare*, and 0.0005 mg mL^{-1} for *M. gordonae* (Figure 1). The DMSO growth control showed that the concentration applied did not affect the growth of the mycobacteria being tested.

The best effective combination of low synergistic combinations of the EOs to achieve a high efficacy against *M. avium* in the checkerboard synergy method was 0.8 mg mL^{-1} (1/2 of the MIC) for *J. communis* EO, 0.006 (1/512 of the MIC) and 0.012 mg mL^{-1} (1/256 of the MIC) for *H. italicum* EO. A combination of 0.8 mg mL^{-1} *J. communis* EO with 0.006 mg *H. italicum* EO represents the MIC for this pair of EOs against *M. avium*. A combination of these EOs only showed an additive effect against *M. intracellulare*, with the lowest concentrations of these combined EOs (MIC of the EO combination) being 0.8 mg mL^{-1} (1/2 of the MIC) for *J. communis* and 1.6 mg mL^{-1} (1/2 × MIC) for *H. italicum*. MIC of the combined EOs against *M. gordonae* was *J. communis* EO in concentrations of 0.1 mg mL^{-1} (1/16 of the MIC) or 0.2 mg mL^{-1} (1/8 of the MIC) and *H. italicum* in concentrations of 0.4 mg mL^{-1} (1/8 of the MIC) or 0.8 mg mL^{-1} (1/4 of the MIC). Nine possible synergistic combinations were found against *M. gordonae*. The combinations of EOs that showed a synergistic inhibitory effect against *M. avium*, also had a synergistic bactericidal effect (MBC of the EO combination, Figure 2). Against *M. intracellulare*, no synergistic or additive bactericidal effect of EO combinations was observed. The combinations of 0.4 mg mL^{-1} *J. communis* EO and 0.025 mg mL^{-1} or 0.8 mg mL^{-1} *H. italicum* EO showed synergistic bactericidal effect against *M. gordonae*. The MBC for amikacin was 0.004 mg mL^{-1} against *M. avium* and *M. intracellulare* and 0.008 mg mL^{-1} against *M. gordonae*.

3.2. Effect of Juniperus communis and Helichrysum italicum Essential Oils on Mycobacterial Biofilm on Stainless Steel Discs in Sterilized Tap Water

As can be seen in Figure 3, *H. italicum* EO was more effective than *J. communis* EO at degrading biofilm formed in STW on stainless steel AISI 316 discs for all treatments of mycobacteria. Almost all of the treatments (excluding the concentration of *J. communis* MIC for *M. avium* and *M. intracellulare*) caused statistically significant biofilm degradation ($p < 0.05$) using both EOs, when compared to the control group. In the control group, the 2 × MIC concentration of *H. italicum* EO led to the most substantial degradation of the biofilm. No statistically significant differences were found in *M. avium* and *M. intracellulare* biofilm degradation with *H. italicum* EO at concentrations of either the MIC and 2 × MIC (Figure 3a,b). In contrast, the *M. gordonae* (Figure 3c) biofilm showed statistically significant biofilm degradation using either the MIC or 2 × MIC of *H. italicum* EO ($p < 0.05$). *J. communis* EO demonstrated a lower effectiveness on biofilm degradation in all treatments and no statistically significant differences were found for any of the mycobacteria.

Subinhibitory synergistic concentrations of *J. communis* and *H. italicum* EO did not degrade biofilms of *M. gordonae* formed on stainless steel discs in STW in a statistically significant manner (Figure 4c). Furthermore, significant degradation of *M. avium* biofilm by *J. communis* and *H. italicum* EOs was observed using concentrations of 0.8 mg mL^{-1} and/or 0.012 mg mL^{-1} (Figure 4a). Meanwhile, a subinhibitory concentration of *H. italicum* EO (1.6 mg mL^{-1}) degraded biofilms formed by *M. intracellulare* ($p < 0.05$; Figure 4b). The combination of subinhibitory concentrations of *J. communis* and *H. italicum* EOs had a significant effect ($p < 0.05$) on the degradation of all mycobacteria biofilms formed on stainless steel discs.

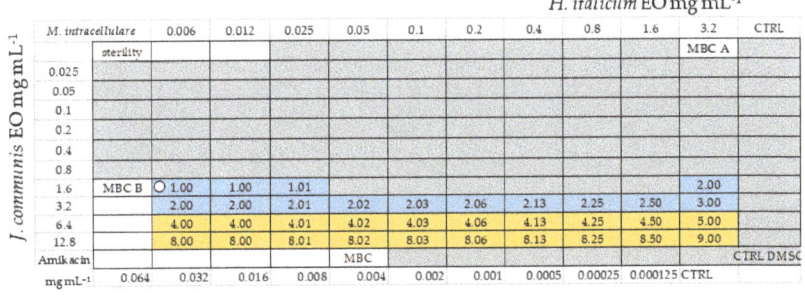

Figure 2. Checkerboard synergy method for the potential interaction of *J. communis* and *H. italicum* EOs on NTM. MBC—minimal inhibitory concentration; FBC—fractional inhibitory concentration; FBC_i—fractional inhibitory concentration index; CTRL—control; EO—essential oil.

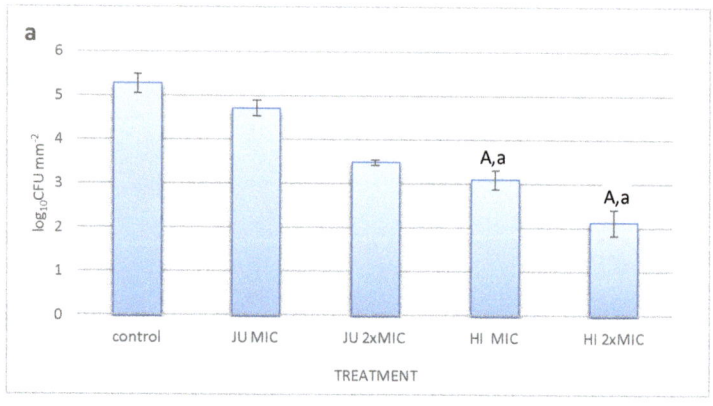
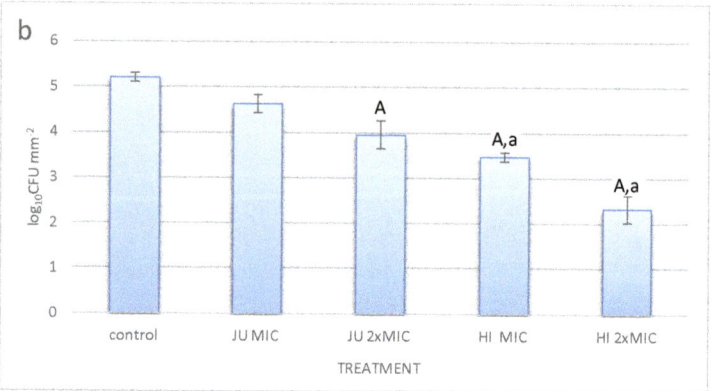
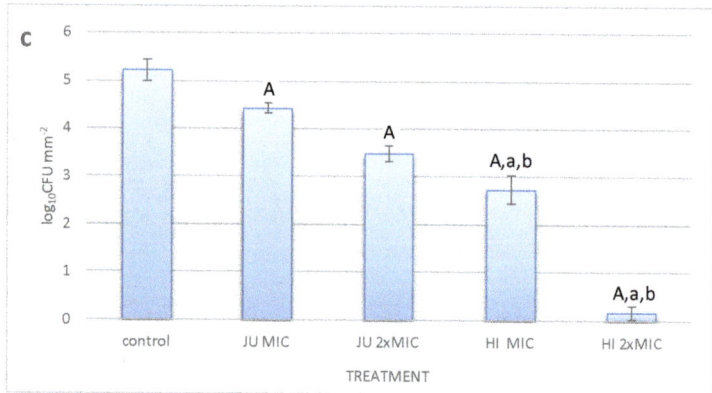

Figure 3. Effect of the MIC and 2 × MIC in mg mL^{-1} of *J. communis* and *H. italicum* EOs on the degradation of biofilms of *M. avium* (**a**), *M. intracellulare* (**b**), and *M. gordonae* (**c**) formed on stainless steel (AISI316) discs. Untreated mycobacterial cells served as controls. MIC—minimum inhibitory concentration; CFU—colony forming unit; JU—*Juniperus communis*; HI—*Helichrysum italicum*. The experiment was repeated three times in duplicate and the mean ± SD is shown. Mean values marked with an uppercase letter A were significantly different compared to the control group. Mean values marked with lowercase letter a represent significant differences within different groups of EOs ($p < 0.05$).

3.3. Percentage of Degradation of Mycobacterial Biofilms on Stainless Steel Discs

Table 1 shows the degradation (shown as percentages) of NTM biofilms grown on stainless steel discs caused by different concentrations of *J. communis* and *H. italicum* EOs, both individually and in combination. *H. italicum* EO at concentrations of 2 × MIC and MIC was more effective at degrading biofilms of all three NTMs compared to *J. communis* EO. A concentration of 1/256 × MIC (0.012 mg mL^{-1}) of *H. italicum* EO caused a higher percentage of *M. avium* biofilm degradation (87.4%) than the MIC and 1/2 × MIC of *J. communis* EO (72.1% and 86.8%). However, subinhibitory concentrations of these EOs in combination caused a very high percentage of biofilm degradation of selected NTMs (>98.2%). *J. communis* EO at a concentration of 1/2 × MIC, plus *H. italicum* EO at a concentration of only 1/256 × MIC (0.012 mg mL^{-1}) or 1/512 × MIC (0.006 mg mL^{-1}) caused a degree of degradation of *M. avium* biofilm comparable to that of 2 × MIC of *J. communis* EO. Subinhibitory concentrations, 1/8 × MIC and 1/2 MIC, of these EOs caused the degradation of 98.9% and 99.9% of three-day-old biofilms of *M. intracellulare* and *M. gordonae*, respectively.

3.4. Cell Viability of Biofilm on Stainless Steel Discs Treated with Juniperus communis and Helichrysum italicum Essential Oils

In order to further investigate the anti-biofilm properties of *J. communis* and *H. italicum* EOs, confocal laser scanning microscopy (CLSM) analyses were performed (Figure 5). Some regions of the biofilm appeared yellow because of overlapping green and red cells.

The CLSM results indicate a strong synergistic effect of *J. communis* and *H. italicum* EOs on biofilm eradication of both bacterial strains. *M. intracellulare* was more sensitive, with more total red fluorescence (154.7 AU) than *M. avium* (137.9 AU). Individual treatment with *H. italicum* EO showed a better anti-biofilm effect than that with *J. communis* EO on both *Mycobacterium* species, although *M. intracellulare* was again the more sensitive species.

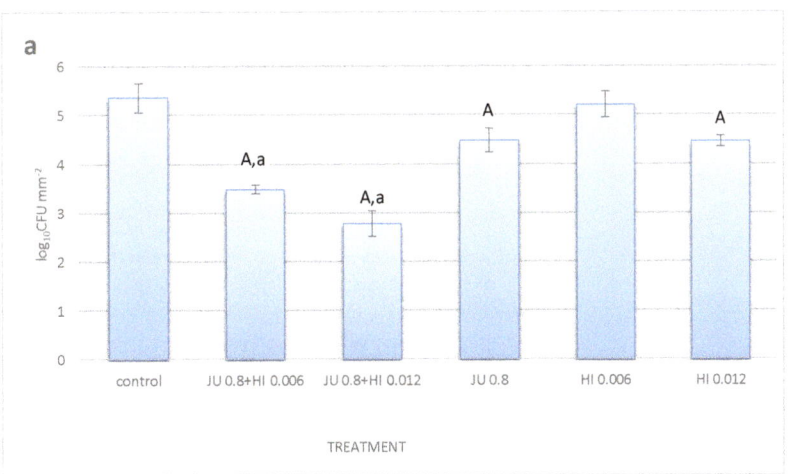

Figure 4. *Cont.*

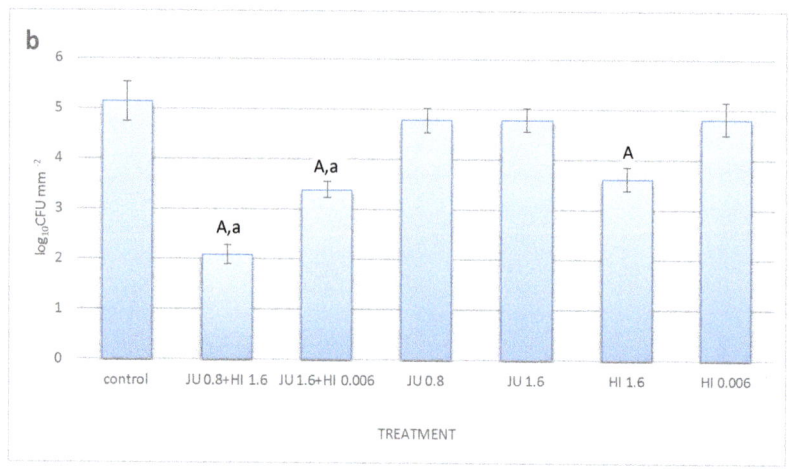

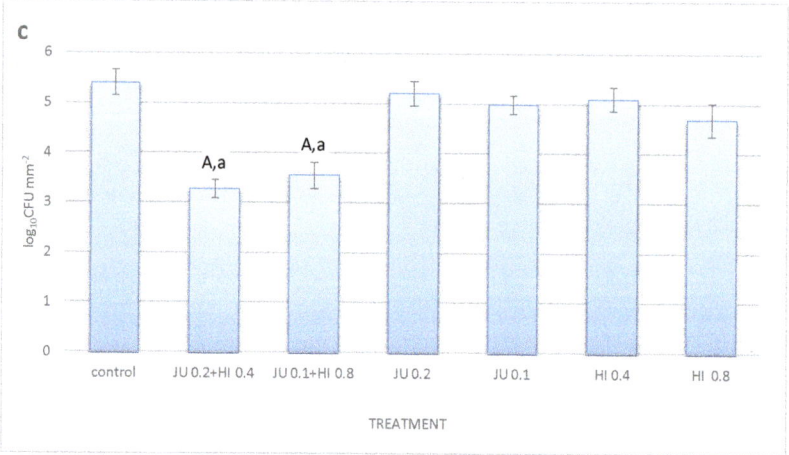

Figure 4. Effect of synergistic or additive concentrations of *J. communis* and *H. italicum* EOs in mg mL^{-1} on biofilm degradation of *M. avium* (**a**), *M. intracellulare* (**b**), and *M. gordonae* (**c**) formed on stainless steel discs. Untreated mycobacterial cells served as controls. MIC—minimum inhibitory concentration; CFU—colony forming unit; JU—*Juniperus communis*; HI—*Helichrysum italicum*. The experiment was repeated three times in duplicate and the mean ± SD is shown. Mean values marked with an uppercase letter A were significantly different compared to the control group. Mean values marked with a lowercase letter a represent significant differences in synergistic and individual groups of EOs ($p < 0.05$).

Table 1. Percentage of degradation (%) of mycobacterial biofilms on stainless steel discs after treatment with *J. communis* EO and/or *H. italicum* EOs.

Treatment	*M. avium*	*M. intracellulare*	*M. gordonae*
H. italicum EO (mg mL^{-1})			
6.4	99.9	99.9	99.9
3.2	99.3	98.2	99.6
1.6	ND	96.9	ND

Table 1. Cont.

Treatment	M. avium	M. intracellulare	M. gordonae
0.8	ND	ND	81.0
0.4	ND	ND	49.7
0.012	87.4	ND	ND
0.006	71.1	52.8	ND
J. communis EO (mg mL^{-1})			
3.2	98.5	94.5	98.2
1.6	72.1	72.5	83.6
0.8	86.8	57.0	ND
0.2	ND	ND	37.2
0.1	ND	ND	61.2
H. italicum EO/*J. communis* EO (mg mL^{-1})			
0.006/0.8	98.7	ND	ND
0.012/0.8	99.4	ND	ND
1.6/0.8	ND	99.9	ND
0.006/1.6	ND	98.2	ND
0.4/0.2	ND	ND	98.9
0.8/0.1	ND	ND	98.6

ND—not determined; EO—essential oil.

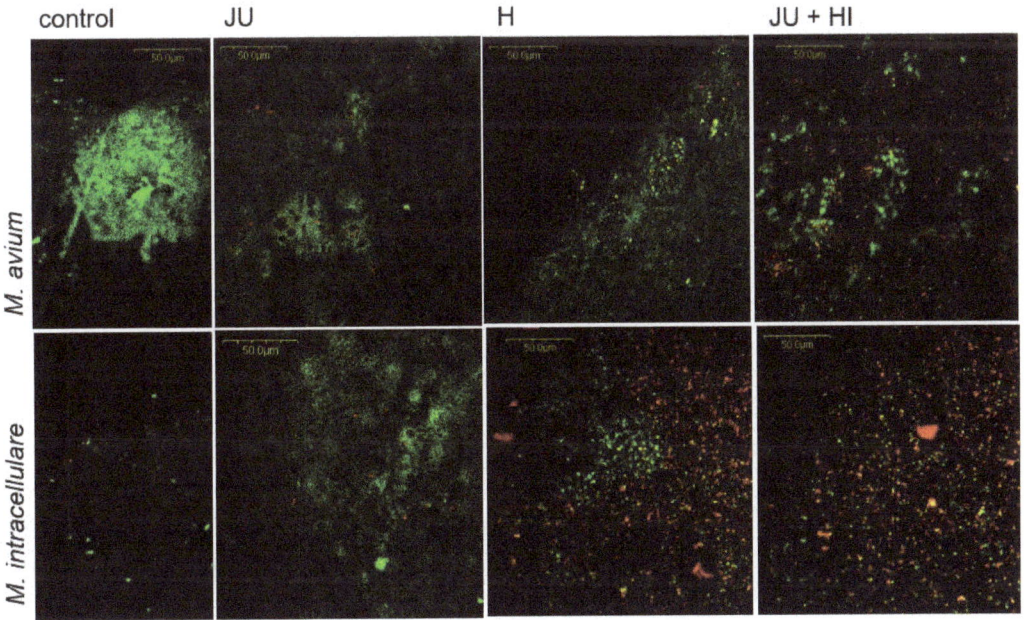

Figure 5. Live/dead stained images of *Mycobacterium* biofilms grown on stainless steel discs, performed by confocal laser scanning microscopy (CLSM) after treatment with *J. communis* (JU) and/or *H. italicum* (HI) EOs. *M. avium* was treated with JU 0.8 mg mL^{-1} and/or HI 0.012 mg mL^{-1}; *M. intracellulare* was treated with JU 0.8 mg mL^{-1} and/or HI 1.6 mg mL^{-1}. Untreated mycobacterial cells served as controls. Performed at 40× magnification.

Lower total fluorescence of the *M. intracellulare* biofilm and a lower number of cells in the biofilm (Figure 6) may indicate both biofilm destruction and cell detachment due to EO action.

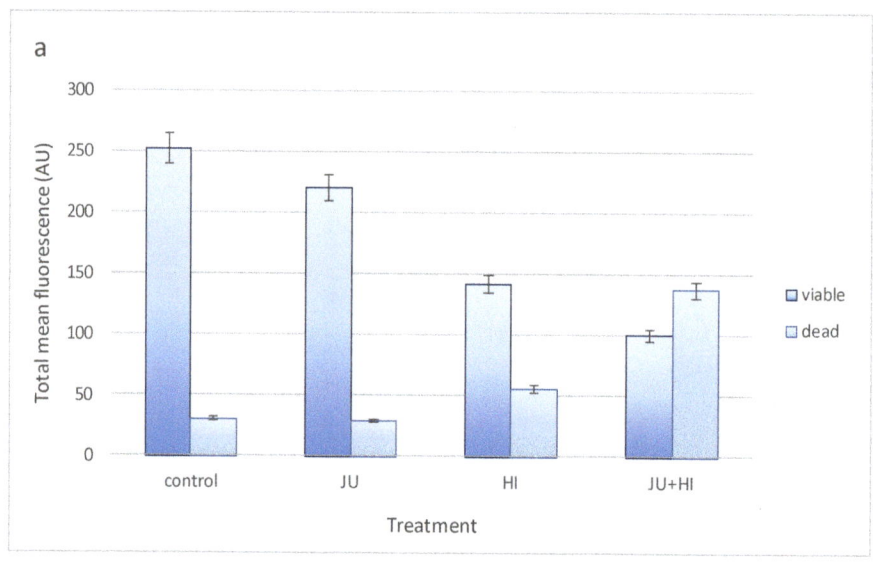

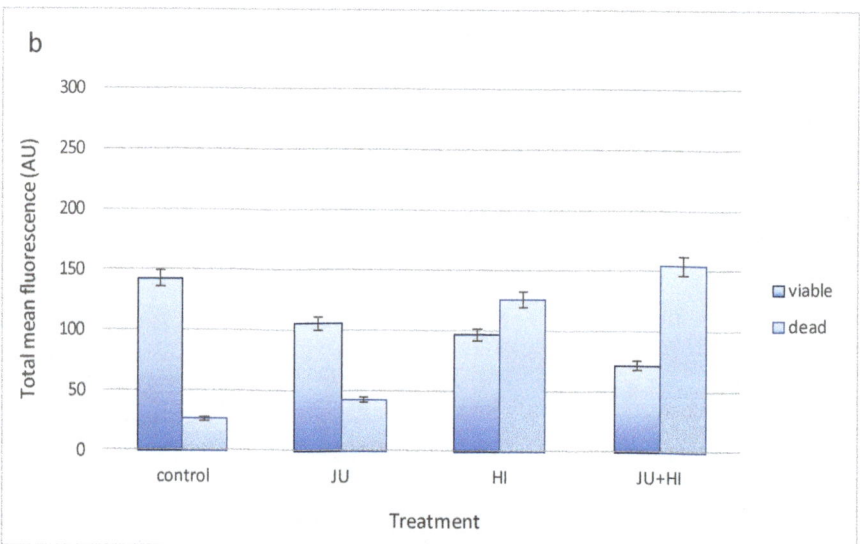

Figure 6. Total mean fluorescence measured for propidium iodide and SYTO® 9 stained biofilms of *M. avium* (**a**) and *M. intracellulare* (**b**) on stainless steel discs, as visualized with confocal laser scanning microscopy (control, three-day-old biofilm of *M. avium* treated for 22 h with 0.8 mg mL^{-1} *J. communis* EO (JU) and/or 0.012 mg mL^{-1} *H. italicum* EO (HI), and three-day-old biofilm of *M. intracellulare* treated for 22 h with 0.8 mg mL^{-1} *J. communis* EO (JU) and/or 1.6 mg mL^{-1} *H. italicum* EO (HI). The experiment was repeated twice and a minimum of three images were analyzed and the mean fluorescence ± SD is shown.

4. Discussion

Mycobacterium avium and other NTMs belong to the specific group of waterborne microorganisms named opportunistic premise plumbing pathogens, which are normal inhabitants of premise plumbing systems and can cause infections in immunocompromised patients [12,40].

Cell wall hydrophobicity and aggregation ability in liquid media are key factors in their pathogenicity and biofilm formation as well as play a crucial role in NTM resistance to disinfectants, acidic environments, and high ambient temperatures. The growth of NTM in the form of biofilms on glass, copper, galvanized steel or plastic results in their resistance to antimicrobials and disinfectants [41,42].

Due to the extreme resistance of OPPP biofilms including those of NTM, new approaches or new substances are needed to fight biofilm formation and destruction. Our previous studies have demonstrated the great potential of EOs as inhibitors of mycobacterial adhesion or biofilm formation on polystyrene as well as inhibitors of adhesion to living cells (amoebae and HeLa cells) [27,32,33,43]. The EOs of *J. communis* and *H. italicum* from coastal regions of Croatia have been shown to be particularly effective. In this study, we used commercial EOs produced from the same manufacturer two years apart, and although deviations in the amount of α-pinene and some other compounds can be seen, all repeated experiments gave the same MIC concentrations and synergistic effects of combinations of these two oils. Obviously, the antibacterial effect against NTM is not a result of a single dominant component, but the effect of the interaction of different components in these oils [27,32].

Haziri et al. [44] found moderate to high antimicrobial activity of *J. communis* EO against *S. aureus*, *E. coli*, and *Hafnia alvei*, while *P. aeruginosa* was shown to be resistant to this oil. Klančnik et al. [24] analyzed the effect of *J. communis* EO on the adhesion of *C. jejuni* to AISI 304 stainless steel. They reported that the adhesion of *C. jejuni* to AISI 304 under the influence of *J. communis* EO was reduced by more than 90%.

Monoterpenes, α and β-pinene, sabinene, and β-myrcene, together make up at least a quarter, and sometimes more than two-thirds of the chemical composition of *J. communis* and *H. italicum* EO, with the remainder consisting of sesquiterpenes, primarily γ-curcumene and neryl acetate. However, when we tested α-pinene as an individual compound against *M. avium* and *M. intracellulare*, its MIC/MBC/MIC values were three times higher than those of the *J. communis* EO and twice as high as those of the *H. italicum* EO [27]. In an experiment with *M. gordonae*, α-pinene had the same MIC value as *J. communis* EO, however, the MBC and MIC values were two and three times higher, respectively. We could assume that the antimycobacterial activity of *J. communis* EO and *H. italicum* EO can be attributed to α-pinene, but it is more likely that it could be due to the synergistic activity of several major compounds within these EOs.

M. avium, *M. intracellulare*, and *M. gordonae* demonstrated an abundant biofilm forming ability on stainless steel in STW. In our previous study, *M. avium* and *M. intracellulare* formed biofilms on polystyrene, but the number of bacteria was lower by two logarithmic units than in this study [32]. *M. avium* produced larger volume biofilms than *M. intracellulare*, which coincides with data from research studies [4]. The highest degree of adhesion of *M. avium* was observed on galvanized stainless steel, followed by stainless steel, polyvinyl chloride, glass, and copper. Factors enhancing the adhesion of *M. avium* to the surface are the roughness and hydrophobicity of the substrate as well as the presence of zinc, calcium, and magnesium [41]. Fast-growing and saprophytic species of *M. chelonae*, *M. fortuitum*, *M. gordonae*, and *M. tarrae* were identified in 90% of the polymicrobial biofilms found in the water supply systems of households and water treatment plants. In polymicrobial biofilms, *M. avium*, *M. intracellulare*, and *M. xenopi*, are predominantly present on faucets and shower heads [14]. It has been observed that *Methylobacterium* spp., like *M. avium*, rapidly forms a biofilm of a characteristic pink color in water supply systems [45].

Esteban et al. [46] studied biofilm formation by unpigmented fast-growing mycobacteria on a plastic surface in three different media. Biofilm formation was monitored at room temperature in Middlebrook 7H9S, STW, and phosphate buffered saline with 5% glucose (PBS 5% GLU). All the examined/analyzed species showed a sigmoid growth curve in 7H9S and STW. In 7H9, they initially had a characteristic lacy growth pattern with a delicate reticulate structure, which was then firmly formed and covered the entire surface by the 28th day of incubation. In STW, they showed the same growth pattern, but the fully developed biofilm was formed only on day 63, while in PBS 5% GLU, they did not manage to cover the entire surface within 69 days. It has long been known that low-nutrient media reduce the amount of biofilm produced by slow-growing NTMs [45]. However, in a study by Esteban et al. [46], STW was observed to be a better biofilm development medium than PBS 5% GLU. The authors concluded that such behavior may be due to a multitude of chemicals present at low levels in STW, serving as nutrients for mycobacteria. Ambient temperature was recognized as another important factor affecting biofilm development. Incubation of cultures was performed at room temperature, naturally present in the environment [46]. Our study into the effects of temperature on the mycobacterial biofilm formation revealed a temperature of 25 °C to be the most favorable for biofilm formation. At this temperature, *J. communis* EO showed the weakest anti-adhesion and antibiofilm activity against NTM on polystyrene [33].

M. gordonae is a saprophytic, environmental NTM. According to our study, *M. gordonae* on stainless steel AISI 316 in STW, after 72 hours, produced a significantly larger volume biofilm than *M. avium* and *M. intracellulare*, which confirmed previous observations found in scientific papers of a significant presence of *M. gordonae* in the biofilm on metal surfaces of water supply systems [13]. NTMs in the aqueous medium showed greater sensitivity to the action of *J. communis* EO and *H. italicum* EO, than was observed in the nutritive liquid medium 7H9S [27]. The reason for this may be that nutrient-rich broth stimulates the multiplication of mycobacteria, which makes them more sensitive to the effect of EOs, or it could be due to the greater solubility of EOs in this nutrient-rich medium. In contrast, an aqueous medium slows down the multiplication of mycobacteria and promotes their resistance.

The degradation of three-day biofilms of *M. avium*, *M. intracellulare*, and *M. gordonae* on AISI 316 was most strongly affected by *H. italicum* EO at a concentration of $2 \times$ MIC. The greatest degree of degradation of biofilm, at this concentration of *H. italicum* EO, was observed in *M. gordonae*, followed by *M. avium*, whereas the most resistant was the biofilm of *M. intracellulare*. Thus, in studies conducted with *M. gordonae* and *M. avium*, we revealed its exceptional ability to form a biofilm. However, the biofilm of *M. gordonae*, in contrast to the biofilm of *M. avium* and *M. intracellulare*, is more sensitive to degradation caused by *H. italicum* and *J. communis* EO activity.

Increased resistance of *M. avium* biofilm was observed by Carter et al. [47] who recently reported that clarithromycin could inhibit *M. avium* if administered before the formation of a biofilm in the respiratory system and becomes ineffective after the formation of a biofilm by this mycobacterium. Due to the altered *M. avium* phenotype in the biofilm, its response to antimicrobial therapy is limited, which is a key problem in the treatment of pulmonary mycobacteriosis caused by this mycobacterium [48]. The most likely explanation for the synergistic action of the EOs is that compounds from each EO have a different target site, combined with improved diffusion and distribution of each EO and components in the bacterial cell, inhibition of common biochemical pathway, inhibition of protective enzymes, and action on the specific resistance mechanism [20,49].

5. Conclusions

Our study showed that the tested EOs, when used at subinhibitory synergistic concentrations, had a greater effect on the degradation of mycobacterial biofilms grown on stainless steel than when they were applied individually at inhibitory concentrations. This allowed for the application of low non-toxic concentrations in biofilm eradication. Synergistic combinations of *J. communis* and *H. italicum* EOs could therefore potentially be applied in new ways to prevent the adhesion and biofilm formation of NTM, not only in the water supply system as a reservoir of NTM and a source of human infections, but also on artificial materials used in medicine or in the case of infections associated with biofilm formation.

Author Contributions: Conceptualization, D.P. and I.G.; Formal analysis, D.P., Z.M., L.K., and I.G.; Methodology, D.P., Z.M., L.K., and I.G.; Investigation, D.P., Z.M., and I.G.; Validation, All authors; Data curation, D.B., D.P., and I.G.; Funding acquisition, I.G., Ž.M., and D.B.; Project administration, I.G., Ž.M., and D.B.; Resources, I.G., Ž.M., and D.B.; Visualization, L.K., I.G., and Ž.M.; Supervision, I.G.; Writing—original draft, D.P., Z.M., Ž.M., D.B., and I.G.; Writing—review and editing, I.G., D.B., and Ž.M. All authors have read and agreed to the published version of the manuscript.

Funding: The research described here was funded by grants from the University of Rijeka (uniri-biomed-18-171, uniri-biomed-18-155-1304, uniri-prirod-18-302).

Institutional Review Board Statement: Not applicable.

Informed Consent Statement: Not applicable.

Data Availability Statement: Not applicable.

Acknowledgments: We are grateful to Meta Sterniš, from the Biotechnical Faculty of the University of Ljubljana for the donation of the stainless steel discs.

Conflicts of Interest: The authors declare no conflict of interest.

References

1. Cambau, E.; Drancourt, M. Steps towards the discovery of *Mycobacterium tuberculosis* by Robert Koch, 1882. *Clin. Microbiol. Infect.* **2014**, *20*, 196–201. [CrossRef]
2. Forbes, B.A.; Hall, G.S.; Miller, M.B.; Novak, S.M.; Rowlinson, M.C.; Salfinger, M.; Somoskovi, A.; Warshauer, D.M.; Wilson, M.L. Practice Guidelines for Clinical Microbiology Laboratories: Mycobacteria. *Clin. Microbiol. Rev.* **2018**, *31*. [CrossRef]
3. Sousa, S.; Bandeira, M.; Carvalho, P.A.; Duarte, A.; Jordao, L. Nontuberculous mycobacteria pathogenesis and biofilm assembly. *Int. J. Mycobacteriol.* **2015**, *4*, 36–43. [CrossRef]
4. Faria, S.; Joao, I.; Jordao, L. General Overview on Nontuberculous Mycobacteria, Biofilms, and Human Infection. *J. Pathog.* **2015**, *2015*, 809014. [CrossRef]
5. Pfyffer, G.E.; Brown-Elliott, B.A.; Wallace, R.J.J. Mycobacterium: General Characteristics, Isolation, and Staining Procedures. In *Manual of Clinical Microbiology*, 8th ed.; Murray, P.R., Ed.; American Society of Microbiology: Washington, DC, USA, 2003; Volume 1, pp. 532–584.
6. Vincent, V.; Brown-Elliott, B.A.; Jost, K.C.; Wallace, R.J.J. Mycobacterium: Phenotypic and Genotypic Identification. In *Manual of Clinical Microbiology*, 8th ed.; Murray, P.R., Ed.; American Society of Microbiology: Washington, DC, USA, 2003; Volume 1, pp. 560–584.
7. Jankovic, M.; Zmak, L.; Krajinovic, V.; Viskovic, K.; Crnek, S.S.; Obrovac, M.; Haris, V.; Jankovic, V.K. A fatal *Mycobacterium chelonae* infection in an immunosuppressed patient with systemic lupus erythematosus and concomitant Fahr's syndrome. *J. Infect. Chemother.* **2011**, *17*, 264–267. [PubMed]
8. Halstrom, S.; Price, P.; Thomson, R. Review: Environmental mycobacteria as a cause of human infection. *Int. J. Mycobacteriol* **2015**, *4*, 81–91. [CrossRef] [PubMed]
9. Nishiuchi, Y.; Iwamoto, T.; Maruyama, F. Infection Sources of a Common Non-tuberculous Mycobacterial Pathogen, *Mycobacterium avium* Complex. *Front. Med.* **2017**, *4*, 27. [CrossRef] [PubMed]
10. Tortoli, E. Clinical manifestations of nontuberculous mycobacteria infections. *Clin. Microbiol. Infect.* **2009**, *15*, 906–910. [CrossRef] [PubMed]
11. De Groote, M.A.; Huitt, G. Infections due to rapidly growing mycobacteria. *Clin. Infect. Dis.* **2006**, *42*, 1756–1763. [CrossRef]
12. Falkinham, J.O.; Pruden, A.; Edwards, M. Opportunistic Premise Plumbing Pathogens: Increasingly Important Pathogens in Drinking Water. *Pathogens* **2015**, *4*, 373–386. [CrossRef] [PubMed]
13. Feazel, L.M.; Baumgartner, L.K.; Peterson, K.L.; Frank, D.N.; Harris, J.K.; Pace, N.R. Opportunistic pathogens enriched in showerhead biofilms. *Proc. Natl. Acad. Sci. USA* **2009**, *106*, 16393–16399. [CrossRef]
14. Richards, J.P.; Ojha, A.K. Mycobacterial Biofilms. *Microbiol. Spectr.* **2014**, *2*, 1–11. [CrossRef] [PubMed]
15. Hall-Stoodley, L.; Keevil, C.W.; Lappin-Scott, H.M. Mycobacterium fortuitum and Mycobacterium chelonae biofilm formation under high and low nutrient conditions. *J. Appl. Microbiol.* **1998**, *85* (Suppl. 1), 60S–69S. [CrossRef] [PubMed]
16. Nikolić, T.; Rešetnik, I. Plant uses in Croatia. *Phytol. Balc.* **2007**, *13*, 229–238.
17. Malenica Staver, M.; Gobin, I.; Ratkaj, I.; Petrović, M.; Vulinović, A.; Dinarina-Sablić, M.; Broznić, D. In vitro antiproliferative and antimicrobial activity of the essential oil from the flowers and leaves of *Helichrysum italicum* (Roth) G. Don growing in Central Dalmatia (Croatia). *J. Essent. Oil Bear. Pl.* **2018**, *21*, 77–91. [CrossRef]
18. Bakkali, F.; Averbeck, S.; Averbeck, D.; Idaomar, M. Biological effects of essential oils—A review. *Food Chem. Toxicol.* **2008**, *46*, 446–475. [CrossRef]

19. Bag, A.; Chattopadhyay, R.R. Evaluation of Synergistic Antibacterial and Antioxidant Efficacy of Essential Oils of Spices and Herbs in Combination. *PLoS ONE* **2015**, *10*, e0131321. [CrossRef] [PubMed]
20. Bassole, I.H.; Juliani, H.R. Essential oils in combination and their antimicrobial properties. *Molecules* **2012**, *17*, 3989–4006. [CrossRef]
21. Dorman, H.J.; Deans, S.G. Antimicrobial agents from plants: Antibacterial activity of plant volatile oils. *J. Appl. Microbiol.* **2000**, *88*, 308–316. [CrossRef]
22. Newton, S.M.; Lau, C.; Wright, C.W. A review of antimycobacterial natural products. *Phytother. Res.* **2000**, *14*, 303–322. [CrossRef]
23. Sawicki, R.; Golus, J.; Przekora, A.; Ludwiczuk, A.; Sieniawska, E.; Ginalska, G. Antimycobacterial Activity of Cinnamaldehyde in a *Mycobacterium tuberculosis*(H37Ra) Model. *Molecules* **2018**, *23*, 2381. [CrossRef]
24. Klančnik, A.; Zorko, Š.; Toplak, N.; Kovač, M.; Bucar, F.; Jeršek, B.; Smole Možina, S. Antiadhesion activity of juniper (*Juniperus communis* L.) preparations against *Campylobacter jejuni* evaluated with PCR-based methods. *Phytother. Res.* **2018**, *32*, 542–550. [CrossRef]
25. Angioni, A.; Barra, A.; Russo, M.T.; Coroneo, V.; Dessiä, S.; Cabras, P. Chemical Composition of the Essential Oils of Juniperus from Ripe and Unripe Berries and Leaves and Their Antimicrobial Activity. *J. Agric. Food Chem.* **2003**, *51*, 3073–3078. [CrossRef]
26. Rezvani, S.; Ali Rezai, M.; Mahmodi, N. Analysis of Essential Oils of *Juniperus polycarpos* and *Juniperus communis*. *Asian J. Chem.* **2007**, *19*, 5019–5022.
27. Peruč, D.; Gobin, I.; Abram, M.; Brozniċ, D.; Svalina, T.; Štifter, S.; Staver, M.M.; Tićac, B. Antimycobacterial potential of the juniper berry essential oil in tap water. *Arh. Hig. Rada. Toksikol.* **2018**, *69*, 46–54. [CrossRef]
28. Mastelic, J.; Politeo, O.; Jerkovic, I. Contribution to the analysis of the essential oil of *Helichrysum italicum* (Roth) G. Don. Determination of ester bonded acids and phenols. *Molecules* **2008**, *13*, 795–803. [CrossRef]
29. Antunes Viegas, D.; Palmeira-de-Oliveira, A.; Salgueiro, L.; Martinez-de-Oliveira, J.; Palmeira-de-Oliveira, R. *Helichrysum italicum*: From traditional use to scientific data. *J. Ethnopharmacol.* **2014**, *151*, 54–65. [CrossRef] [PubMed]
30. Mancini, E.; De Martino, L.; Marandino, A.; Scognamiglio, M.R.; De Feo, V. Chemical composition and possible in vitro phytotoxic activity of *Helichrsyum italicum* (Roth) Don ssp. italicum. *Molecules* **2011**, *16*, 7725–7735. [CrossRef]
31. Jerkovic, I.; Marijanovic, Z.; Kus, P.M.; Tuberoso, C.I. Comprehensive Study of Mediterranean (Croatian) Propolis Peculiarity: Headspace, Volatiles, Anti-Varroa-Treatment Residue, Phenolics, and Antioxidant Properties. *Chem. Biodivers.* **2016**, *13*, 210–218. [CrossRef]
32. Peruč, D.; Tićac, B.; Abram, M.; Brozniċ, D.; Štifter, S.; Staver, M.M.; Gobin, I. Synergistic potential of *Juniperus communis* and *Helichrysum italicum* essential oils against nontuberculous mycobacteria. *J. Med. Microbiol.* **2019**, *68*, 703–710. [CrossRef]
33. Peruc, D.; Ticac, B.; Broznic, D.; Maglica, Z.; Sarolic, M.; Gobin, I. Juniperus communis essential oil limit the biofilm formation of *Mycobacterium avium* and *Mycobacterium intracellulare* on polystyrene in a temperature-dependent manner. *Int. J. Environ. Health Res.* **2020**, 1–14. [CrossRef]
34. Sarker, S.D.; Nahar, L.; Kumarasamy, Y. Microtitre plate-based antibacterial assay incorporating resazurin as an indicator of cell growth, and its application in the in vitro antibacterial screening of phytochemicals. *Methods* **2007**, *42*, 321–324. [CrossRef]
35. Andrejak, C.; Almeida, D.V.; Tyagi, S.; Converse, P.J.; Ammerman, N.C.; Grosset, J.H. Characterization of mouse models of *Mycobacterium avium* complex infection and evaluation of drug combinations. *Antimicrob. Agents Chemother.* **2015**, *59*, 2129–2135. [CrossRef] [PubMed]
36. Vasiljević, B.; Knežević-Vučković, J.; Mitić-Ćulafić, D.; Orčić, D.; Franišković, M.; Srdic-Rajic, T.; Jovanović, M.; Nikolić, B. Chemical characterization, antioxidant, genotoxic and in vitro cytotoxic activity assessment of *Juniperus communis* var. saxatilis. *Food Chem. Toxicol.* **2018**, *112*, 118–125. [CrossRef] [PubMed]
37. White, R.L.; Burgess, D.S.; Manduru, M.; Bosso, J.A. Comparison of three different in vitro methods of detecting synergy: Time-kill, checkerboard, and E test. *Antimicrob. Agents Chemother.* **1996**, *40*, 1914–1918. [CrossRef] [PubMed]
38. Balouiri, M.; Sadiki, M.; Ibnsouda, S.K. Methods for in vitro evaluating antimicrobial activity: A review. *J. Pharm. Anal.* **2016**, *6*, 71–79. [CrossRef] [PubMed]
39. Teanpaisan, R.; Kawsud, P.; Pahumunto, N.; Puripattanavong, J. Screening for antibacterial and antibiofilm activity in Thai medicinal plant extracts against oral microorganisms. *J. Tradit. Complement. Med.* **2017**, *7*, 172–177. [CrossRef] [PubMed]
40. Falkinham, J.O. Surrounded by mycobacteria: Nontuberculous mycobacteria in the human environment. *J. Appl Microbiol.* **2009**, *107*, 356–367. [CrossRef]
41. Falkinham, J.O. *Mycobacterium avium* complex: Adherence as a way of life. *AIMS Microbiol.* **2018**, *4*, 428–438. [CrossRef]
42. Steed, K.A.; Falkinham, J.O., 3rd. Effect of growth in biofilms on chlorine susceptibility of *Mycobacterium avium* and *Mycobacterium intracellulare*. *Appl. Environ. Microbiol.* **2006**, *72*, 4007–4011. [CrossRef]
43. Peruč, D.; Gobin, I.; Brozniċ, D.; Malenica Staver, M.; Tićac, B. Influence of essential oil *Helichrysum italicum* (Roth) G. Don on the formation of non-tuberculous mycobacterial biofilm. *Med. Flum.* **2018**, *54*, 282–289. [CrossRef]
44. Haziri, A.; Faiku, F.; Mehmeti, A.; Govori, S.; Abazi, S.; Daci, M.; Haziri, I.; Bytyqi-Damoni, A.; Mele, A. Antimicrobial properties of the essential oil of *Juniperus communis (L.)* growing wild in east part of Kosovo. *Am. J. Pharmacol. Toxicol.* **2013**, *8*, 128–133. [CrossRef]
45. Munoz Egea, M.C.; Ji, P.; Pruden, A.; Falkinham Iii, J.O. Inhibition of Adherence of *Mycobacterium avium* to Plumbing Surface Biofilms of Methylobacterium spp. *Pathogens* **2017**, *6*, 42. [CrossRef]

46. Esteban, J.; Martin-de-Hijas, N.Z.; Kinnari, T.J.; Ayala, G.; Fernandez-Roblas, R.; Gadea, I. Biofilm development by potentially pathogenic non-pigmented rapidly growing mycobacteria. *BMC Microbiol.* **2008**, *8*, 184. [CrossRef] [PubMed]
47. Carter, G.; Wu, M.; Drummond, D.C.; Bermudez, L.E. Characterization of biofilm formation by clinical isolates of *Mycobacterium avium*. *J. Med. Microbiol.* **2003**, *52*, 747–752. [CrossRef]
48. Yamazaki, Y.; Danelishvili, L.; Wu, M.; Hidaka, E.; Katsuyama, T.; Stang, B.; Petrofsky, M.; Bildfell, R.; Bermudez, L.E. The ability to form biofilm influences *Mycobacterium avium* invasion and translocation of bronchial epithelial cells. *Cell Microbiol.* **2006**, *8*, 806–814. [CrossRef] [PubMed]
49. Langeveld, W.T.; Veldhuizen, E.J.; Burt, S.A. Synergy between essential oil components and antibiotics: A review. *Crit. Rev. Microbiol.* **2014**, *40*, 76–94. [CrossRef] [PubMed]

Review

Chitosan-Coating Effect on the Characteristics of Liposomes: A Focus on Bioactive Compounds and Essential Oils: A Review

Carine Sebaaly [1,*], Adriana Trifan [2,*], Elwira Sieniawska [3] and Hélène Greige-Gerges [1]

[1] Bioactive Molecules Research Laboratory, Department of Chemistry and Biochemistry, Faculty of Sciences, Section II, Lebanese University, Jdaidet el-Matn B.P. 90656, Lebanon; hgreige@ul.edu.lb
[2] Department of Pharmacognosy, Faculty of Pharmacy, Grigore T. Popa University of Medicine and Pharmacy Iasi, 700115 Iasi, Romania
[3] Department of Pharmacognosy, Medical University of Lublin, 20-093 Lublin, Poland; esieniawska@pharmacognosy.org
* Correspondence: c.sebaaly@ul.edu.lb (C.S.); adriana.trifan@umfiasi.ro (A.T.); Tel.: +40-232301815 (A.T.)

Abstract: In recent years, liposomes have gained increasing attention for their potential applications as drug delivery systems in the pharmaceutic, cosmetic and food industries. However, they have a tendency to aggregate and are sensitive to degradation caused by several factors, which may limit their effectiveness. A promising approach to improve liposomal stability is to modify liposomal surfaces by forming polymeric layers. Among natural polymers, chitosan has received great interest due to its biocompatibility and biodegradability. This review discussed the characteristics of this combined system, called chitosomes, in comparison to those of conventional liposomes. The coating of liposomes with chitosan or its derivatives improved liposome stability, provided sustained drug release and increased drug penetration across mucus layers. The mechanisms behind these results are highlighted in this paper. Alternative assembly of polyelectrolytes using alginate, sodium hyaluronate, or pectin with chitosan could further improve the liposomal characteristics. Chitosomal encapsulation could also ensure targeted delivery and boost the antimicrobial efficacy of essential oils (EOs). Moreover, chitosomes could be an efficient tool to overcome the major drawbacks related to the chemical properties of EOs (low water solubility, sensitivity to oxygen, light, heat, and humidity) and their poor bioavailability. Overall, chitosomes could be considered as a promising strategy to enlarge the use of liposomes.

Keywords: chitosan; coating; essential oils; liposomes; mechanism; polyelectrolyte

1. Introduction

Liposomes are spherical vesicles comprising a central aqueous compartment surrounded by a membrane constituted mainly of phospholipids and cholesterol in some cases. They are biocompatible, biodegradable, non-immunogenic and non-toxic [1]. In their original form, liposomes have a tendency to aggregate and fuse, which leads to drug leakage during storage [2]. This poor stability in an aqueous medium has major consequences on their shelf life [3]. The pH, bile salts and enzymes in the gastrointestinal (GI) tract can destabilize the liposome membrane [4]. In fact, the acidic pH of the stomach and the lipases hydrolyze the ester bonds of phospholipids that form liposomes. The bile salts act as surfactants leading to liposome membrane solubilization [5]. Liposomes are also prone to rapid elimination from the circulation system after intravenous injection [6]. In order to overcome these problems, covering the liposome's surface with polymers has been developed. The coating of liposomes with polyethylene glycol (PEG) reduced their uptake by the mononuclear phagocyte system, resulting in a prolonged blood circulation time of liposomes [7]. The surface modification of liposomes with PEG can be achieved by physically adsorbing the polymer onto the surface of vesicles, by anchoring the polymer in the liposomal membrane via a cross-linked lipid, such as distearoylphosphatidylethanolamine

(DSPE) during liposome preparation, or by covalently attaching reactive groups onto the surface of preformed liposomes [7]. Stealth liposomes provided delayed and targeted drug delivery, enhancing the effectiveness of the transported drug and reducing its side effects [8]. PEGylated liposomes have reached clinical usage, such as DOXIL®, originally developed by Sequus Pharmaceuticals in 1995, for the intravenous administration of the anticancer drug doxorubicin for the management of advanced ovarian cancer, multiple myeloma and Kaposi's sarcoma [9].

The use of natural polymers received increasing attention, particularly chitosan, which is isolated from crustacean exoskeletons, squid pen and fungi. Chitosan, a linear cationic polysaccharide composed of β-(1,4)-linked-2-amino-2-deoxy-D-glucopyranose (glucosamine) and 2-acetamido-2-deoxy-D-glucopyranose (N-acetylglucosamine), is obtained by alkaline or enzymatic deacetylation of chitin [10]. The chitin and chitosan structures are presented in Figure 1.

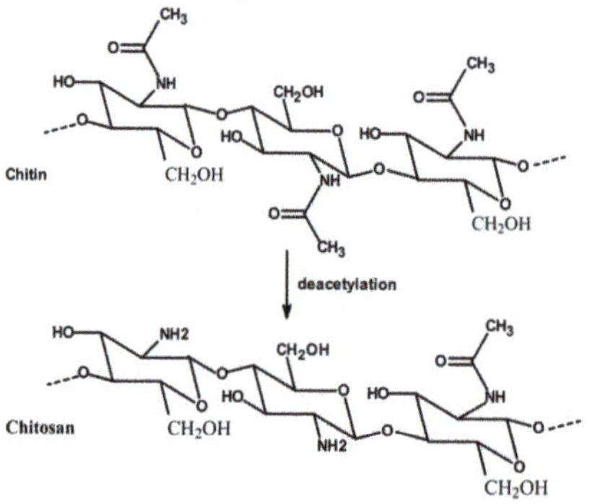

Figure 1. Chitosan product from chitin deacetylation.

The degree of deacetylation (DD) is defined as the glucosamine/N-acetylglucosamine ratio; in other words, DD is the percentage of glucosamine units present in the copolymer chain. Chitosan is soluble in an acidic aqueous medium. Under acidic pH, the amino groups in the chitosan chain become protonated, and the polymer dissolves in aqueous media. Its solubility is related to the DD, molecular weight (MW) and distribution of the acetyl and amino groups along the chain [11]. For example, the increase in chitosan MW from 5 to 50 kDa led to a significant decrease in chitosan aqueous solubility from 123.2 to 0.4 mg/mL [12]. Solubility at neutral pH has been claimed for chitosan with a DD of around 50% [13]. For very high DD (>75%), protonated charge condensation occurs in the chitosan solution due to large charge density, which leads to electrostatic repulsion and high solubility [14]. Indeed, the degree of deacetylation showed a great effect on pKa values, which were increased from 6.17 to 6.51, with the degree of deacetylation decreasing from 94.6 to 73.3% [11]. The distribution of acetyl groups along the chain may influence the solubility of the polymer and also the inter-chain interactions due to the hydrogen bonds and the hydrophobic character of the acetyl group [13].

Chitosan has been considered as a biomaterial for drug delivery systems, as it possesses low toxicity, high biocompatibility [15], and in vivo biodegradability via lysozymes and human chitinases [16]. In addition, it exhibits numerous biological activities, including mucoadhesive [17], antioxidant [18], antimicrobial activity against Gram-positive and Gram-negative bacteria [19], wound healing capacity [20], and the in vitro and in vivo ability to complex genetic material [21]. Thus, a great interest has been shown for its applications in areas such as hematology, immunology, wound healing, drug delivery, food packaging and cosmetics.

On the other hand, the chitosan structure can be modified through its amino and hydroxyl groups. The preparation of chitosan derivatives has been carried out to improve chitosan properties, including solubility and bring new functional properties and promising applications. The aim of the chemical modifications of chitosan and the resulted structures used in the liposome coating are presented in Table 1.

Table 1. Chemical structures of chitosan and its derivatives and role of chitosan modification in liposome coating.

Chitosan Derivatives	Chemical Structure	Aim of Chitosan Derivatization	Ref
Chitosan		- Improve chitosan properties	[22]
Glycol chitosan		- Target acidic tumor microenvironment - Improve anticancer drug efficacy	[23]
Methylated N-(4-N,N-dimethylaminobenzyl) chitosan (TMBz-chitosan)	The methylation could also occur at the primary amino group of chitosan	- Provide the hydrophobic moiety to improve the hydrophobic interaction with the cell membrane	[24,25]
N-dodecyl chitosan		- Improve the liposome stability by anchoring the liposome bilayer by the long alkyl chain	[26]
N-[(2-hydroxy-3-trimethylamine) propyl] chitosan chloride (HPTMA-chitosan)			
N-dodecyl-chitosan N-[(2-hydroxy-3-trimethylamine) propyl]chloride (N-dodecyl-chitosan-HPTMA)		- Improve the stability of coated liposomes - Increase chitosan solubility	[26]

Table 1. *Cont.*

Chitosan Derivatives	Chemical Structure	Aim of Chitosan Derivatization	Ref
N-trimethyl chitosan		- Improve chitosan solubility over a wide pH range - Improve liposomal stability	[27,28]
PEGylated octadecyl-quaternized lysine modified chitosan		- Provide amphiphilic character and steric stabilizations	[22]
Pelargonic chitosan (n=7) Lauric chitosan (n=10)		- Coat positively charged liposomes with mucoadhesive properties. - The side groups introduced into the polysaccharide chains provide additional steric stabilization for liposomes in solutions	[29]
Thioglycolic acid chitosan (TGA-chitosan)		- Improve the mucoadhesive property and enhance oral bioavailability of peptides	[30]
Thioglycolic acid 6-mercaptonicotinamide-conjugate chitosan (TGA-MNA-chitosan)		- Thioglycolic acid chitosan was S-protected via conjugation with 6,6'-dithionicotinamide resulting in a derivative being less prone to oxidation and exhibiting higher mucoadhesive properties	[30]

Chitosan has been known to coat the surface of negatively charged liposomes due to electrostatic interactions between negatively charged phospholipids and positive charges of primary amino groups of chitosan [31]. Other mechanisms, such as hydrogen bonding between the polysaccharide and the phospholipid head groups, can also be implicated in the chitosan coating process [32]. Figure 2 illustrates the combined system named chitosome.

This review is focused on the effect of chitosan coating on liposomal characteristics. The method used to prepare drug-loaded chitosomes is presented. Conventional liposomes, chitosan- and modified chitosan-coated liposomes are compared for their characteristics, including particle size, zeta potential, polydispersity index (pdI), morphology, encapsulation efficiency (EE), stability, drug release, pharmacokinetics and pharmacodynamics. Literature data concerning the comparison between both systems are resumed into different tables (Tables 2–12). Mechanisms controlling vesicle stability, drug release and mucoadhesivity are also highlighted in this paper. In addition, a section deals with a multilayer coating of polyelectrolytes using alginate, sodium hyaluronate or pectin with chitosan on the liposome surface. The last section is dedicated to chitosomal encapsulation of essential oils (EOs) and its perspectives for the clinical development of novel therapeutic agents with increased stability and prolonged release.

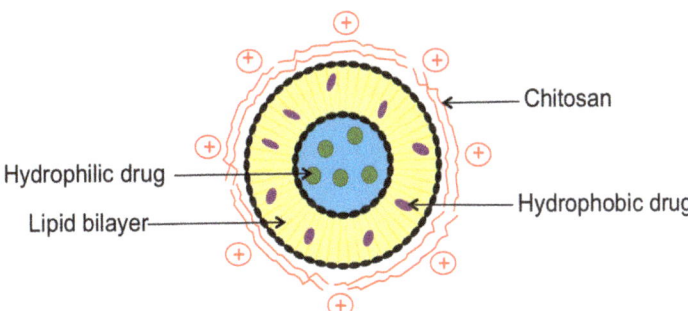

Figure 2. Schematic representation of drug-loaded chitosomes.

2. Chitosomes Preparation Method

Chitosan-coated liposomes are being prepared by a dropwise addition of a defined volume of chitosan solution to the same volume of liposome suspension and kept under stirring for 1 or 2 h. Chitosan should be dissolved either in acetic acid solution adjusted to pH 4–5, hydrogen chloride (HCl) solution or phosphate-buffered saline (PBS) buffer (pH 7.4), and incubated overnight at room temperature [33–35].

3. Comparison between Conventional Liposomes and Chitosomes

A comparison between chitosan- or chitosan derivative-coated liposomes and conventional liposomes encapsulating various drugs is detailed below. Tables 2–5 summarize the characteristics of conventional liposomes and chitosomes loading natural bioactive molecules (plant extracts, EOs, vitamins), antimicrobials, drugs of different classes (anticancer, anti-inflammatory, anesthetic, anti-histaminic, diuretic and immunosuppressive), macromolecules (proteins, deoxyribonucleic acid (DNA)) and active peptides, respectively. Chitosan coating effect is discussed in the following paragraphs regarding the particles size, zeta potential, pdI, morphology, EE, stability, drug release, pharmacokinetics and pharmacodynamics behavior of drugs.

3.1. Particles Size

In contrast to a single previous study focusing on the encapsulation of EOs in lipid vesicles and where liposomes of micrometric size were obtained [36], the coating of liposomes with chitosan produced an increase in liposome size (Tables 2–5). The increase was probably due to the bridging between chitosan and liposomes [37,38]. Liposome size depends on chitosan concentration. The particle size of polymer-coated liposomes increased with increasing chitosan concentration from 0.05 to 1.2% (*w/v*), forming thicker coating layers with a higher concentration of chitosan [4,5,12,28,35,38–44,46,47]. However, extensive aggregation occurred at low chitosan concentration ranging from 0.025 to 0.2% (*w/v*) regarding phospholipid concentration [48,49]. When liposome surfaces are not saturated with chitosan, liposomes associate with each other due to charge neutralization as surface charge consists of both partially negative and positive charges. Moreover, when there is excess chitosan, bridging flocculation caused by the interaction between the extended chitosan segments on the liposome surfaces will lead to particle–polymer–particle bridges. Hence, the stability of chitosomes relies on a sufficient chitosan concentration [49].

Additionally, the effect of different chitosan MW (65, 140, 680, 1000 kDa) on the size of insulin-loaded liposomes was investigated, and no significant differences were observed [38]. However, chitosomes prepared with trimethyl chitosan of high MW (HMW of 450 kDa) exhibited greater mean size than those prepared with low MW (LMW of 100 kDa), which can be explained by the presence of long-chain molecules of trimethyl chitosan leading to high viscosity and more adsorbed polymer [28].

Moreover, the composition of lipid vesicles, especially the phospholipid type used, may also affect the chitosome size. Conventional liposomes composed of Epikuron 170 have a smaller size than those composed of Epikuron 200. Liposomes obtained from Epikuron 170 composed of 70% phosphatidylcholine, 10% phosphatidylethanolamine, 3% phosphatidylinositol, 3% phosphatidic acid and 4% lysophosphatidylcholine absorbed more chitosan than those prepared with Epikuron 200 composed of 92% phosphatidylcholine and 3% lysophosphatidylcholine [40]. In addition, the size of uncharged liposome types tested (egg phosphatidylcholine (EPC) and distearoylphatidylcholine (DSPC)) is minimally affected by chitosan compared to negatively charged vesicles (EPC/phosphatidylglycerol (PG) and DSPC/PG) that become substantially larger as the chitosan/lipid ratio increases [32].

The liposome preparation method could affect chitosome size. Chitosomes loading curcumin prepared by ethanol injection method (EIM) were slightly larger than those prepared by thin-film hydration method (TFH) for the entire chitosan concentration range (0.1 to 0.5%) [43].

3.2. Zeta Potential

Several studies have investigated the effect of chitosan or chitosan derivatives on the Zeta potential values of the liposomes. The presence of polymer coating on the liposome surface is confirmed by the inversion of the Zeta potential from negative to positive values between uncoated and coated systems (Tables 2–5). Since chitosan carried a high positive charge, the adsorption of chitosan increased the density of positive charge and made the Zeta potential positive [4,36,42,50].

Moreover, Zeta potential values increased when the chitosan concentration increased from 0.1 to 0.3% (w/v), then it reached a relatively constant value, indicating the saturated adsorption of chitosan to liposomes [12,28,35,40,42,47–49,51–53]. It is important to mention that the modification of the surface of the liposome by another polymer, such as PEG, also changes the Zeta potential by varying polymer to lipid ratio from 1 to 10%(w/w) depending on the experimental protocol used based on a supercritical CO_2 assisted process. In the first method, the PEG dissolved in water was premixed in an ethanolic lipid solution (ethanol/water ratio 80/20 (v/v)), and the final solution was fed to supercritical assisted apparatus, while in the second method, PEG was dissolved in a separate aqueous solution and the two feeding solutions (aqueous and lipidic) were fed separately to the process. The authors explained the variations of Zeta potential between the two experimental protocols by the fact that PEG exhibits a better coverage of the liposome surface using the first method, which allows the addition of different amounts of PEG, resulting in a variety of surface charge [8].

It should be noted that the DD plays an important role in the effect of different chitosan MW on the zeta potential of the liposomes. The DD (85%) of HMW of chitosan (150 kDa) was slightly higher (80%) than that of LMW of chitosan (22 kDa), the number of protonated amine groups on HMW chitosan was higher than that on LMW chitosan, resulting in high positive zeta potential value [54].

3.3. Homogeneity

Although chitosan coating broadened the mean vesicle diameter [49], the pdI values remained below or close to 0.5, indicating an acceptable degree of polydispersity (Tables 2–5). The pdI values of chitosomes loading curcumin prepared by EIM were smaller than those prepared by TFH for the entire chitosan concentration range (0 to 0.5%) [43].

3.4. Morphology

Transmission electron microscopy was used to visualize conventional liposomes and chitosomes. Both systems were spherical. The existence of chitosan surrounding the liposomes has been well visualized on chitosomes surface [15,33,37,40,43,44,47,51,52,55,56]. No significant morphological differences, except size, between liposomes with or without chitosan coating were observed [35,44,55]. This was explained by strong adsorption between the polymer and the liposomal bilayer [35]. However, some aggregations were observed after coating [44,46,55,57].

3.5. Encapsulation Efficiency

Drug EE is calculated as the ratio of drug content within the liposomes to the total drug content of the suspension. The comparison of EE values between drug-loaded liposomes and chitosomes is discussed in this section and presented in Tables 2–5.

Different results were obtained in the literature concerning the chitosan coating effect on drug EE in liposomes. This discrepancy may be due to drug physicochemical properties (solubility, partition coefficient, ionization), its location in vesicles and orientation inside the liposomal membrane, as well as the medium pH. For example, many studies demonstrated that chitosan coating decreased the EE of drugs, mostly having positive charges at pH range between 4 and 7.4 compared to uncoated liposomes as presented in Tables 2–5 [5,34,35,37,38,40,42,48,56–59]. It was explained as a consequence of positively charged chitosan and positively charged drug competing for the negatively charged phospholipids [34,37,40,48].

However, other studies showed an increase in the EE of other drugs in the presence of chitosan at a pH range between 4 and 7.4 [4,32,43,44,49,55,60–63]. This may be due to the surface properties following the addition of chitosan during preparation which created the ionic interaction between positive chitosan and negative drug in solution producing high drug loading [4,55,60,61]. In addition, the coating enlarged EE, probably due to polyphenols interaction with chitosan [62]. Conceivably, the chitosan layer prevented carotenoid or curcumin leakage from the bilayer core [44,64].

The drug EE in chitosomes may also be affected by chitosan concentration, chitosan MW and liposomal preparation method. A further increase in chitosan concentration resulted in a non-significant change in drug EE [37,41]. This may be explained by the fact that the adsorptive layer has already been formed, and thus chitosan surrounds liposomes from the outside [37,40,41]. In addition, insulin EE in chitosomes was slightly increased with an increase in chitosan MW from 65 to 1000 kDa [38]. Curcumin EE in liposomes prepared by EIM (54.7%) was higher than that obtained in the liposomes prepared by TFH (42.6%) under the same conditions [43].

3.6. Chitosomes Stability

This section is dedicated to literature data related to the stability of conventional liposomes and chitosomes (in suspensions or dried forms) over time under various conditions, such as storage temperature, chitosan concentration and medium composition. The mechanism controlling vesicle stability in the presence of chitosan is explained below.

Table 2. Comparison of size, surface charge, homogeneity and drug encapsulation efficiency (EE) between liposomes and chitosomes loading natural bioactive molecules. The liposomal composition is indicated in the table in molar ratio except when * exists, indicating a weight ratio (w/w).

Natural Molecules	Liposomes a. Composition b. Preparation Method	Chitosan or Chitosan Derivative a. Concentration (% w/v) b. MW (kDa) c. DD (%) d. Chitosan Type	Size (nm) CH-LP	Size (nm) UN-LP	Zeta Potential (mV) CH-LP	Zeta Potential (mV) UN-LP	pdI CH-LP	pdI UN-LP	EE CH-LP	EE UN-LP	Ref
Artemisia afra	a. DSPC:DSPE 94:6 b. REV+sonication	a. 0.15 b. LMW c. NR d. Chitosan	1079 ± 62	8269 ± 79	22.8	9.0	0.798	0.429	NR	18.7	[36]
Berberine hydrochloride	a. EPC:CHO:DHP 1:0.242:0.036 * b. TFH+sonication	a. 0.1; 0.3 b. NR c. >90 d. Chitosan	194 ± 3–264 ± 8	142 ± 5	24.1–29.3	−26.8	0.34–0.53	0.27	78.4–81.6	83.2	[5]
Black mulberry extract	a. Lecithin (2% w/v) b. Homogenization	a. 0.4 b. NR c. 80 d. Chitosan	473 ± 12.7	173 ± 1.2	41.8	−32.4	NR	NR	NR	NR	[65]
Carotenoids: lutein; β-carotene; lycopene; canthaxanthin	a. EPC:Tween-80 NR b. TFH+sonication	a. 0.05; 0.1; 0.15 b. 200 c. 85 d. Chitosan	78–83 ± 0.1 76–78 ± 0.1 72–75 ± 0.1 125–130 ± 1.4	77 ± 0.1 75 ± 0.1 70 ± 0.1 120 ± 1.4	9.3–20 9.3–20 9.3–20 9.3–20	−5.3 −5.3 −5.3 −5.3	0.17–0.22 0.2–0.25 0.23–0.25 0.3–0.32	0.15 0.18 0.22 0.32	87–92 86–88 76–85 59–65	87 86 75 58	[44]
Coenzyme Q10	a. SPC:CHO 83:17 * b. EIM+sonication	a. 0.1; 0.2; 0.5; 1 b. 100; 450 c. >85 d. N-trimethyl chitosan	193–331 245–354	136	4.1–24.1 8.1–25.1	−8.7	NR	NR	98	98	[28]
	a. EPC:CHO 2:1 b. EIM	a. 0.1–0.5 b. 30 c. 88 d. Chitosan	123 ± 0.8–204 ± 0.6	101.4 ± 5	30.1–32.1	−14.1	0.185–0.216	0.247	64.93	54.7	[43]
Curcumin	a. EPC:CHO 2:1 b. TFH+sonication	a. 0.1–0.5 b. 30 c. 88 d. Chitosan	104 ± 1–192 ± 0.8	115.7 ± 2.3	30.4–43	−20.1	0.218–0.281	0.388	NR	42.6	

Table 2. Cont.

Natural Molecules	Liposomes a. Composition b. Preparation Method	Chitosan or Chitosan Derivative a. Concentration (% w/v) b. MW (kDa) c. DD (%) d. Chitosan Type	Size (nm)		Zeta Potential (mV)		pdI		EE		Ref
			CH-LP	UN-LP	CH-LP	UN-LP	CH-LP	UN-LP	CH-LP	UN-LP	
	a. PC:CHO 5:1 * b. EIM	a. 1 b. 28 c. 89 d. Chitosan	332.7 ± 53.8	93.2 ± 8.2	67.1	−24.3	NR	NR	52.08	41.42	[66]
		a. 0.0025 b. NR c. 80 d. N-dodecyl chitosan	140.3	51.7	31.6	−39	NR	NR	NR	NR	[26]
	a. EPC:DHP:CHO NR b. NR	a. 0.0025 b. NR c. 80 d. HPTMA-chitosan	76.3	51.7	32	−39	NR	NR	NR	NR	
		a. 0.0025 b. NR c. 80 d. N-dodecyl chitosan-HPTMA	73.1	51.7	32.3	−39	NR	NR	NR	NR	
	a. EPC: Phosphatidic acid 6.5:3.5 b. REV	a. 0.1 b. NR c. NR d. Chitosan	300	129	33	−49	0.1	0.095	NR	NR	[67]
	a. SPC:CHO 20:2 * b. TFH+ extrusion	a. 0.5 b. 200 c. >85 d. N-trimethyl chitosan	657.7	221.4	15.6	−9.6	0.37	0.198	92.6	86.6	[27]
Eucalyptus globulus	a. DSPC:DSPE 94:6 b. REV+sonication	a. 0.15 b. LMW c. NR d. Chitosan	885 ± 119	9914 ± 224	13.0	−14.9	0.678	0.585	NR	69.2	[36]
	a. Lipoid S75 1% * b. High-pressure homogenizer	a. 0.1 b. NR c. 79 d. Chitosan	173 ± 0.1	84 ± 0.1	63	−49	0.4	0.3	86.6	85.4	[68]
Grape seed extract		a. 1 b. NR c. 79 d. Chitosan	160.3 ± 0.1	86.5 ± 0.1	64.9	−42.5	NR	NR	99.5	88.2	[62]

Table 2. Cont.

Natural Molecules	Liposomes a. Composition b. Preparation Method	Chitosan or Chitosan Derivative a. Concentration (% w/v) b. MW (kDa) c. DD (%) d. Chitosan Type	Size (nm)		Zeta Potential (mV)		pdI		EE		Ref
			CH-LP	UN-LP	CH-LP	UN-LP	CH-LP	UN-LP	CH-LP	UN-LP	
Melaleuca alternifolia	a. DSPC:DSPE 94:6 b. REV+sonication	a. 0.15 b. LMW c. NR d. Chitosan	5781 ± 51	9280 ± 654	30.0	1.4	0.845	0.491	NR	41.7	[36]
Resveratrol	a. EPC 2%(w/v) b. TFH+ sonication	a. 0.1; 0.3; 0.5 b. NR c. NR d. Chitosan	279.8–558.3 ± 0.2	212.8 ± 0.01	26.3–39.2	−9.4	NR	NR	81.3	83.9	[42]
Rosmarinic acid esters	a. Lecithin 1%(w/v) b. Homogenization	a. 0.2 b. 205 c. 91.8 d. Chitosan	205.1	87.8	66.3	−37.8	NR	NR	NR	NR	[69]
Vitamin E	a. PC:CHO 20:80; 40:60; 60:40; 80:20 b. Sonication	a. 0.1 b. 4 c. > 90 d. Chitosan	144–531 ± 5	133–357 ± 5	53.5	−29.5	NR	NR	55.4–99.8	NR	[70]

Table 3. Comparison of size, surface charge, homogeneity and drug EE between liposomes and chitosomes loading antimicrobials. The liposomal composition is indicated in the table in molar ratio except when * exists, indicating a weight ratio (w/w).

Antimicrobials	Liposomes a. Composition b. Preparation Method	Chitosan or Chitosan Derivative a. Concentration (% w/v) b. MW (kDa) c. DD (%) d. Chitosan Type	Size (nm)		Zeta Potential (mV)		pdI		EE		Ref
			CH-LP	UN-LP	CH-LP	UN-LP	CH-LP	UN-LP	CH-LP	UN-LP	
Clotrimazole	a. Lipoid S100 200 mg b. TFH+ sonication	a. 0.1; 0.3; 0.6 b. NR c. 92 d. Chitosan	135 ± 21–190 ± 8	107	25.9–43.8	−1.6	0.27–0.29	0.34	NR	16.5	[17]
Dicloxacillin	a. Lipoid S100: CHO:Tween-80 0.9:0.3:0.1 b. TFH+sonication	a. 1 b. NR c. NR d. Chitosan	263.4 ± 19.1	178.5 ± 13.6	15.7	−12.7	0.411	0.247	62	38	[60]

Table 3. Cont.

Antimicrobials	Liposomes a. Composition b. Preparation Method	Chitosan or Chitosan Derivative a. Concentration (% w/v) b. MW (kDa) c. DD (%) d. Chitosan Type	Size (nm)		Zeta Potential (mV)			pdI			EE		Ref
			CH-LP	UN-LP	CH-LP	UN-LP		CH-LP	UN-LP		CH-LP	UN-LP	
Nisin Nisin silica	a. Lecithin:CHO 20:4 * b. TFH+ Homogenization	a. 0.1 b. NR c. NR d. Chitosan	134 ± 1.34 149 ± 1.34	NR	−42 −44	NR		0.27 0.283	NR		60 72	NR	[71]
Triazavirin	a. SPC-CHO 85:15 * b. TFH+ extrusion	a. 0.275 b. 190 c. 95 d. Pelargonic chitosan	188 ± 3	147 ± 3	20.4	30.2		0.16	0.13		NR	77.9	[29]
		a. 0.275 b. 190 c. 95 d. Lauric chitosan	192 ± 4	147 ± 3	18.9	30.2		0.18	0.13		NR	77.9	
Vancomycin hydrochloride	a. Lecithin:CHO 32.5:5 * b. REV	a. 0.4 b. NR c. NR d. Chitosan	220.4 ± 3.6	NR	25.7	NR		0.21	NR		32.6	40	[56]

Table 4. Comparison of size, surface charge, homogeneity and drug EE between liposomes and chitosomes loading drugs of different classes. The liposomal composition is indicated in the table in molar ratio except when * exists, indicating a weight ratio (w/w).

Drugs	Liposomes a. Composition b. Preparation Method	Chitosan or Chitosan Derivative a. Concentration (% w/v) b. MW (kDa) c. DD (%) d. Chitosan Type	Size (nm)		Zeta Potential (mV)		pdI		EE		Ref
			CH-LP	UN-LP	CH-LP	UN-LP	CH-LP	UN-LP	CH-LP	UN-LP	
Atenolol	a. Lipoid S100 20 mg b. EIM	a. 0.1; 0.6 b. NR c. NR d. Chitosan	240 ± 4–250 ± 1.2	89 ± 3.5	27	−20	NR	0.223	24.6–25.7	21.6	[63]

Table 4. Cont.

Drugs	Liposomes a. Composition b. Preparation Method	Chitosan or Chitosan Derivative a. Concentration (% w/v) b. MW (kDa) c. DD (%) d. Chitosan Type	Size (nm)		Zeta Potential (mV)		pdI		EE		Ref
			CH-LP	UN-LP	CH-LP	UN-LP	CH-LP	UN-LP	CH-LP	UN-LP	
Butyric acid	a. PC:CHO 20:5 * b. TFH+ sonication	a. 0.1 b. NR c. NR d. Chitosan	132.2 ± 2.3	92.1 ± 4.1	15.3	−9.3	0.22	0.18	NR	NR	[72]
Cyclospori A	a. EPC:CHO: Pluronic F 127 28:5:11 b. TFH+ extrusion	a. 0.04 b. 200 c. 90 d. Chitosan	207.8 ± 12.2	165.2 ± 9.2	41.7	−7.6	0.187	0.132	82	85.1	[59]
Diclofenac sodium	a. HSPC:PS:CHO 3:0.1:1 b. EIM	a. 0.1; 0.25; 0.5 b. 540 c. 97 d. Chitosan	82.4 ± 2.2– 392.3 ± 12.5	69 ± 3.1	−0.7– 10.1	−26.1	NR	NR	99.6– 100	99.6	[12]
Docetaxel	a. Lipoid S100: CHO:Tween-80: SDC:DCP 0.9:0.3:0.1:0.1:0.1 b. TFH+ sonication	a. 1 b. NR c. NR d. Chitosan	328.6 ± 9.1	238 ± 14.2	9.6	−5.5	0.581	0.413	76.5	58.7	[55]
Doxorubicin	a. HSPC:CHO NR b. TFH+ extrusion	a. NR b. NR c. NR d. Glycol chitosan	142.7 ± 2.7	123.7 ± 1.4	−14.3– 9.1	−25	0.068	0.04	90	90	[23]
Epirubicin	a. PC:CHO 50:15 * b. TFH+ sonication	a. 12.5; 33; 75; 200 mg b. 80 c. 92 d. Chitosan	180–262 ± 6.5	148 ± 3	21.1–25.4	−4.7	NR	NR	NR	NR	[47]
Fexofenadine	a. DPPC:DPPG: CHO 8:1:2.25 b. TFH+ extrusion	a. 0.1 b. NR c. NR d. Chitosan	716 ± 14.2	359 ± 5.5	11.8	−110	0.1	<0.1	66.1	65.9	[73]

Table 4. Cont.

Drugs	Liposomes a. Composition b. Preparation Method	Chitosan or Chitosan Derivative a. Concentration (% w/v) b. MW (kDa) c. DD (%) d. Chitosan Type	Size (nm)		Zeta Potential (mV)		pdI		EE		Ref
			CH-LP	UN-LP	CH-LP	UN-LP	CH-LP	UN-LP	CH-LP	UN-LP	
Flurbiprofen	a. EPC:solutol HS15 7.5:1 b. Modified EIM	a. 0.05; 0.1; 0.2 b. 50 c. 95 d. Chitosan	123.3 ± 1.7–213.9 ± 16.5	107.7 ± 2.8	8.4–28.6	−22.9	NR	NR	90.2–92.5	85.5	[61]
Furosemide	a. SPC:CHO 10:1 b. TFH+ sonication	a. 0.5 b. NR c. NR d. Chitosan	115.4 ± 2.86	49.8 ± 0.85	32.4	−13.5	NR	NR	71.1	42.6	[4]
Lidocaine	a. Lecithin:SDC 15% * b. TFH+ sonication+ extrusion	a. 0.1–0.5 b. 150 c. 90 d. Chitosan	202 ± 9.7–468.6 ± 14.4	178.6 ± 10.6	−12.2–46.6	−30.3	0.19–0.94	0.26	42.7–80.2	82.3	[48]
Mitoxantrone	a. SPC:CHO 5:1 b. TFH+ sonication	a. 0.1; 0.3; 0.6; 1.2 b. 70 c. 92 d. Chitosan	120–154	115	20–35	−30.4	NR	NR	93.5–96.5	97.4	[35]
Paclitaxel	a. Lecithin:CHO: SA:polyacrylic acid 1.225:0.575:0.1 * b. TFH+sonication	a. 0.1 b. 50 c. NR d. Chitosan	215 ± 17	152 ± 12	27.9	−37.6	NR	NR	70.9	77.1	[74]
Prednisolone	a. SPC:CHO 6:3 * b. TFH+ sonication	a. 2 b. NR c. NR d. Chitosan	235.8 ± 0.1	99.9 ± 0.2	35.3	−33.1	NR	NR	92.8	94.2	[58]

Table 5. Comparison of size, surface charge, homogeneity and drug EE between liposomes and chitosomes loading macromolecules and active peptides. The liposomal composition is indicated in the table in molar ratio except when * exists, indicating a weight ratio (w/w).

Macromolecules/ Active Peptides	Liposomes a. Composition b. Preparation Method	Chitosan or Chitosan Derivative a. Concentration (% w/v) b. MW (kDa) c. DD (%) d. Chitosan Type	Size (nm)		Zeta Potential (mV)		pdI		EE		Ref
			CH-LP	UN-LP	CH-LP	UN-LP	CH-LP	UN-LP	CH-LP	UN-LP	
Anti-sense oligodeoxynucleotides	a. SPC:CHO 20:5 * b. TFH+sonication	a. 0.05–1 b. 100 c. 90 d. Chitosan	65.6 ± 14.9–95.2 ± 2.7	55.7 ± 2.69	3.8–17.2	−11.7	0.181–0.701	0.426	NR	NR	[53]
Bovine serum albumin (BSA)	a. EPC:sodium oleate 10:2 b. TFH+ sonication	a. 1.25–20 mM b. 276 c. 94 d. TMBz-chitosan	108.2 ± 24–128 ± 15	107.6 ± 36	−23.3–5.3	−27.1	0.29–0.47	0.32	NR	50.1	[25]
Calcitonin	a. DPPC:DPPE-MCC 3:0.3 b. TFH+ extrusion	a. 0.2 b. 150 c. NR d. TGA-chitosan	709.2 ± 36	174.8 ± 0.9	43.5	−39.8	0.34	0.19	NR	NR	[30]
		a. 0.2 b. 150 c. NR d. TGA-MNA-chitosan	604.8 ± 29.6	174.8 ± 0.9	27.9	−39.8	0.91	0.19	NR	NR	
DNA	a. Phospholipon 80:DCP:CHO 5:1:4 b. REV	a. 0.1 b. 300 c. 87 d. Chitosan	346 ± 4–554 ± 10	441 ± 41	22	−52	0.19–0.37	0.47	84–87	NR	[39]
Extracellular proteins	a. Lecithin 100 mg b. EIM	a. 0.3 b. NR c. NR d. Chitosan	1200	500	NR	NR	NR	NR	70	80	[57]
Insulin	a. Lecithin:CHO 4:1 b. REV	a. 0.1–0.5 b. 65; 140; 680; 1000 c. 90 d. Chitosan	199.7–206.2	168.6	4.9–6.7	−2.9	0.132–0.246	0.143	69.7–75.9	81.6	[38]

Table 5. Cont.

Macromolecules/Active Peptides	Liposomes a. Composition b. Preparation Method	Chitosan or Chitosan Derivative a. Concentration (% w/v) b. MW (kDa) c. DD (%) d. Chitosan Type	Size (nm)		Zeta Potential (mV)		pdI		EE		Ref
			CH-LP	UN-LP	CH-LP	UN-LP	CH-LP	UN-LP	CH-LP	UN-LP	
Leuprolide	a. Epikuron 170: CHO 6:1 * Epikuron 200: CHO 6:1 * a. TFH+sonication	a. 0.1; 0.2; 0.5; 1 b. 1000 c. >90 d. Chitosan	60–140 75–120	15 54	10–40 5–20	−29.6 5	NR	NR	62.4 49.1	73.1 58.5	[40]
Salmon protein hydrolysates	a. MFGM Phospholac 700 3;5;10%(w/v) b. Heating+ Homogenization	a. 0.2–0.6 b. NR c. NR d. Chitosan	200	100	40	−55	0.2–0.7	<0.19	40–70	NR	[49]
siRNA-H1F1-α siRNA-VEGF	a. HSPC:DCP: CHO 1.0.1:1 b. TFH+ sonication	a.1 b. 75 c. 75–85 d. Chitosan	641.7 ± 25.2 609.4 ± 69.6	167 ± 14.9 159.3 ± 15.1	24.1 27	−23.1 −24.1	NR	NR	NR	NR	[75]
Substance P	a. Lecithin:CHO 20:3.3 * b. TFH+ sonication	a. 0.1 b. NR c. 88 d. Chitosan	243 ± 24	151 ± 27	32	−49	0.3	0.2	66	81.3	[34]

3.6.1. Physical Stability: Mechanism Controlled by Chitosan Concentration

Stability studies were conducted to compare the size, homogeneity, zeta potential and drug EE for both conventional liposomes and chitosomes in aqueous suspension. Many studies (Table 6) reported similar stability for both systems without significant changes in their physicochemical characteristics. By comparing the liposomal composition, the presence of saturated phospholipids [12,73,76] and the addition of cholesterol (40% mol) lead to a decrease in both bilayer hydration and effective size of the polar head group. Subsequently, bilayer defects are reduced, enhancing lateral packing of acyl chains, lowering thereby the leakage of liposomal contents and increasing liposomal stability. This could explain the similar stability for both systems.

However, other studies found that chitosan coating improved liposomes stability (Table 6). This is ascribed to the presence of a chitosan layer forming a wall that hinders swelling and release of encapsulated materials [5]. Second, electrostatic interaction and a weak hydrophobic force between chitosan and lipid bilayer suppressed lipid molecules mobility and kept the structural integrity of lipid membranes [44]. Moreover, the presence of surfactants like sodium oleate, dihexadecylphosphate, dicetylphosphate (DCP) or tween-80 in some studies (Table 6) can explain the decrease in the liposomal stability because surfactants increase the bilayer deformability.

It is worthy to note that chitosan concentration seems to be the main factor controlling liposomal stability. Increasing chitosan concentration led to an increase in liposomal stability [5,44]. However, an excess of chitosan may promote the flocculation and coagulation process of the liposomes [42,45,49]. A proposed mechanism (Figure 3) explained the chitosomal stability controlled by the so-called chitosan saturation concentration, which is the minimum polymer concentration required to cover the oppositely charged particles. According to Laye's explanation [3], the addition of chitosan to the liposomes below and above the saturation concentration can both lead to liposomal dispersions destabilization. At insufficient polymer concentrations, the anionic phospholipid molecules of liposomes may be bounded to the cationic chitosan molecules to form coacervates rather than chitosan molecules wrapping themselves around the liposome surface. At excess polymer concentrations, the exclusion of polymer molecules from a narrow region surrounding the particle surfaces generates an attractive force strong enough to overcome the intermolecular repulsive forces and to bring the particles together, making the liposomes susceptible to bridging flocculation [3].

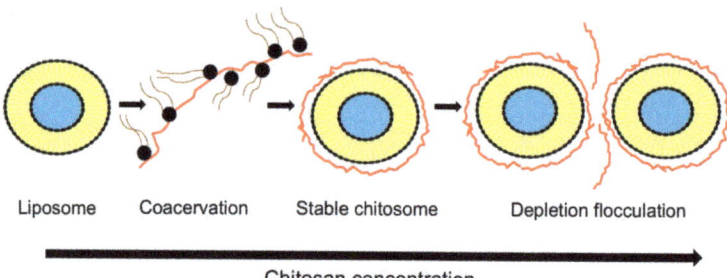

Figure 3. Proposed mechanism of liposome stability controlled by chitosan concentration.

The storage temperature influenced vesicle stability. Low-temperature achieved better stability for both systems. This could be explained by the low permeability of coating layers at refrigeration temperature, the inhibition of aggregation (low molecular mobility) and the retardation of oxidative degradation of unsaturated fatty acids of phospholipid bilayers [5,12,48,49].

Physical stability of liposomes was also evaluated by measuring particle size change after freeze-drying followed by rehydration (FD-RH) (Table 6). Chitosan improved the stability by protecting the liposomes against severe physical stress (−70 °C) [35,49]. Using chitosan as a cryoprotectant, along with surface coating, liposomes could achieve better stability and the desired physicochemical characteristics for a prolonged duration.

Modified chitosan effect on the stability of the liposomes was investigated. The side groups introduced into the polysaccharide chains play an important role in stabilizing the liposomes [26,29], as reported in Table 6.

3.6.2. Mechanism Controlled by Medium Composition

Lecithin includes unsaturated double bonds, which are prone to oxidation, thus contributing to the instability of the liposomal lipid bilayers. Transition metals, such as ferrous iron, can induce oxidation in liposomes by interacting with residual lipid hydroperoxides to produce free reactive radicals [77]. The stability of liposomes and chitosomes were tested in the presence of ferrous iron in order to determine the lipid hydroperoxides formation. Being a specific volatile oxidation product of polyunsaturated fatty acids like linoleic acid, hexanal determined by gas chromatography was also used as lipid oxidation indicator. Results showed that uncoated liposomes were highly prone to lipid oxidation since the formation of hexanal and lipid hydroperoxides occurred rapidly. However, chitosan coating inhibited lipid oxidation, hence improving the oxidative stability to some extent due to its ability to repel pro-oxidants metals from the liposome surface [68,69]. In addition, the combination of antioxidants, such as rosmarinic acid and chitosan coating, resulted in greater inhibition of lipid oxidation in liposomes [69].

Moreover, measurement of malonaldehyde (MDA), an oxidation product of phospholipids, can give useful information regarding the stability of liposomes/chitosomes. The release of MDA was lower in the case of chitosomes encapsulating *Chrysanthemum* EO vs. noncoated liposomes [78]. It has been demonstrated that a chitosan coating was able to protect phospholipid membranes from oxidation during different temperature storage; still, the increase of storage temperature increased the speed of phospholipids oxidation [78].

Furthermore, conventional liposomes are sensitive to damage caused by harsh chemical and enzymatic GI environments, resulting in reduced oral bioavailability [5]. Chitosan's effect on liposome stability in simulated gastric (SGF) and intestinal (SIF) fluid is presented in Table 6. The chitosan layer improved liposomes stability in SGF [5,74], explained by enhanced interactions between chitosan and liposome surface under low pH in SGF (pH 1.2) due to amino groups protonation in chitosan (pKa 6.5). The molecular configuration of chitosan also became more expanded, leading to a stronger affinity for the liposome surface. However, chitosomes were less stable than liposomes in SIF (pH 6.8) [5,59] due to a decrease in the number of charged cationic groups in chitosan at the medium pH, resulting in weaker electrostatic interactions between chitosan and liposomes surface, thus an increase in the diameter of the liposome. Moreover, SIF constituents, such as bile salts, act as surfactants promoting lipid solubilization for conventional liposomes and chitosomes. Pancreatic lipases have a digestive action on phospholipids, also contributing to destabilization of the liposomal system [5].

Table 6. Comparison of stability between drug-loaded liposomes and drug-loaded chitosomes under various conditions. The liposomal composition is indicated in the table in molar ratio except when * exists, indicating a weight ratio (w/w).

Drug/EO	Liposomes a. Composition b. Preparation Method	Chitosan or Chitosan Derivative a. Concentration (% w/v) b. MW (kDa) c. DD (%) d. Chitosan Type	Storage Conditions a. Temperature b. Time c. Medium	Stability: Chitosomes and Liposomes	Ref
Berberine hydrochloride	a. EPC:CHO:DHP 1:0.242:0.036 * b. TFH + sonication	a. 0.1; 0.3 b. NR c. >90 d. Chitosan	a. 4, 25 °C b. 30 days c. Aqueous suspension	- Chitosomes displayed better stability at 4, and 25 °C since the changes in size, zeta potential and drug EE were less than those in uncoated ones - The changes in size, Zeta potential and leakage ratio at 25 °C for both systems were higher than that at 4 °C - 0.3% chitosomes were more stable than 0.1% chitosomes due to the thicker coating layer.	[5]
			a. 37 °C b. 24 h c. SGF (pH 1.2); SIF (pH 7.4)	- The changes in size and zeta potential of coated liposomes were less than those for uncoated ones in SGF - In SIF, uncoated liposome size increased by 1.6-fold, while that of chitosomes increased by 6.2- and 4.2-fold for 0.1 and 0.3% chitosan, respectively	
Black mulberry extract	a. Lecithin 2% (w/v) b. Homogenization	a. 0.4 b. NR c. 80. d. Chitosan	a. 37 °C b. 2 h c. SGF (pH 2)	- The percentage recovery of anthocyanins in chitosomes (3.7%) was higher than that in liposomes (2.1%) after incubation in SGF	[65]
BSA	a. EPC:sodium oleate 10:2 b. TFH + sonication	a. 20 mM b. 276 c. 94 d. TMBz-chitosan	a. 37 °C b. 60 min c. SIF (pH 7.5)	- TMBz chitosan-coated liposomes protected BSA from pancreatin degradation in SIF more than conventional liposomes due to the interaction between positively charged derivative and negatively charged BSA	[25]
Calcitonin	a. DSPC:CHO: DCP 8:1:2 b. TFH + extrusion	a. 0.6 b. 150; 22 c. >85; 80 d. Chitosan	a. 37 °C b. 60 min c. Tris-HCl buffer (pH 8)	- LMW chitosomes had more efficiency to protect calcitonin from trypsin degradation than HMW chitosomes	[54]

Table 6. Cont.

Drug/EO	Liposomes a. Composition b. Preparation Method	Chitosan or Chitosan Derivative a. Concentration (% w/v) b. MW (kDa) c. DD (%) d. Chitosan Type	Storage Conditions a. Temperature b. Time c. Medium	Stability: Chitosomes and Liposomes	Ref
Carotenoids: lutein; β-carotene; lycopene; canthaxanthin	a. EPC:Tween-80 NR b. TFH + sonication	a. 0.05; 0.1; 0.15 b. 200 c. 85 d. Chitosan	a. 37; 65; 90 °C b. 390 min c. Aqueous suspension	- Chitosan coating increased carotenoid retention rates in liposomes by 8–15% after coating - When heating at 37 and 65 °C, the retaining capacity of liposomes showed chitosan concentration dependency. The higher the chitosan concentration was, the stronger the thermal resistance of chitosomes - Whatever the heating conditions were, liposomes exhibited the strongest retaining ability to lutein, followed by β-carotene, lycopene and canthaxanthin	[44]
Chrysanthemum sp.	a. Lecithin:CHO 5:1 b. TFH + extrusion	a. 0.025; 0.05; 0.075; 0.1 mg/mL b. NR c. NR d. Chitosan	a. 4; 12; 25; 37 °C b. 15 days c. NR	- MDA content was lower in case of EO chitosomes compared to EO loaded liposomes	[78]
	a. EPC:CHO 2:1 b. EIM and TFH + sonication	a. 0.1 b. 30 c. 88 d. Chitosan	a. 4; 25 °C b. 40 days c. Aqueous suspension	- Both systems prepared either by EIM or TFH were stable at both temperatures since no changes in mean size and pdI values were observed after 40 days	[43]
Curcumin	a. PC:CHO 5:1 * b. EIM	a. 1 b. 28 c. 89 d. Chitosan	a. 4; 25; 30; 40; 50; 60; 70; 80; 90 °C b. 40 days c. Aqueous suspension	- 90.68% of curcumin remained encapsulated in chitosomes compared to 26.03% in liposomes after 40 days at 4 °C - The remaining percentage of curcumin decreased to 75.77% when chitosomes were stored at 25 °C - Chitosomes showed the highest remaining percentage of curcumin at various temperatures tested up to 90 °C compared to liposomes and free curcumin	[66]
	a. EPC:DHP:CHO NR b. NR	a. 0.0025 b. NR c. 80 d. Chitosan; N-dodecyl chitosan; HPTMA-chitosan; N-dodecyl chitosan-HPTMA	a. NR b. NR c. Triton X100 pH 7.4	- Alkyl anchors (N-dodecyl chitosan; N-dodecyl chitosan-HPTMA chloride) showed better stability compared to native chitosan and uncoated liposomes since the disruption process by triton X100 was slowed down considerably in the presence of these polymers on liposomes	[26]

Table 6. Cont.

Drug/EO	Liposomes a. Composition b. Preparation Method	Chitosan or Chitosan Derivative a. Concentration (% w/v) b. MW (kDa) c. DD (%) d. Chitosan Type	Storage Conditions a. Temperature b. Time c. Medium	Stability: Chitosomes and Liposomes	Ref
Diclofenac sodium	a. HSPC:PS:CHO 3:0.1:1 b. EIM	a. 0.25; 0.5 b. 540 c. 97 d. Chitosan	a. 4; 25 °C b. 30 days c. Aqueous suspension	- Both chitosomes and liposomes were stable at 4 °C without significant changes in their size, Zeta potential and EE - At 25 °C, chitosomes with both concentrations used showed better stability than liposomes in terms of size and EE	[12]
DNA	a. Phospholipon 80:DCP:CHO 5:1:4 b. REV	a. 0.1 b. 300 c. 87 d. Chitosan	a. 37 °C b. 1, 2 h c. SGF (pH 1.2); SIF (pH 6.8)	- Chitosomes protected the DNA from the endonuclease digestion after incubation in both SGF and SIF. However, conventional liposomes were less protective in SIF	[39]
Epirubicin	a. PC:CHO 50:15 * b. TFH + sonication	a. 12.5; 33; 75; 200 mg b. 80 c. 92 d. Chitosan	a. 4; 25; 37 °C b. 30 days c. Aqueous suspension	- Chitosomes showed better stability after 30 days of storage at 4 and 25 °C with no significant changes in size, contrary to conventional liposomes - Both systems were unstable at 37 °C with a significant increase in vesicle size	[47]
Extracellular proteins	a. Lecithin 100 mg b. EIM	a. 0.3 b. NR c. NR d. Chitosan	a. 4 °C b. 60 days c. Aqueous suspension	- Chitosomes improved liposome stability since more than 70% and 50% of extracellular proteins remained encapsulated after 2 months at 4 °C in coated and noncoated liposomes, respectively	[57]
Fexofenadine	a. DPPC:DPPG: CHO 8:1:2.25 b. TFH+ extrusion	a. 0.1 b. NR c. NR d. Chitosan	a. 4; 25 °C b. 180 days c. Freeze-dried powder	- Under different tested conditions, drug leakage was lower than 10%, and the size change was minimal for both systems	[73]
Glucose	a. DPPC 0.27 M b. ISCRPE	a. 0.005 b. NR c. 70–90 d. Chitosan	a. 25 °C b. 30 days c. Aqueous suspension	- Both systems were stable since the loss in glucose EE from chitosomes over time was almost similar to that in liposomes	[76]
Grape seed extract	a. Lipoid S75 1% (w/w) b. High-pressure homogenizer	a. 0.1 b. NR c. 79 d. Chitosan	a. 25 °C b. 98 days c. Aqueous suspension	- Both systems were stable since no significant changes in size and zeta potential were observed	[68]

Table 6. Cont.

Drug/EO	Liposomes a. Composition b. Preparation Method	Chitosan or Chitosan Derivative a. Concentration (% w/v) b. MW (kDa) c. DD (%) d. Chitosan Type	Storage Conditions a. Temperature b. Time c. Medium	Stability: Chitosomes and Liposomes	Ref
Insulin	a. Lecithin:CHO 4:1 b. REV	a. 1 b. NR c. 79 d. Chitosan	a. 25 °C b. 15 days c. Aqueous suspension	- Both systems were stable since no significant changes in size and zeta potential were observed	[62]
		a. 0.1–0.5 b. 65; 140; 680; 1000 c. 90 d. Chitosan	a. 37 °C b. NR c. Tris-HCl buffered saline (pH 2 and 7.4)	- Chitosan coating reduced peptic and tryptic digestion of insulin compared to uncoated liposomes - This protective action in chitosomes was enhanced by the increase in chitosan MW and concentration	[38]
Lidocaine	a. Lecithin:SDC15% * b. TFH + sonication+ extrusion	a. 0.3; 0.5 b. 150 c. 90 d. Chitosan	a. 4; 25 °C b. 90 days c. Aqueous suspension	- Elastic chitosomes with both chitosan concentrations used were more stable than uncoated ones for 3 months at 4 and 25 °C, where a slow increase in size and drug leakage ratio were observed - No significant difference in size and drug leakage ratio between elastic liposomes coated with 0.3 and 0.5% chitosan after 3 months; - A better stability was obtained at 4 °C since the changes in size and leakage ratio were less than those obtained at 25 °C	[48]
Mitoxantrone	a. SPC:CHO 5:1 b. TFH + sonication	a. 0.1; 0.3; 0.6; 1.2 b. 70 c. 92 d. Chitosan	a. −70 °C b. NR c. FD-RH	- Uncoated liposomes showed higher size after FD-RH compared to chitosomes, indicating the protective effect of chitosan-coating during FD-RH - As chitosan concentration increased from 0 to 0.3%, liposomes showed fewer changes in their size after FD-RH	[35]
Paclitaxel	a. Lecithin:CHO:SA 1.225:0.575:0.1 * b. TFH + sonication	a. 0.1 b. 50 c. NR d. Chitosan	a. 4; 25 °C b. 180 days c. Aqueous suspension	- Both systems were stable at 4 and 25 °C since no significant changes were observed in size, zeta potential and EE after storage	[74]
			a. 37 °C b. 2 h, 6 h c. SGF (pH 1.2); SIF (pH 6.8)	- Chitosomes were more stable than liposomes in both SGF and SIF since no changes in size, zeta potential and EE were obtained	

Table 6. Cont.

Drug/EO	Liposomes a. Composition b. Preparation Method	Chitosan or Chitosan Derivative a. Concentration (% w/v) b. MW (kDa) c. DD (%) d. Chitosan Type	Storage Conditions a. Temperature b. Time c. Medium	Stability: Chitosomes and Liposomes	Ref
Resveratrol	a. EPC 2% (w/v) b. TFH + sonication	a. 0.1; 0.3; 0.5 b. NR c. NR d. Chitosan	a. 25 °C b. 7 days c. Aqueous suspension	- Chitosan improved liposomes stability since the size increase after storage was lower than that of uncoated liposomes - 0.1% chitosan coating displayed very little change in size compared to high chitosan concentrations (0.3 and 0.5%)	[42]
Rosmarinic acid esters	a. Lecithin 1% (w/v) b. Homogenization	a. 0.2 b. 205 c. 91.8	a. 55 °C b. 14 days c. pH 3	- Chitosomes were more stable than liposomes, where chitosomes size increased by 1-fold after storage compared to 1.5-fold for uncoated ones	[69]
Salmon protein hydrolysates	a. MFGM Phosphlac 700 3; 5; 10% (w/v) b. Heating+ Homogenization	a. 0.4; 0.6 b. NR c. NR d. Chitosan	a. 4; 20 °C b. 30 days c. Aqueous suspension; and FD-RH	- Both systems were stable at 4 °C without significant changes in their size - A better stability at 4 °C for both systems. - The excess of chitosan (0.6%) resulted in more drug loss after 1 month at 20 °C compared to 0.4% chitosan - Conventional liposomes exhibited larger size and higher drug loss compared to chitosomes after FD-RH - No significant difference in drug loss between liposomes coated with either 0.4 or 0.6% chitosan after FD-RH	[49]
Substance P	a. Lecithin:CHO 20:3.3 * b. TFH + sonication	a. 0.1 b. NR c. 88 d. Chitosan	a. 37 °C b. 24 h c. PBS (pH 7.4)	- Both systems were stable since the mean size and pdI did not increase over time	[34]
Triazavirin	a. SPC:CHO 85:15 * b. TFH+ extrusion	a. 0.275 b. 190 c. 95 d. Pelargonic chitosan	a. 4 °C b. 90 days c. Aqueous suspension	- Unmodified liposomes were proved to be unstable after one month of storage - Coating of liposomes with pelargonic chitosan extended the shelf life of liposomes up to 3 months at 4 °C compared to uncoated ones since the size and pdI was almost unchanged	[29]
Vitamin E	a. PC:CHO 60:40 b. Sonication	a. 0.1 b. 4 c. >90 d. Chitosan	a. 4; 25 °C b. 84 days c. Aqueous suspension	- After 12 weeks of storage at 4 °C, 97% of vitamin E remained encapsulated in chitosomes compared to 60.76% in liposomes - When chitosomes were stored at 25 °C, the stability of vitamin E decreased to 31.2%	[70]

3.7. Drug Release

Studies were conducted to compare the drug release rate from conventional liposomes and chitosomes. In vitro drug release from both systems was generally performed in PBS at pH 7.4 and 37 °C by dialysis technique. Both liposomes and chitosomes showed a two-stage profile release, an initial rapid release followed by a sustained release. The initial burst drug release can be attributed to the immediate release of surface-associated drugs. The sustained release of encapsulated drug results from drug diffusion from lipid bilayer and the adhesive chitosan layer for chitosomes [29,55,56,60]. Liposomes coated with chitosan [12,34,35,47,48,55,56,60,74,79] or modified chitosan [22,29] released the drug in a retarded and slower manner compared to noncoated liposomes. This was attributed to the existence of the chitosan layer, which delayed the drug diffusion into the medium [34,35,47,55,56,60].

In fact, the biphasic pattern of drug release is also obtained in simulated GI fluid. The deposition of chitosan on the liposome surface displayed a lower level of drug release in both SGF and SIF compared to uncoated liposomes [5,44,49,58]. Several factors controlled the drug release rate, especially the medium composition, polymer ionization and dissolution in the medium and drug ionization depending on the medium pH and the pKa value of the drug. For example, the drug release rate from both systems was enhanced in SIF relatively to SGF due to the decrease in the protonation of amino groups of chitosan in a high-pH medium [5,44,49]. This confirmed the mechanism by which the medium composition affects the vesicle stability described previously (Section 3.6.2 mechanism controlled by medium composition) and subsequently the drug release rate. Otherwise, the aqueous solubility of chitosan and its derivatives depends on the pH of the buffer solution. Since the octadecyl-quaternized lysine-modified chitosan derivative is much easier dissolved in acidic solution [22], the calcein release rate from octadecyl-quaternized lysine-modified chitosomes is higher at low pH 5.7 (90% after 14 h) than that at pH 8 (70%). In addition, due to the dissolution of N-trimethyl chitosan chloride in water, and a relatively weak electrostatic interaction between liposome and polymers, a similar curcumin release profile was demonstrated between uncoated and N-trimethyl chitosan-coated liposomes [27].

Moreover, the in vitro release data of grape-seed polyphenols performed in acetate buffer at pH 3.8 at 25 °C [62], quercetin performed in acetate buffer at pH 5.5 and PBS pH 7.4 [80], and curcumin in PBS pH 7 at 23 °C and 60 °C [66] from the liposomes and chitosomes were analyzed using various mathematical models, including the zero-order equation, first-order, Baker–Lonsdale, Higuchi, Hixson–Crowell or Korsmeyer–Peppas models to determine the kinetics and the mechanism of drug release from different formulations. The regression analysis was performed, and the model that best fit the release data was chosen on the basis of the highest correlation coefficient R^2 [62,80]. The models of controlled release mechanisms for the liposomes coated with chitosan are in agreement with the release behavior of uncoated liposomes. The Korsmeyer–Peppas model was reported as the optimal model for the different formulations containing quercetin [80]. In contrast, the coefficients of correlation were equal for both Higuchi and Peppas equations (R^2 = 0.972) for uncoated and chitosan-coated liposomal formulations containing grape-seed polyphenols [62]. In addition, the release of curcumin from liposomes and chitosomes mostly followed the Higuchi model at 23 °C and the Peppas model at 60 °C [66]. It is important to mention that both Higuchi and Peppas equations indicate a diffusion-driven release of drugs from uncoated and coated liposomes. In addition, the diffusional exponent n determined from Korsmeyer–Peppas model indicates the mechanism of drug release, where a value of n equal 0.45 (or 0.5 in some studies [62]), indicates a Fickian diffusion, while a value of n between 0.45 and 0.89 indicates a non-Fickian (anomalous) release, which refers to a combination of both diffusion and erosion of the polymeric chain. When $n \geq 0.89$, the release by the erosion of polymeric chain is the major mechanism [80]. The diffusional exponent n was 0.74 and 0.61 for uncoated and chitosan-coated liposomes loading quercetin, respectively [80], and in the range of 0.64 and 0.81 for both systems loading curcumin at both temperatures (23 and 60 °C) [66], indicating an anomalous release of quercetin [80] and curcumin [66]. However, a Fickian diffusion was reported for polyphenols from chitosomes (n = 0.502), while an anomalous transport from uncoated liposomes (n = 0.518) [62]. When an ionic polymer, such as positively charged chitosan, interacts with a released compound having an opposite charge, such as gallic acid, this results in retention via ionic bonds. This can be the reason for the difference in the release behavior of coated and uncoated liposomes [62].

Other factors, such as polymer concentration, chitosan MW and temperature, also influenced the drug release behavior. Increasing the concentration of chitosan from 0.1 to 0.6% *w/v* [5,17,37] or modified chitosan from 0.05 to 0.4% [22] resulted in a decrease in drug release percentage compared to uncoated liposomes. The thicker coatings (0.3 and 0.6% *w/v*) cause an obstacle for drug release [17]. It was also demonstrated that the drug release rate was not affected when chitosan content reaches saturation. Thus, no significant difference in lidocaine release profile was obtained from 0.3 and 0.5% *w/v* chitosan-coated elastic liposomes [48].

Additionally, a high MW of chitosan-coated liposomes showed a slower release rate of cyclosporine A than that obtained with a low MW of chitosan-coated liposomes [79] as a stronger outer coating membrane forms with a high MW of polymers.

Another factor influencing the release was the temperature. Temperature increase from 23 to 60 °C resulted in a fast curcumin release rate from both curcumin-loaded liposomes and chitosomes with a low release rate obtained in chitosomes at tested temperatures [66].

3.8. Pharmacokinetic Studies: Conventional Liposomes and Chitosomes

The pharmacokinetic parameters (T_{max}, C_{max}, AUC, $T_{1/2}$) of many drugs obtained by in vivo studies were improved for chitosan-coated liposomes compared to free drug or drug-loaded conventional liposomes (Table 7). Chitosomes showed the greatest absorption, the slowest elimination, longer retention time, and enhanced bioavailability compared to drug-loaded liposomes.

Table 7. Drug pharmacokinetic behavior: conventional liposomes and chitosomes. The liposomal composition is indicated in the table in molar ratio except when * exists, indicating a weight ratio (w/w).

Drug	Liposomes A. Composition B. Preparation Method	Chitosan or Chitosan Derivative a. Concentration (% w/v) b. MW (kDa) c. DD (%) d. Chitosan Type	Pharmacokinetic Behavior	Ref
Berberine Hydrochloride	a. EPC:CHO:DHP 1:0.242:0.036 b. TFH+ sonication	a. 0.1; 0.3 b. NR c. >90 d. Chitosan	- Pharmacokinetics parameters (AUC, T_{max}, C_{max}) for berberine hydrochloride-loaded chitosomes after oral administration to rabbits were higher than those obtained with uncoated liposomes	[5]
	a. DPPC:DCP 4:1 DPPC:SA 4:1 b. TFH	a. 1.5 b. 150 c. 85 d. Chitosan	- The area under the plasma calcium concentration curve was 2.4 and 2.8 times higher for chitosomes than for positively and negatively charged uncoated liposomes, respectively, after oral administration to rats	[81]
	a. DSPC:DCP:CHO 8:2:1 b. TFH+ sonication	a. 0.3 b. 150 c. 85 d. Chitosan	- The area under plasma calcium concentration obtained after oral administration to rats increased with decreasing liposomes size	[82]
Calcitonin	a. DSPC:DCP:CHO 8:2:1 b. TFH+ extrusion	a. 0.6 b. 150; 22 c. >85; 80 d. Chitosan	- After oral administration to rats, calcitonin-loaded chitosomes prepared with LMW chitosan showed more pharmacological effectiveness in decreasing blood calcium concentration than did HMW chitosomes	[54]
	a. DPPC:DPPE-MCC 3:0.3 b. TFH+ extrusion	a. 0.2 b. 150 c. NR d. TGA chitosan; TGA-MNA-chitosan	- The highest reduction in blood calcium level after oral administration to rats was achieved for TGA-MNA-chitosan-coated liposomes	[30]
Curcumin	a. SPC:CHO 20:2 b. TFH+ extrusion	a. 0.5 b. 200 c. >85 d. N-trimethyl chitosan chloride	- After oral administration to rats, curcumin incorporated into N-trimethyl chitosan-coated liposomes exhibited different pharmacokinetic parameters (C_{max}, $T_{1/2}$, AUC), the greatest absorption, the slowest elimination and enhanced bioavailability compared to curcumin-loaded liposomes	[27]
Cyclosporin A	a. EPC:CHO:Pluronic F 127 28:5:11 b. TFH+ extrusion	a. 0.4 b. 200 c. 90 d. Chitosan	- Pharmacokinetic analysis after oral administration to rats showed that C_{max} and AUC of deformable liposomes were 1.73- and 1.84-fold higher than those of chitosomes, respectively	[39]

Table 7. Cont.

Drug	Liposomes A. Composition B. Preparation Method	Chitosan or Chitosan Derivative a. Concentration (% w/v) b. MW (kDa) c. DD (%) d. Chitosan Type	Pharmacokinetic Behavior	Ref
Docetaxel	a. Lipoid S100:CHO: Tween-80:SDC:DCP 0.9:0.3:0.1:0.1:0.1 b. TFH+ sonication	a. 1 b. NR c. NR d. Chitosan	- After intraperitoneal administration to rats, the pharmacokinetic parameters (AUC, C_{max}, mean residence time) were higher in deformable chitosomes than in deformable liposomes	[55]
Fexofenadine	a. DPPC:DPPG:CHO 8:1:2.25 b. TFH+ extrusion	a. 0.1 b. NR c. NR d. Chitosan	- Bioavailability of fexofenadine was increased up to 34.7% via intranasal administration of chitosomes in rats compared to uncoated liposomes (24.5%)	[73]
Vancomycin hydrochloride	a. Lecithin:CHO 32.5:5 * b. REV	a. 0.4 b. NR c. NR d. Chitosan	- After intravenous injection to mice, chitosomes loading vancomycin hydrochloride showed a longer retention time and higher AUC values compared to vancomycin hydrochloride injection and vancomycin hydrochloride-loaded liposomes	[56]

3.9. Pharmacodynamics: Conventional Liposomes and Chitosomes

In the section below, the in vitro and in vivo biological effects of drug- or EO-loaded chitosomes and liposomes are reported (Tables 8–12). Chitosan-coating of liposomes improved numerous biological activities, including antimicrobial activity, mucoadhesive property, cytotoxic effect against cancer cell lines, anti-inflammatory, analgesic and suppression of gene expression.

3.9.1. Antimicrobial Property

Although humans developed medications for many contagious diseases, the antimicrobial and antiviral activities of synthetic and natural substances still attract much attention. In the area of antibiotic resistance, new antimicrobials are highly desired but not easy to obtain. Therefore, efforts are undertaken to increase or tailor antimicrobial activity by formulations. The antimicrobial properties of chitosan alone or blended with other natural polymers are well-known. Its activity against Gram-positive and Gram-negative bacteria results from the polycationic structure of chitosan [19]. In addition, chitosomes, even non-loaded with any drug, can exert antimicrobial activity, which was proven for *Staphylococcus epidermidis* and *Staphylococcus aureus*. The activity was dependent on the type of bacteria and the formulation, and *S. epidermidis* was susceptible to lower concentrations of chitosan (0.03%, 0.1% and 0.3%) [83]. For this reason, antimicrobial activity measured for chitosomes loaded with drugs can be considered as a synergistic activity of the drug itself and chitosan. What is more, chitosomes are able to assure the prolonged release of the drug, as it was shown for metronidazole. The antimicrobial efficacy of chitosomes combined with the antifungal potential of the entrapped metronidazole was effective against *Candida albicans* and could offer improved efficacy in the treatment of mixed or complex vaginal infections [84]. Similar enhanced controlled release and antimicrobial effects against multidrug-resistant foodborne pathogens were observed for nisin entrapped in chitosomes. The inhibition of *S. aureus*, *Enterococcus faecalis* and *Listeria monocytogenes* growth were better for nisin-loaded chitosomes than free or liposomal-nisin [85]. The findings indicate the possible applications of chitosomes as external use antimicrobial formulations.

It was established for the first time that polymer-coating could enhance the stability of the liposomal formulations entrapping EOs, this study being a stepping-stone in the development of EOs as antimicrobial agents [36]. Thus, *Artemisia afra*, *Eucalyptus globulus* and *Melaleuca alternifolia* EOs were encapsulated within polymeric liposomal systems. First, synergistic to additive interactions were shown for *E. globulus* and *M. alternifolia* liposomal formulations against *Escherichia coli*, *Staphylococcus aureus*, *Pseudomonas aeruginosa* and *Candida albicans*. Further, chitosan-coating of the liposomes improved their surface stability and prolonged the EOs release, thus extending their antimicrobial activity [36]. The antimicrobial activity of EOs and other bioactive molecules in both systems is summarized in Table 8.

Table 8. Antimicrobial activity of bioactive molecules: conventional liposomes and chitosomes. The liposomal composition is indicated in the table in molar ratio except when * exists, indicating a weight ratio (w/w).

Drug/EO	Liposomes a. Composition b. Preparation Method	Chitosan a. Concentration (% w/v) b. MW (kDa) c. DD (%)	Antibacterial Activity	Ref
Artemisia afra, Eucalyptus globulus, Melaleuca alternifolia	a. DSPC:DSPE 94:6 b. REV+sonication	a. 0.15 b. NR c. NR	- A. afra chitosomes displayed lower MIC values compared to liposomes and unencapsulated EO against Staphyloccocus aureus, Escherichia coli, Pseudomonas aeruginosa, and Candida albicans, indicating that polymer coating overcomes the increased EO volatility - E. globulus chitosomes displayed lower MIC values compared to liposomes and unencapsulated EO against C. albicans - M. alternifolia chitosomes showed similar MIC compared to liposomes against S. aureus, E. coli, P. aeruginosa, and C. albicans	[36]
Chrysanthemum sp.	a. Lecithin:CHO 5:1 b. TFH+extrusion	a. 0.0025–0.01 b. NR c. NR	- EO chitosomes reduced Campylobacter jejuni viability in chicken compared to liposomes due to the antibacterial properties of the chitosan coating	[78]
Dicloxacillin	a. Lipid S100:CHO:Tween-80 0.9:0.3:0.1 b. TFH+sonication	a. 1 b. NR c. NR	- Dicloxacillin-loaded liposomes exhibited a significantly wider zone of S. aureus inhibition compared to dicloxacillin or dicloxacillin-loaded chitosomes, probably due to liposome flexibility and relatively small size compared to chitosomes	[60]
Metronidazole	a. SPC b. TFH	a. 0.17 b. NR c. 77	- Metronidazole loading chitosan-coated liposomes exhibited growth inhibition against C. albicans (MIC 0.11–0.22 mg/mL), whereas control carbopol-loaded liposomes and plain liposomes, as well as the metronidazole control solution, showed no inhibition	[84]
Nisin	a. Lecithin NR + tripolyphosphate as crosslinker (0.1% w/v) b. Stirring+sonication	a. 0.3–0.9 b. NR c. NR	Chitosomes controlled S. aureus, E. faecalis and L. monocytogenes growth better than free or liposomal-nisin	[85]
Nisin silica	a. Lecithin:CHO 20:4 * b. TFH+homogenization	a. 0.1 b. NR c. NR	- Chitosan-coated nisin-silica liposomes displayed better antibacterial activity against L. monocytogenes in cheese models compared to chitosan-coated nisin liposomes and uncoated ones	[71]

3.9.2. Mucoadhesive Property

The mucoadhesive property of chitosomes was the most studied one among other activities. It was carried out *in vitro* by incubating a mucin solution with a liposomal or chitosomal suspension at 37 °C for 1 h. Using a colorimetric method, the amount of free mucin in the supernatant obtained by centrifugation of the suspension is used to calculate the amount of adsorbed mucin on particle surface from the difference between total and free mucin. Mucin adsorption percent was then calculated as the ratio between the adsorbed mucin and the total amount of mucin used. Mucoadhesivity was also performed in vivo, where the liposomal or chitosomal suspension was administered orally to rats. The intestinal were removed from scarified rats and divided into segments (duodenum, jejunum and ileum). Confocal laser scanning microscopy was performed to visualize the mucopenetrative behaviors of liposomes across the intestinal mucosa. Mucus is a viscous coating on many epithelial surfaces and consists mainly of water (up to 95% weight), inorganic salts, carbohydrates, lipids and glycoproteins, termed mucins. Mucins are hydrosoluble and responsible for the gel-like properties of mucus [86]. The mucoadhesive property of chitosomes is mainly due to the electrostatic interaction between the amine group (NH_3^+) of chitosan and the carboxylate (COO^-) or sulfonate (SO_3^-) group of mucin [43] as well as by other non-covalent bonds, such as hydrogen and hydrophobic bonds (from the remaining acetyl group on chitosan molecules) [54]. Several factors, such as zeta potential, liposomes size, the polymer used, chitosan concentration and chitosan MW, may influence the chitosome's mucoadhesive property. A linear correlation was demonstrated between the mucin percent absorbed on the vesicles and their corresponding zeta potential values (Figure 4) [32].

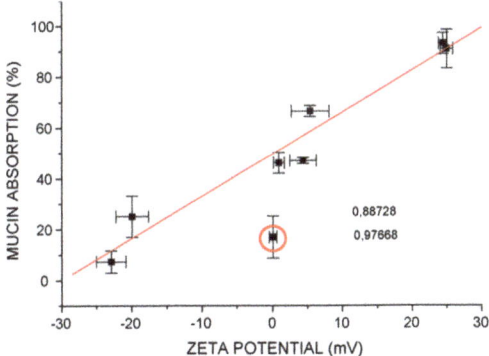

Figure 4. Effect of vesicle zeta potential on the mucoadhesive properties of chitosomes [32].

Small chitosome size showed high mucoadhesion [82]. Low chitosan concentration also favors mucoadhesivity [17]. In order for mucoadhesion to take place, the wetting and swelling of the polymer should enable an intimate contact with the mucosal tissue, followed by the interpenetration of the polymer chains and entanglement between the polymer and mucin chains [17]. Thiolated chitosans have stronger mucoadhesive properties than non-modified chitosan [17,30]. However, excessive water uptake will lead to overhydration forming slippery mucilage and less adhesiveness [87]. The slow swelling behavior of S-protected thiomers via conjugation of thiolated chitosan with 6-mercaptonicotinamide can avoid overhydration and loss of adhesiveness, resulting in a prolonged mucoadhesion [30,87]. Overall, chitosan-coated liposomes were proved to enhance the mucoadhesive property of several bioactive molecules when compared to conventional liposomes (Table 9).

Table 9. Drug mucoadhesive property: conventional liposomes and chitosomes. The liposomal composition is indicated in the table in molar ratio except when * exists, indicating a weight ratio (w/w).

Drug	Liposomes a. Composition b. Preparation Method	Chitosan or Chitosan Derivative a. Concentration (% w/v) b. MW (kDa) c. DD (%) d. Chitosan Type	Mucoadhesive Property	Ref
Atenolol	a. Lipoid S100 20 mg b. EIM	a. 0.6 b. NR c. NR d. Chitosan	- Chitosomes have higher mucoadhesive strength performed on pork intestines (≈35%) compared to uncoated liposomes (10%)	[63]
Calcitonin	a. DPPC:DCP 4:1 DPPC:SA 40:1 b. TFH	a. 1.5 b. 150 c. 85 d. Chitosan	- The mucoadhesive percentage was as follows: chitosomes> noncoated positively charged liposomes> noncoated negatively charged liposomes	[81]
Calcitonin	a. DSPC:DCP:CHO 8:2:1 b. TFH+ sonication	a. 0.3 b. 150 c. 85 d. Chitosan	- Small-sized liposomes (200 nm) and chitosomes (400 nm) showed high penetration into intestinal mucosa, while such behavior was not observed for large vesicles (3810 nm) even when coated with chitosan (4130–4640 nm)	[82]
Clotrimazole	a. Lipoid S100 200 mg b. TFH+ sonication	a. 0.1; 0.3; 0.6 b. NR c. 92 d. Chitosan	- Mucin studies revealed that coating with low chitosan concentration (0.1%) increased the system's mucoadhesive potential compared to coating with high chitosan concentrations (0.3 and 0.6%)	[17]
Curcumin	a. EPC:CHO 2:1 b. EIM and TFH+ sonication	a. 0.1 b. 30 c. 88 d. Chitosan	- Mucin adsorption was improved after chitosan coating with a value of 33.60 and 56.47%, respectively, for curcumin-loaded liposomes and curcumin-loaded chitosomes	[43]
Cyclosporin A	a. EPC:CHO:Pluronic F 127 28:5:11 b. TFH+ extrusion	a. 0.4 b. 200 c. 90 d. Chitosan	- After oral administration to rats, chitosomes were trapped by mucus and remained in the upper portion of the intestinal tract with limited penetration ability. However, deformable liposomes were found throughout the intestinal tract and were able to penetrate the mucus layers to reach the epithelial surface	[59]
DiI	a. DSPC:DCP:CHO 8:2:1 b. TFH+ sonication	a. 0.6 b. 150 c. 85 d. Chitosan	- Both liposomes and chitosomes were retained in the stomach at 40% in fed rats after 1 h oral administration, and intestinal transition was reduced compared to fasted rats	[88]

Table 9. *Cont.*

Drug	Liposomes a. Composition b. Preparation Method	Chitosan or Chitosan Derivative a. Concentration (% w/v) b. MW (kDa) c. DD (%) d. Chitosan Type	Mucoadhesive Property	Ref
Fexofenadine	a. DPPC:DPPG:CHO 8:1:2.25 b. TFH+ extrusion	a. 0.1 b. NR c. NR d. Chitosan	- Mucoadhesive property was improved after chitosan coating with 30 and 90% for fexofenadine-loaded liposomes chitosomes, respectively	[73]
Rifampicin	a. EPC:CHO 2:1 EPC:PG:CHO 9:1:5 DSPC:CHO 2:1 DSPC:PG:CHO 9:1:5 b. TFH+ sonication	a. 0.001–0.66 b. NR c. 87 d. Chitosan	- The mucoadhesive percentage was in the following order: chitosomes> noncoated uncharged liposomes> noncoated negatively charged liposomes	[32]
Triazavirin	a. SPC:CHO 85:15 * b. TFH+ extrusion	a. 0.275 b. 190 c. 95 d. Pelargonic chitosan; lauric chitosan	- Unmodified chitosomes showed 1.3 and 1.6 times higher mucoadhesive properties than pelargonic- and lauric chitosan-coated liposomes, respectively	[29]

3.9.3. Permeability and Drug Penetration Effect

Chitosomes exhibited higher permeability and drug penetration into the skin than liposomes (Table 10). The increased skin drug permeation with chitosan coating could be explained by the tendency of positively charged chitosan to electrostatically interact with the negatively charged lipid present in the lipid layer of the stratum corneum to open the epidermal tight junctions and to promote the drug delivery [42,48]. In addition, chitosomes exhibited potential ocular applications by increasing transcorneal drug penetration, compared to uncoated liposomes or commercially available eye drops with no ocular irritation [12,37,79]. The penetration enhancing effect of chitosomes into the cornea was higher with HMW of chitosan [28] but did not increase with the excess amount of chitosan [12]. The main findings concerning the permeation enhancing effect of chitosomes in comparison to liposomes are shown in Table 10.

Table 10. Permeability and drug penetration studies: conventional liposomes and chitosomes. The liposomal composition is indicated in the table in molar ratio except when * exists, indicating a weight ratio (w/w).

Drug	Liposomes a. Composition b. Preparation Method	Chitosan or Chitosan Derivative a. Concentration (% w/v) b. MW (kDa) c. DD (%) d. Chitosan Type	Permeability and drug Penetration Effect	Ref
Anti-sense oligodeoxynucleotides	a. SPC:CHO 20:5 * b. TFH+ sonication	a. 0.05–1 b. 100 c. 90 d. Chitosan	- Chitosomes significantly enhanced COS7 cells uptake of anti-sense oligodeoxynucleotides compared to the nucleotide alone or nucleotide-loaded liposomes	[53]
BSA	a. EPC:sodium oleate 10:2 b. TFH+ sonication	a. 20 mM b. 276 c. 94 d. TMBz-chitosan	- Compared to BSA-loaded liposomes, TMBz chitosan-coated liposomes enhanced BSA permeability across Caco-2 cell monolayers	[25]
Calcein	a. PC:CHO 3:1 * PC:Folate:PEG:CHO 1:1:1:1 * b. TFH+ sonication	a. 0.5 b. 50 c. NR d. Octadecyl-quaternized lysine modified chitosan	- Octadecyl-quaternized lysine-modified chitosan-coated deformable liposomes showed higher calcein delivery to MCF-7 cells compared to traditional liposomes	[22]
Calcitonin	a. DPPC:DPPE-MCC 3:≤0.3 b. TFH+ extrusion	a. 0.2 b. 150 c. NR d. TGA chitosan; TGA-MNA-chitosan	- Calcitonin permeation enhancing effect through intestinal mucus was more pronounced for modified chitosomes than uncoated liposomes with 1.8-, 2.7- and a 3.8-fold increase for uncoated liposomes, TGA chitosan-coated liposomes and TGA-MNA-chitosan-coated liposomes, respectively, compared to a calcitonin buffer solution	[30]
Ciprofloxacin hydrochloride	a. PC:SA 10:0.5 PC:DCP 10:1 b. TFH	a. 0.3 b. NR c. 85 d. Chitosan	- Chitosomes exhibited high drug levels in the external eye of albino rabbits compared to uncoated liposomes and the commercially available eye drop, with no ocular irritation	[37]
Coenzyme Q10	a. SPC:CHO 83:17 * b. EIM+ sonication	a. 0.5 b. 100; 450 c. >85 d. Trimethyl chitosan	- Trimethyl chitosan with HMW (450 kDa) led to higher precorneal retention times than that of LMW (100 kDa) and liposomes	[28]
Cyclosporin A	a. HSPC:PS:CHO 4:0.1:1 b. EIM	a. 0.25 b. 540 c. 94 d. Chitosan	- After topical instillation in rabbits, cyclosporin A concentrations in cornea, conjunctiva and sclera were higher in chitosomes than in liposomes	[79]

Table 10. Cont.

Drug	Liposomes a. Composition b. Preparation Method	Chitosan or Chitosan Derivative a. Concentration (% w/v) b. MW (kDa) c. DD (%) d. Chitosan Type	Permeability and drug Penetration Effect	Ref
Diclofenac sodium	a. HSPC:PS:CHO 3:0.1:1 b. EIM	a. 0.25; 0.5 b. 540 c. 97 d. Chitosan	- Diclofenac sodium-loaded chitosomes improved the transcorneal drug penetration rate compared to uncoated liposomes or commercially available eye drops with no ocular irritation	[12]
Flurbiprofen	a. EPC:solutol HS15 7.5:1 b. Modified EIM	a. 0.1 b. 50 c. 95 d. Chitosan	- The apparent permeability coefficient of flurbiprofen-loaded deformable chitosomes evaluated using isolated rabbit corneas was 1.29-fold greater than that of uncoated flurbiprofen-loaded deformable liposomes	[61]
Furosemide	a. SPC:CHO 10:1 b. TFH+ sonication	a. 0.5 b. NR c. NR d. Chitosan	- Chitosomes increased the apical to basolateral permeability of furosemide by 8-fold through Caco-2 cells compared to furosemide loaded liposomes and furosemide solution	[4]
Lidocaine	a. Lecithin:SDC 15% * b. TFH+ sonication+ extrusion	a. 0.3 b. 150 c. 90 d. Chitosan	- Chitosan-coated elastic liposomes significantly improved lidocaine hydrochloride skin permeation compared to elastic liposome and chitosan solution	[48]
Resveratrol	a. EPC 2% * b. TFH+ sonication	a. 0.1 b. NR c. NR d. Chitosan	-Resveratrol permeated skin animal with 40.42 and 30.84% for chitosomes and liposomes, respectively	[42]

3.9.4. Cytotoxicity

Chitosomes proved a high cell attraction which potentially increased the cellular drug uptake leading to drug cytotoxicity as demonstrated by MTT assay [55]. Table 11 reported an enhanced cytotoxic effect on several cancer cell lines for various drug-loaded chitosomes or -modified chitosomes when compared to drug-conventional liposomes and free drugs. It is important to note that the cell viability decreased with increasing chitosan concentration [79]. In addition, the pH affects the surface charge of glycol chitosomes leading to an improvement in their antitumor efficacy compared to uncoated liposomes (Table 11) [23].

3.9.5. Other Biological Effects

The coating of the liposomes with chitosan and its derivatives confers not only high mucoadhesion capacity, antimicrobial activity and enhanced carrier permeability but also enhanced other biological activities, including anti-inflammatory, immune-stimulatory effect, analgesic and suppression of gene expression as reported in Table 12.

Table 11. Cytotoxicity and anticancer effect of drugs: conventional liposomes and chitosomes. The liposomal composition is indicated in the table in molar ratio except when * exists, indicating a weight ratio (w/w).

Drug	Liposomes a. Composition b. Preparation Method	Chitosan or Chitosan Derivative a. Concentration (% w/v) b. MW (kDa) c. DD (%) d. Chitosan Type	Cytotoxicity and Anticancer Effects of Drugs	Ref
Butyric acid	a. PC:CHO 20:5 * b. TFH+ sonication	a. 0.1 b. NR c. NR d. Chitosan	- Chitosomes displayed higher cytotoxicity against human hepatoblastoma HepG2 cells with an IC50 value of 1.6 mM after 72 h of incubation than uncoated liposomes (2.7 mM) and free butyric acid (4.5 mM)	[72]
Cyclosporin A	a. HSPC:PS:CHO 4:0.1:1 b. EIM	a. 0.25; 0.5; 1; 2 b. 540 c. 94 d. Chitosan	- Chitosomes and liposomes loading cyclosporin A demonstrated low toxicity to rabbit conjunctival epithelium cells	[79]
Docetaxel	a. Lipoid S100:CHO:Tween-80:SDC:DCP 0.9:0.3:0.1:0.1:0.1 b. TFH+ sonication	a. 1 b. NR c. NR d. Chitosan	- Uncoated deformable liposomes displayed 52% of human colon cancer HT-29 cell growth, and cell viability was greatly reduced by 80% in deformable chitosomes, indicating enhanced cytotoxic activity for deformable chitosomes	[55]
Doxorubicin	a. HSPC:CHO NR b. TFH+ extrusion	a. NR b. NR c. NR d. Glycol chitosan	- Glycol chitosan-coated doxorubicin-loaded liposomes resulted in a 64% reduction in HT1080 cells viability at pH 6.5 and less than 15% reduction at pH 7.4 compared to uncoated liposomes exhibiting less than 20% reduction in viability regardless of pH	[23]
Doxorubicin	a. HSPC:CHO NR b. TFH+ extrusion	a. NR b. NR c. NR d. Glycol chitosan	- Hematoxylin and eosin-stained tumor sections excised from tumor-bearing mice following intravenous injection of free doxorubicin and doxorubicin-loaded liposomes and glycol chitosan-coated doxorubicin-loaded liposomes showed the strongest antitumor effect for glycol chitosan-coated doxorubicin-loaded liposomes	[23]
Furosemide	a. SPC:CHO 10:1 b. TFH+ sonication	a. 0.5 b. NR c. NR d. Chitosan	- Chitosomes showed less cytotoxicity toward Caco-2 cells than uncoated ones	[4]
Paclitaxel	a. Lecithin:CHO:SA 1.225:0.575:0.1 b. TFH+ sonication	a. 0.1 b. 50 c. NR d. Chitosan	- Chitosomes enhanced paclitaxel-induced cytotoxicity in human cervical cancer cells compared to paclitaxel loaded-liposomes	[74]
Rifampicin	a. EPC:CHO 2:1 EPC:PG:CHO 9:1:5 DSPC:CHO 2:1 DSPC:PG:CHO 9:1:5 b. TFH+ sonication	a. 0.001–0.66 b. NR c. 87 d. Chitosan	-The toxicity of rifampicin-loaded liposomes towards A549 epithelial cells was lower compared to the free drug for all the vesicles types (negatively charged and non-charged ones), especially chitosan-coated ones	[32]
si RNA-VEGF si RNA-H1F1-α	a. HSPC:CHO 1:1 HSPC:DCP:CHO1:0.1:1 HSPC:SA:CHO1:0.1:1 b. TFH+ sonication	a.1 b. 75 c. 75–85 d. Chitosan	- Chitosomes showed 96% of MCF7 cancer cell viability. However, anionic and cationic liposomes showed reduced cell viability of 76.27 and 67.79%, respectively	[75]

Table 11. Cont.

Drug	Liposomes a. Composition b. Preparation Method	Chitosan or Chitosan Derivative a. Concentration (% w/v) b. MW (kDa) c. DD (%) d. Chitosan Type	Cytotoxicity and Anticancer Effects of Drugs	Ref
Substance P	a. Lecithin:CHO 20:3.3 * b. TFH+ sonication	a. 0.1 b. NR c. 88 d. Chitosan	-Both chitosomes and liposomes loading substance P showed no toxic effect on keratinocytes at different tested concentrations	[34]

Table 12. Other biological effects of drugs: conventional liposomes and chitosomes. The liposomal composition is indicated in the table in molar ratio except when * exists, indicating a weight ratio (w/w).

Drug	Liposomes a. Composition b. Preparation Method	Chitosan or Chitosan Derivative a. Concentration (% w/v) b. MW (kDa) c. DD (%) d. Chitosan Type	Other Biological Effects	Ref
Butyric acid	a. PC:CHO 20:5 * b. TFH+ sonication	a. 0.1 b. NR c. NR d. Chitosan	- Chitosomes showed higher anti-inflammatory effects by reducing IL-8, IL-6, TNF-α and TGF-β expression in HepG2 cells compared to free butyric acid and butyric acid-loaded liposomes at different tested concentrations	[72]
Extracellular proteins	a. Lecithin 100 mg b. EIM	a. 0.3 b. NR c. NR d. Chitosan	Nonspecific immune parameters myeloperoxidase, respiratory burst, hemagglutination, hemolytic, antiprotease activity and bacterial agglutination activity were tested after parenteral immunization in fish and rabbits. The specific antibody level was also measured. Chitosomes showed significantly higher specific and nonspecific immune responses than the liposomes	[57]
Lidocaine	a. Lecithin:SDC 15% * b. TFH+ sonication+ extrusion	a. 0.3 b. 150 c. 90 d. Chitosan	- Chitosan-coated elastic lidocaine loaded liposomes revealed greater suppression of formalin-induced nociceptive behavior in mice transdermally treated, thus a better analgesic effect compared to elastic liposome and chitosan solution	[48]

Table 12. Cont.

Drug	Liposomes a. Composition b. Preparation Method	Chitosan or Chitosan Derivative a. Concentration (% w/v) b. MW (kDa) c. DD (%) d. Chitosan Type	Other Biological Effects	Ref
si RNA-VEGF si RNA-H1F1-α	a. HSPC:CHO 1:1 HSPC:DCP:CHO 1:0.1:1 HSPC:SA:CHO 1:0.1:1 b. TFH+ sonication	a. 1 b. 75 c. 75–85 d. Chitosan	- VEGF and HIF1-α protein levels in cells treated with anionic liposomes were significantly lower than those treated with cationic and chitosan-coated ones. - In vitro codelivery of siVEGF and siHIF1-α in breast cancer cells using chitosomes significantly inhibited VEGF (89%) and HIF1-α (62%) protein expression compared to other liposome formulations.	[75]

4. Multilayer Coating of Polyelectrolytes on the Liposomes

A few studies have developed a polyelectrolyte delivery system (PDS) based on liposomes coated with alternating layers of polysaccharides, such as chitosan, alginate, hyaluronate or pectin [64,78,80,89,90]. PDS is represented in Figure 5, in which positively charged chitosan was self-assembly coated onto the anionic liposome surface, and negatively charged alginate, hyaluronate or pectin was then deposited on the outer layer of cationic liposomes.

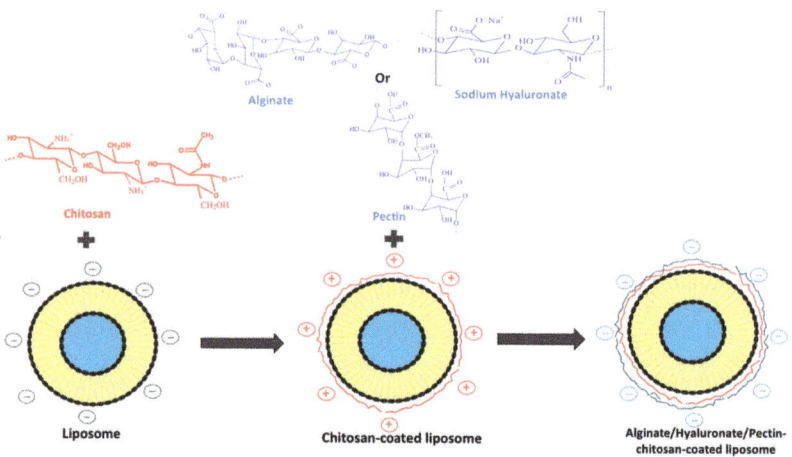

Figure 5. Preparation of polyelectrolyte delivery system layer-by-layer self-assembly of chitosan and alginate/hyaluronate/pectin onto the liposome.

The effect of alternating layers of cationic and anionic polysaccharides on the liposome surface is presented in this section. The characteristics of PDS in comparison to chitosomes and conventional liposomes are presented in Table 13. The adsorbed polymers on the liposomal surface caused a negative zeta potential, an increase in the membrane thickness [89,90], in size [64,78,80,89,90], and in drug EE, which increased with increasing layers of polyelectrolytes [89].

Table 13. Comparison of size, zeta potential, stability and drug release between polyelectrolyte delivery system (PDS), chitosomes and conventional liposomes. The liposomal composition is indicated in the table in molar ratio except when * exists, indicating a weight ratio (w/w).

Liposome a. Composition b. Preparation Method c. Drug/EO	Chitosan a. Concentration (% w/v) b. MW (kDa) c. DD (%)	a. Anionic Polysaccharide b. Concentration (% w/v) c. MW (kDa)	Size (nm) a. PDS b. CH-LP c. UN-LP	Zeta Potential (mv) a. PDS b. CH-LP c. UN-LP	Drug Release	Ref
a. DPPC:CHO: DDAB NR b. TFH+ extrusion c. BSA	a. 0.1 b. 91.11 c. 85	a. Alginate b. 0.1 c. 12	a. 345 ± 10.9 b. NR c. 180 ± 10.5	a. 36.6 b. NR c. 35.4	- BSA released from uncoated liposomes is faster than from PDS - The increase in coating thickness by increasing polyelectrolyte layers number decreased protein release rate	[89]
a. Lecithin:CHO 5:1 b. TFH+extrusion c. Chrysanthemum sp.	a. 0.0025–0.01 b. NR c. NR	a. Pectin b. 0.0025–0.01 c. NR	a. 642 ± 7–3235 ± 7 b. 530 ± 5–793 ± 7.5 c. 98 ± 6–231 ± 9	a. −19.3 – −13.5 b. 34.2–45.4 c. −37.6 – −27.7	- PDS strongly reduced the leakage of EO from the liposomes - Liposomes exhibited the highest release rate (88.2%), followed by chitosomes (60.2%), and lastly, by triple layer liposomes (25.2%)	[78]
a. Lipoid S75 1, 2, 5% * b. High shear disperser + microfluidization c. Hibiscus extract	a. 1 b. NR c. 79	a. Pectin b. 0.005–0.1 c. 55	a. 98–343 b. 60–150 c. 32–46	a. −25 b. 78 c. −29	NR	[91]
a. SPC:CHO: Tween-80 6:1:1.8 * b. TFH+ high-pressure microfluidization c. Medium-chain fatty acids	a. 0.05–2 b. 50 c. NR	a. Alginate b. 0.1–2 c. 12	a. 170 ± 28–3229 ± 203 b. 124 ± 19–255 ± 35 c. 89	a. 1.5–16.1 b. −1.1–3.1 c. −6.3	- In SGF, all liposomes formulations showed low medium-chain fatty acids release rates (29.8 and 20.4% for the liposomes and PDS, respectively) - In SIF, liposomes exhibited the highest medium-chain fatty acids (79.8%) release rate compared to PDS (56.9%)	[90]
a. EPC:CHO: DHP 10:2.5:1 b. TFH+ sonication c. Quercetin	a. 0.1 b. 50–190 c. NR	a. Sodium hyaluronate b. 0.1 c. 490	a. 528 ± 29 b. NR c. 121 ± 2.2	a. −50 b. NR c. −38.2	- Uncoated liposomes exhibited the highest quercetin released amount after 24 h (62% at pH 5.5 and 50% at pH 7.4) - Quercetin exhibited a sustained release as the number of polyelectrolyte layers increased up to 5 (below 20% at both pH)	[80]

Table 13. Cont.

Liposome a. Composition b. Preparation Method c. Drug/EO	Chitosan a. Concentration (% w/v) b. MW (kDa) c. DD (%)	a. Anionic Polysaccharide b. Concentration (% w/v) c. MW (kDa)	Size (nm) a. PDS b. CH-LP c. UN-LP	Zeta Potential (mv) a. PDS b. CH-LP c. UN-LP	Drug Release	Ref
a. SPC:CHO:Tween-80 6:1:1.8 * b. TFH+ high-pressure microfluidization c. Vitamin C	a. 0.6 b. 50 c. NR	a. Alginate b. 0.5 c. 12	a. 1809 ± 210 b. 1098 ± 46 c. 601 ± 76	a. -25.2 b. 24.5 c. -12.5	In SGF, all liposome formulations showed low vitamin C release rates (25, 27 and 14% for the liposomes, chitosomes and PDS, respectively). In SIF, PDS exhibited the slowest vitamin release rate (10%) compared to chitosomes (30%) and liposomes (82%)	[64]

It has been reported that the addition of polyelectrolyte layer improved liposomal stability. For example, triple-layer liposomes composed of chitosan and pectin-loading hibiscus extract were more stable than the liposomes after 30 days of storage at 25 °C with the highest stability obtained with PDS [91]. In addition, triple-layer liposomes containing Chrysanthemum sp. exhibited better stability after 60 days at different temperatures (4, 12, 25 and 37 °C) in terms of particle size, pdI and zeta potential than conventional liposomes and chitosomes [78]. Liposomes modified by chitosan and alginate were stable after 12 months at room temperature without significant changes in their size [89]. PDS systems were not only proved to be stable at aqueous suspensions but also in lyophilized forms. The lyophilization of PDS in the presence of sucrose maintained their size and zeta potential values as those before lyophilization [89].

It is important to note that medium composition (pH and NaCl concentration) affected the PDS stability. PDS size increased significantly from 170 nm at pH 1.5 to 410 nm at pH 5 then decreased to 235 nm at pH 9. However, uncoated liposomes maintained stable at different pH. In SGF, both liposomes and PDS showed a slight change in size for 120 min. In SIF (pH 7.4), compared to the liposomes (from 107 to 114 nm), PDS size increased significantly from 335 to 620 nm over 15 min of digestion and decreased to 530 nm at the end of digestion [90]. In addition, high NaCl concentration (200 mM) at pH 5.5 induced more alteration of PDS than chitosomes and uncoated liposomes in appearance and mean diameter, but the cores (liposomes) of these systems were maintained stable [64]. The following mechanism explained the PDS stability affected by the medium composition. At low pH conditions (pH 1.5), outer-layer alginate shrank and converted into an insoluble so-called alginic acid skin which protected chitosan from dissolution. With pH value increase (even in SIF conditions), there was a decrease in the number of charged cationic groups on chitosan. Thus, the electrostatic interaction between the carboxyl group of alginate and the amino group of chitosan was weaker, medium gradually entered into the particles, and the mean diameter increased. The subsequent decrease in mean diameter could be due to some of the alginate being progressively dissolved. In addition, in SIF conditions, this decrease in the size was explained by the higher affinity of chitosan to bile salts ions than to the liposomes [90]. This was supported by the influence of ionic concentration in the medium on the PDS stability. At pH 5.5 and in the presence of low ionic NaCl concentration, the carboxyl group of alginate was ionized, and the amine group of chitosan was protonated. Interaction in the polyionic complex could govern the alginate–chitosan-coated liposomes to swell water to fill the void regions of the polymer network between alginate and chitosan. When they encountered electrolyte solutions, such as high NaCl concentrations, the equilibrium state was provoked. Ions competed with polymers to interact with water, electrostatic interaction and steric force were weakened, resulting in the erosion of alginate–chitosan-coated liposomes and phase separation between water and particles [64].

In addition, the concentration of anionic polysaccharides affects the PDS stability, where both a higher and lower addition of pectin to chitosan-coated liposomes above or below the concentration of saturation resulted in the destabilization of the liposomes via bridging flocculation [91]. The temperature also affects the PDS stability. PDS size decreased after 1 h at 70 °C due to the degradation of the outer layer alginate at high-temperature. The following increase of particle size may be due to the increased propensity for inter-chain cross-linking of chitosan under the influence of heating [90]. Moreover, PDS composed of 2 polyelectrolytes layers were stable after 3 weeks at 25 °C, whereas a size increase and flocculation were obtained for those composed of 3 to 5 polyelectrolytes layers [80].

PDS delayed the release of encapsulated contents in SGF and SIF compared to chitosomes and conventional liposomes due to several possible mechanisms as follows: (a) there was a physical barrier (shrunken alginate network at low pH and insoluble chitosan layers at high pH) formed on the liposome surface and then enzyme (pancreatic lipase, phospholipase A2, and cholesterol esterase) was restricted to contact with the liposomal phospholipids; (b) electrostatic bridges existing between the phospholipids and polymers reduced the lipid bilayer permeability [90]; (c) formation of a denser shell through the ionic interaction of the two polymers [80].

In vitro skin permeability studies showed that negatively charged sodium hyaluronate-chitosan-coated liposomes and positively charged chitosomes have similar skin permeability, which was superior to uncoated liposomes. This was explained by the ability of hyaluronate to increase the stratum corneum hydration due to its water uptake properties [80].

5. Encapsulation of Essential Oils: Chitosomes vs. Liposomes. Novel Formulation Strategies for Old Antimicrobials

In the last decades, a growing interest in using plant-based antimicrobials has been known a rise, and special attention was given to EOs. EOs are products obtained from aromatic plants by physical processes of distillation or pressing [92]. They contain volatile compounds stored in plant's specialized structures to offer protection against various insults, including pathogen (bacteria, fungi, viruses) attacks [93]. EOs are complex mixtures of small lipophilic molecules, of which one up to three compounds constitute the main phytochemical markers; still, other minor compounds contribute by phyto-synergic interactions to the overall bioactivity of EOs [94,95].

Isolation of EOs from plant matrices is classically achieved by hydrodistillation (steam or water distillation), but other methods, such as cold and hot expression, microwave-, ultrasonic-solvent free and supercritical fluid extraction, are also employed [96,97].

Generally, EOs constituents are regarded as safe (GRAS) by the FDA, a status that permitted the use of EOs as flavoring agents in food and as additives to cosmetics, perfumes, and cleaning products [94]. In addition, the combination of orange essential oil and trehalose was found to have a great impact on barrier protection against UV-vis radiation. This synergistic effect is potentially useful in using these films as protectants for food packaging and improvers of shelf life and food quality [98]. More, EOs possess a broad-spectrum of significant biological activities with applications in medical and pharmaceutical sectors, but also in agriculture as crop protectants [99–101]. Moreover, their potent and broad-spectrum antimicrobial effects have generated impressive reports in the scientific literature. Thus, several mechanisms of activity have been proposed for EOs and their constituents, including disruption of the phospholipid bilayer of cell membranes, inhibition of efflux pumps, impairment of metabolic pathways, inactivation of genetic material, and anti-quorum sensing effects [102–107]. Compared to antimicrobial drugs, EOs act concurrently towards different microbial targets due to their multicomponent nature, which constitutes an advantage in tackling microbial resistance [108]. In addition to their broad antimicrobial spectrum, EOs have antioxidant, immunomodulatory, anti-inflammatory, and wound healing effects, which highlight them as candidates for the clinical development of novel antimicrobial agents [102,109].

EOs constituents are extremely sensitive to oxygen, light, heat, and humidity. In addition, their low water solubility and bioavailability hamper the clinical use of EOs. Therefore, encapsulation has been widely used to overcome such limitations but also to ensure targeted delivery and to boost the antimicrobial efficacy of EOs [92,107,110,111].

Among the nanoformulated delivery systems, the ability of liposomes to entrap EOs is commonly reported in the literature [112–114].

This section is intended to shed light on the advantages of combining liposomes with the primary chitosan coating (chitosomes) as well as secondary coatings (alginate, hyaluronate, pectin) to overcome the drawbacks of conventional liposomal formulations (aggregations and fusion followed by leakage of their content during storage). Although the application of chitosomes for EOs encapsulation is still in its infancy, it deserves attention.

Considering the antimicrobial propensities of chitosan, such systems are promising tools for the increase of EOs antimicrobial efficacy. Chitosomes could allow targeted delivery of EOs, but also could avail their release, prolonging their bioactivity. They could also reduce the side effects of EOs upon local and systemic administration to humans.

Therefore, the elucidation of their mechanisms of activity and toxicity in biological systems could pave the way for their use in clinical antimicrobial chemotherapy. Moreover, these formulations might modify the sensory properties of foods and drinks and allow their application as preservatives in the food industry.

Still, EOs chemical composition must be well-characterized, and their encapsulation into chitosomes should focus on these particularities for the development of sound therapeutic approaches.

6. Conclusions

Chitosan has emerged as an important biomaterial for drug delivery. The characteristics of drug-loaded chitosomes and conventional liposomes were compared in this review. The addition of a chitosan layer on the liposome surface resulted in a liposomal size increase and inversion of Zeta potential from negative to positive values. Both size and Zeta potential increased as the chitosan concentration increased until reaching a saturated value. Chitosomes showed an acceptable degree of polydispersity and did not affect the liposome morphology. The chitosan or chitosan derivatives layer improved liposomes stability, even in GI fluid, as well as against severe physical stress during freeze-drying. The results of many studies suggested a sustained drug release from chitosomes, an enhanced mucoadhesivity and skin drug penetration compared to uncoated liposomes. Chitosomes enhanced drug bioavailability as well as their biological effect. The mechanisms controlling drug EE, vesicle stability and drug release in chitosomes depend on many factors, such as physicochemical drug characteristics, medium pH, chitosan MW and chitosan concentration that should be taken into consideration in chitosomal preparation. Chitosan should be added at a saturated concentration to ensure vesicle stability, where coacervates and bridging flocculation may occur, respectively, below this concentration and in the presence of excess chitosan concentration. Moreover, the primary amino groups of chitosan protonated at acidic pH electrostatically interacted with negatively charged phospholipids on the liposome surface, showing higher stability and lower drug release rate for various drugs used compared to those obtained at high pH values.

The addition of polyelectrolytes, such as alginate, sodium hyaluronate and pectin, could further enhance the efficacy of chitosomes due to the formation of a denser shell through the ionic interaction of the two polymers, keeping in mind the effect of the medium pH and polyanionic acid concentration on this interaction. Covering the surface of the liposome with chitosan could be, therefore, considered as a promising strategy to enlarge liposomal applications in areas such as hematology, immunology, pharmaceutics, drug delivery, food packaging and cosmetics.

Author Contributions: The writing-original draft preparation was done by the corresponding author C.S. The co-corresponding author A.T. has also contributed in writing and editing this review especially the part concerning the antimicrobials and essential oils. E.S. helped in editing this review. The conceptualization and the supervision of this review was done by H.G.-G. All authors have read and agreed to the published version of the manuscript.

Funding: This research received no external funding.

Acknowledgments: Authors would like to thank the Agence Universitaire de la Francophonie, Projet de Coopération Scientifique Inter-Universitaire (2018–2020) for supporting the project. This work was supported by a grant from the Romanian Ministry of Education and Research, CNCS-UEFISCDI, project number PN-III-P1-1.1-TE-2019-1894, within PNCDI III.

Conflicts of Interest: The authors declare no conflict of interest.

Abbreviations

AUC	area under curve
BSA	bovine serum albumin
Caco-2	human colorectal adenocarcinoma

CH-LP	chitosan-coated liposomes
CHO	cholesterol
Cmax	maximum plasma concentration
DCP	dicetylphosphate
DD	degree of deacetylation
DDAB	dimethyldioctadecyl-ammonium bromide
DHP	dihexadecylphosphate
DiI	1,1′-dioctadecyl-3,3,3′,3′-tetramethylindo carbocyanine perchlorate
DPPC	L-α-dipalmitoylphosphatidylcholine
DPPE-MCC	1,2-dipalmitoylsn-glycero-3-phosphoethanolamine-N-[4-(p maleimidomethyl) cyclohexane-carboxamide];
DSPC	distearoylphosphatidylcholine
EO	essential oil
EPC	egg phosphatidylcholine
FD-RH	freeze-drying followed by rehydration
GI	gastro-intestinal
H1F1-α; hypoxia inducible factor 1	
HMW	high molecular weight
DSPE	distearoylphosphatidylethanolamine
EE	encapsulation efficiency
EIM	ethanol injection method
EO	essential oil
EPC	egg phosphatidylcholine
FD-RH	freeze-drying followed by rehydration
GI	gastro-intestinal
H1F1-α; hypoxia inducible factor 1	
HCl	hydrogen chloride
HMW	high molecular weight
HPTMA	N-[(2-hydroxy-3-trimethylamine) propyl] chloride
HSPC	hydrogenated soy phosphatidylcholine
IC_{50}	half inhibitory concentration
ISCRPE	improved supercritical reverse-phase evaporation method
LMW	low molecular weight
MDA	malonaldehyde
MFGM	milk fat globule membrane
MTT	3-(4,5-dimethylthiazol-2-yl)-2,5-diphenyl tetrazolium bromide
MW	molecular weight
NR	not reported
PBS	phosphate-buffered saline
PC	phosphatidylcholine
pdI	polydispersity index
PDS	polyelectrolyte delivery system
PEG	polyethylene glycol
PG	phosphatidylglycerol
PS	phosphatidylserine
Ref	references
REV	reverse phase evaporation
SA	stearylamine
SDC	sodium deoxycholate
SGF	simulated gastric fluid
SIF	simulated intestinal fluid
SPC	soy phosphatidylcholine
TFH	thin film hydration
UN-LP	uncoated liposomes
VEGF	vascular endothelial growth factor

References

1. Anwekar, H.; Patel, S.; Singhai, A.K. Liposome as drug carriers. *Int. J. Pharm. Life Sci.* **2011**, *2*, 945–951.
2. Barba, A.A.; Bochicchio, S.; Bertoncin, P.; Lamberti, G.; Dalmoro, A. Coating of Nanolipid Structures by a Novel Simil-Microfluidic Technique: Experimental and Theoretical Approaches. *Coatings* **2019**, *9*, 491. [CrossRef]
3. Laye, C.; McClements, D.J.; Weiss, J. Formation of Biopolymer-Coated Liposomes by Electrostatic Deposition of Chitosan. *J. Food Sci.* **2008**, *73*, N7–N15. [CrossRef]
4. Vural, I.; Sarisozen, C.; Olmez, S.S. Chitosan coated furosemide liposomes for improved bioavailability. *J. Biomed. Nanotechnol.* **2011**, *7*, 426–430. [CrossRef]
5. Nguyen, T.X.; Huang, L.; Liu, L.; Abdalla, A.M.E.; Gauthier, M.; Yang, G. Chitosan-coated nano-liposomes for the oral delivery of berberine hydrochloride. *J. Mater. Chem. B* **2014**, *2*, 7149–7159. [CrossRef] [PubMed]
6. Sercombe, L.; Veerati, T.; Moheimani, F.; Wu, S.Y.; Sood, A.K.; Hua, S. Advances and Challenges of Liposome Assisted Drug Delivery. *Front. Pharmacol.* **2015**, *6*, 286. [CrossRef]
7. Immordino, M.L.; Dosio, F.; Cattel, L. Stealth liposomes: Review of the basic science, rationale, and clinical applications, existing and potential. *Int. J. Nanomed.* **2006**, *1*, 297–315.
8. Trucillo, P.; Reverchon, E. Production of PEG-coated liposomes using a continuous supercritical assisted process. *J. Supercrit. Fluids* **2021**, *167*, 105048. [CrossRef]
9. Patel, J. Liposomal doxorubicin: Doxil®. *J. Oncol. Pharm. Pr.* **1996**, *2*, 201–210. [CrossRef]
10. Dash, M.; Chiellini, F.; Ottenbrite, R.M.; Chiellini, E. Chitosan—A versatile semi-synthetic polymer in biomedical applications. *Prog. Polym. Sci.* **2011**, *36*, 981–1014. [CrossRef]
11. Wang, Q.Z.; Chen, X.G.; Liu, N.; Wang, S.X.; Liu, C.S.; Meng, X.H.; Liu, C.G. Protonation constants of chitosan with different molecular weight and degree of deacetylation. *Carbohydr. Polym.* **2006**, *65*, 194–201. [CrossRef]
12. Li, N.; Zhuang, C.; Wang, M.; Sun, X.; Nie, S.; Pan, W. Liposome coated with low molecular weight chitosan and its potential use in ocular drug delivery. *Int. J. Pharm.* **2009**, *379*, 131–138. [CrossRef] [PubMed]
13. Rinaudo, M. Chitin and chitosan: Properties and applications. *Progr. Polym. Sci.* **2006**, *31*, 603–632. [CrossRef]
14. Roy, J.; Salaün, F.; Giraud, S.; Ferri, A. Solubility of chitin: Solvents, solution behaviors and their related mechanisms. In *Solubility of Polysaccharides*; IntechOpen: London, UK, 2017. [CrossRef]
15. Filipović-Grcić, J.; Skalko-Basnet, N.; Jalsenjak, I. Mucoadhesive chitosan-coated liposomes: Characteristics and stability. *J. Microencapsul.* **2001**, *18*, 3–12. [CrossRef] [PubMed]
16. Muzzarelli, R.A. Human enzymatic activities related to the therapeutic administration of chitin derivatives. *Cell. Mol. Life Sci.* **1997**, *53*, 131–140. [CrossRef] [PubMed]
17. Joraholmen, M.W.; Vanic, Z.; Tho, I.; Skalko-Basnet, N. Chitosan-coated liposomes for topical vaginal therapy: Assuring 2 localized drug effect. *Int. J. Pharm.* **2014**, *472*, 94–101. [CrossRef] [PubMed]
18. Ngo, D.H.; Kim, S.K. Antioxidant effects of chitin, chitosan, and their derivatives. *Adv. Food. Nutr. Res.* **2014**, *73*, 15–31. [CrossRef] [PubMed]
19. Kong, M.; Chen, X.G.; Xing, K.; Park, H.J. Antimicrobial properties of chitosan and mode of action: A state of the art review. *Int. J. Food Microbiol.* **2010**, *144*, 51–63. [CrossRef]
20. Dai, T.; Tanaka, M.; Huang, Y.-Y.; Hamblin, M.R. Chitosan preparations for wounds and burns: Antimicrobial and wound-healing effects. *Expert Rev. Anti Infect. Ther.* **2011**, *9*, 857–879. [CrossRef]
21. Raftery, R.; O'Brien, F.J.; Cryan, S.-A. Chitosan for Gene Delivery and Orthopedic Tissue Engineering Applications. *Molecules* **2013**, *18*, 5611–5647. [CrossRef]
22. Wang, H.; Zhao, P.; Liang, X.; Gong, X.; Song, T.; Niu, R.; Chang, J. Folate-PEG coated cationic modified chitosan—Cholesterol liposomes for tumor-targeted drug delivery. *Biomaterials* **2010**, *31*, 4129–4138. [CrossRef]
23. Yan, L.; Crayton, S.H.; Thawani, J.P.; Amirshaghaghi, A.; Tsourkas, A.; Cheng, Z. A pH-Responsive Drug-Delivery Platform Based on Glycol Chitosan-Coated Liposomes. *Small* **2015**, *11*, 4870–4874. [CrossRef]
24. Kowapradit, J.; Opanasopit, P.; Ngawhirunpat, T.; Apirakaramwong, A.; Rojanarata, T.; Ruktanonchai, U.; Sajomsang, W. Methylated N-(4-N,N-Dimethylaminobenzyl) Chitosan, a Novel Chitosan Derivative, Enhances Paracellular Permeability Across Intestinal Epithelial Cells (Caco-2). *AAPS PharmSciTech* **2008**, *9*, 1143–1152. [CrossRef] [PubMed]
25. Kowapradit, J.; Apirakaramwong, A.; Ngawhirunpat, T.; Rojanarata, T.; Sajomsang, W.; Opanasopit, P. Methylated N-(4-N,N-dimethylaminobenzyl) chitosan coated liposomes for oral protein drug delivery. *Eur. J. Pharm. Sci.* **2012**, *47*, 359–366. [CrossRef]
26. Karewicz, A.; Bielska, D.; Loboda, A.; Gzyl-Malcher, B.; Bednar, J.; Jozkowicz, A.; Dulak, J.; Nowakowska, M. Curcumin-containing liposomes stabilized by thin layers of chitosan derivatives. *Colloids Surf. B Biointerfaces* **2013**, *109*, 307–316. [CrossRef] [PubMed]
27. Chen, H.; Wu, J.; Sun, M.; Guo, C.; Yu, A.; Cao, F.; Zhao, L.; Tan, Q.; Zhai, G. N-trimethyl chitosan chloride-coated liposomes for the oral delivery of curcumin. *J. Liposome Res.* **2012**, *22*, 100–109. [CrossRef] [PubMed]
28. Zhang, J.; Wang, S. Topical use of Coenzyme Q10-loaded liposomes coated with trimethyl chitosan: Tolerance, precorneal retention and anti-cataract effect. *Int. J. Pharm.* **2009**, *372*, 66–75. [CrossRef] [PubMed]

29. Kozhikhova, K.V.; Ivantsova, M.N.; Tokareva, M.I.; Shulepov, I.D.; Tretiyakov, A.V.; Shaidarov, L.V.; Rusinov, V.L.; Mironov, M.A. Preparation of chitosan-coated liposomes as a novel carrier system for the antiviral drug Triazavirin. *Pharm. Dev. Technol.* **2018**, *23*, 334–342. [CrossRef]
30. Gradauer, K.; Barthelmes, J.; Vonach, C.; Almer, G.; Mangge, H.; Teubl, B.; Roblegg, E.; Dünnhaupt, S.; Fröhlich, E.; Bernkop-Schnürch, A.; et al. Liposomes coated with thiolated chitosan enhance oral peptide delivery to rats. *J. Control. Release* **2013**, *172*, 872–878. [CrossRef]
31. Bozzuto, G.; Molinari, A. Liposomes as nanomedical devices. *Int. J. Nanomed.* **2015**, *10*, 975–999. [CrossRef]
32. Zaru, M.; Manca, M.L.; Fadda, A.M.; Antimisiaris, S.G. Chitosan-coated liposomes for delivery to lungs by nebulization. *Colloids Surf. B. Biointerfaces* **2009**, *71*, 88–95. [CrossRef] [PubMed]
33. Lee, C.M.; Kim, D.W.; Lee, K.Y. Effects of chitosan coating for liposomes as an oral carrier. *J. Biomed. Sci.* **2011**, *17*, 211–216.
34. Mengoni, T.; Adrian, M.; Pereira, S.; Santos-Carballal, B.; Kaiser, M.; Goycoolea, F.M. A Chitosan—Based Liposome Formulation Enhances the In Vitro Wound Healing Efficacy of Substance P Neuropeptide. *Pharmaceutics* **2017**, *9*, 56. [CrossRef]
35. Zhuang, J.; Ping, Q.; Song, Y.; Qi, J.; Cui, Z. Effects of chitosan coating on physical properties and pharmacokinetic behavior of mitoxantrone liposomes. *Int. J. Nanomed.* **2010**, *5*, 407–416. [CrossRef]
36. Van Vuuren, S.F.; Du Toit, L.C.; Parry, A.; Pillay, V.; Choonara, Y.E. Encapsulation of Essential Oils within a Polymeric Liposomal Formulation for Enhancement of Antimicrobial Efficacy. *Nat. Prod. Commun.* **2010**, *5*, 1401–1408. [CrossRef] [PubMed]
37. Abdelbary, G. Ocular ciprofloxacin hydrochloride mucoadhesive chitosan-coated liposomes. *Pharm. Dev. Technol.* **2009**, *16*, 44–56. [CrossRef]
38. Wu, Z.-H.; Ping, Q.-N.; Wei, Y.; Lai, J.-M. Hypoglycemic efficacy of chitosan-coated insulin liposomes after oral administration in mice. *Acta Pharmacol. Sin.* **2004**, *25*, 966–972.
39. Channarong, S.; Chaicumpa, W.; Sinchaipanid, N.; Mitrevej, A. Development and Evaluation of Chitosan-Coated Liposomes for Oral DNA Vaccine: The Improvement of Peyer's Patch Targeting Using a Polyplex-Loaded Liposomes. *AAPS PharmSciTec.* **2010**, *12*, 192–200. [CrossRef]
40. Guo, J.; Ping, Q.; Jiang, G.; Huang, L.; Tong, Y. Chitosan-coated liposomes: Characterization and interaction with leuprolide. *Int. J. Pharm.* **2003**, *260*, 167–173. [CrossRef]
41. Liu, N.; Park, H.-J. Factors effect on the loading efficiency of Vitamin C loaded chitosan-coated nanoliposomes. *Colloids Surf. B Biointerfaces* **2010**, *76*, 16–19. [CrossRef]
42. Park, S.N.; Jo, N.R.; Jeon, S.H. Chitosan-coated liposomes for enhanced skin permeation of resveratrol. *J. Ind. Eng. Chem.* **2014**, *20*, 1481–1485. [CrossRef]
43. Shin, G.H.; Chung, S.K.; Kim, J.T.; Joung, H.J.; Park, H.J. Preparation of Chitosan-Coated Nanoliposomes for Improving the Mucoadhesive Property of Curcumin Using the Ethanol Injection Method. *J. Agric. Food Chem.* **2013**, *61*, 11119–11126. [CrossRef] [PubMed]
44. Tan, C.; Feng, B.; Zhang, X.; Xia, W.; Xia, S. Biopolymer-coated liposomes by electrostatic adsorption of chitosan (chitosomes) as novel delivery systems for carotenoids. *Food Hydrocoll.* **2016**, *52*, 774–784. [CrossRef]
45. Tan, H.W.; Misran, M. Characterization of fatty acid liposome coated with low-molecular-weight chitosan. *J. Liposome Res.* **2012**, *22*, 329–335. [CrossRef]
46. Venturini, M.; Mazzitelli, S.; Mičetić, I.; Benini, C.; Fabri, J.; Mucelli, S.P.; Benetti, F.; Nastruzzi, C. Analysis of Operating Conditions Influencing the Morphology and In vitro Behaviour of Chitosan Coated Liposomes. *J. Nanomed. Nanotechnol.* **2014**, *5*, 1–8. [CrossRef]
47. Wang, Y.; Tu, S.; Li, R.; Yang, X.; Liu, L.; Zhang, Q. Cholesterol succinyl chitosan anchored liposomes: Preparation, characterization, physical stability, and drug release behavior. *Nanomed. Nanotechnol. Biol. Med.* **2010**, *6*, 471–477. [CrossRef]
48. Li, L.; Zhang, Y.; Han, S.; Qu, Z.; Zhao, J.; Chen, Y.; Chen, Z.; Duan, J.; Pan, Y.; Tang, X. Penetration enhancement of lidocaine hydrochlorid by a novel chitosan coated elastic liposome for transdermal drug delivery. *J. Biomed. Nanotechnol.* **2011**, *7*, 704–713. [CrossRef] [PubMed]
49. Li, Z.; Paulson, A.T.; Gill, T.A. Encapsulation of bioactive salmon protein hydrolysates with chitosan-coated liposomes. *J. Funct. Foods* **2015**, *19*, 733–743. [CrossRef]
50. Diebold, Y.; Jarrín, M.; Sáez, V.; Carvalho, E.L.S.; Orea, M.; Calonge, M.; Seijo, B.; Alonso, M.J. Ocular drug delivery by liposome–chitosan nanoparticle complexes (LCS-NP). *Biomaterials* **2007**, *28*, 1553–1564. [CrossRef] [PubMed]
51. Mady, M.M.; Darwish, M.M.; Khalil, S.; Khalil, W.M. Biophysical studies on chitosan-coated liposomes. *Eur. Biophys. J.* **2009**, *38*, 1127–1133. [CrossRef] [PubMed]
52. Mady, M.M.; Darwish, M.M. Effect of chitosan coating on the characteristics of DPPC liposomes. *J. Adv. Res.* **2010**, *1*, 187–191. [CrossRef]
53. Wang, W.-X.; Gao, J.-Q.; Liang, W.-Q. Chitosan-coated liposomes for intracellular oligonucleotides delivery: Characteristics and cell uptake behavior. *Drug Deliv.* **2010**, *18*, 208–214. [CrossRef] [PubMed]
54. Thongborisute, J.; Tsuruta, A.; Kawabata, Y.; Takeuchi, H. The effect of particle structure of chitosan-coated liposomes and type of chitosan on oral delivery of calcitonin. *J. Drug Target.* **2006**, *14*, 147–154. [CrossRef] [PubMed]
55. Alshraim, M.O.; Sangi, S.; Harisa, G.I.; Alomrani, A.H.; Yusuf, O.; Badran, M.M. Chitosan-Coated Flexible Liposomes Magnify the Anticancer Activity and Bioavailability of Docetaxel: Impact on Composition. *Molecules* **2019**, *24*, 250. [CrossRef] [PubMed]

56. Yang, Z.; Liu, J.; Gao, J.; Chen, S.; Huang, G. Chitosan coated vancomycin hydrochloride liposomes: Characterizations and evaluation. *Int. J. Pharm.* **2015**, *495*, 508–515. [CrossRef] [PubMed]
57. Behera, T.; Swain, P.; Sahoo, S. Antigen in chitosan coated liposomes enhances immune responses through parenteral immunization. *Int. Immunopharmacol.* **2011**, *11*, 907–914. [CrossRef]
58. Ben, M.S.; Marina, K.; Mukund, G.S. Eudragit S-100 Encapsulated Chitosan Coated Liposomes Containing Prednisolone for Colon Targeting: In vitro, Ex vivo and In vivo Evaluation. *J. Young Pharm.* **2019**, *11*, 7–11. [CrossRef]
59. Chen, D.; Xia, D.; Li, X.; Zhu, Q.; Yu, H.; Zhu, C.; Gan, Y. Comparative study of Pluronic® F127-modified liposomes and chitosan-modified liposomes for mucus penetration and oral absorption of cyclosporine A in rats. *Int. J. Pharm.* **2013**, *449*, 1–9. [CrossRef]
60. Alshamsan, A.; Aleanizy, F.S.; Badran, M.; Alqahtani, F.Y.; Alfassam, H.; Almalik, A.; Alosaimy, S. Exploring anti-MRSA activity of chitosan-coated liposomal dicloxacillin. *J. Microbiol. Methods* **2019**, *156*, 23–28. [CrossRef]
61. Chen, H.; Pan, H.; Li, P.; Wang, H.; Wang, X.; Pan, W.; Yuan, Y. The potential use of novel chitosan-coated deformable liposomes in an ocular drug delivery system. *Colloids Surf. B Biointerfaces* **2016**, *143*, 455–462. [CrossRef]
62. Gibis, M.; Ruedt, C.; Weiss, J. In vitro release of grape-seed polyphenols encapsulated from uncoated and chitosan-coated liposomes. *Food Res. Int.* **2016**, *88*, 105–113. [CrossRef]
63. Karn, P.R.; Vanić, Z.; Pepić, I.; Škalko-Basnet, N. Mucoadhesive liposomal delivery systems: The choice of coating material. *Drug Dev. Ind. Pharm.* **2010**, *37*, 482–488. [CrossRef] [PubMed]
64. Liu, W.; Liu, W.; Ye, A.; Peng, S.; Wei, F.; Liu, C.; Han, J. Environmental stress stability of microencapsules based on liposomes decorated with chitosan and sodium alginate. *Food Chem.* **2016**, *196*, 396–404. [CrossRef] [PubMed]
65. Gültekin-Özgüven, M.; Karadağ, A.; Duman, S.; Özkal, B.; Özçelik, B. Fortification of dark chocolate with spray dried black mulberry (Morus nigra) waste extract encapsulated in chitosan-coated liposomes and bioaccessability studies. *Food Chem.* **2016**, *201*, 205–212. [CrossRef] [PubMed]
66. Liu, Y.; Liu, D.; Zhu, L.; Gan, Q.; Le, X. Temperature-dependent structure stability and in vitro release of chitosan-coated curcumin liposome. *Food Res. Int.* **2015**, *74*, 97–105. [CrossRef]
67. Cuomo, F.; Cofelice, M.; Venditti, F.; Ceglie, A.; Miguel, M.; Lindman, B.; Lopez, F. In-vitro digestion of curcumin loaded chitosan-coated liposomes. *Colloids Surf. B Biointerfaces* **2018**, *168*, 29–34. [CrossRef]
68. Gibis, M.; Rahn, N.; Weiss, J. Physical and Oxidative Stability of Uncoated and Chitosan-Coated Liposomes Containing Grape Seed Extract. *Pharmaceutics* **2013**, *5*, 421–433. [CrossRef] [PubMed]
69. Panya, A.; Laguerre, M.; LeComte, J.; Villeneuve, P.; Weiss, J.; McClements, D.J.; Decker, E.A. Effects of Chitosan and Rosmarinate Esters on the Physical and Oxidative Stability of Liposomes. *J. Agric. Food Chem.* **2010**, *58*, 5679–5684. [CrossRef]
70. Liu, N.; Park, H.-J. Chitosan-coated nanoliposome as vitamin E carrier. *J. Microencapsul.* **2009**, *26*, 235–242. [CrossRef]
71. Cui, H.Y.; Wu, J.; Li, C.Z.; Lin, L. Anti-listeria effects of chitosan-coated nisin-silica liposome on Cheddar cheese. *J. Dairy Sci.* **2016**, *99*, 8598–8606. [CrossRef] [PubMed]
72. Quagliariello, V.; Masarone, M.; Armenia, E.; Giudice, A.; Barbarisi, M.; Caraglia, M.; Barbarisi, A.; Persico, M. Chitosan-coated liposomes loaded with butyric acid demonstrate anticancer and anti-inflammatory activity in human hepatoma HepG2 cells. *Oncol. Rep.* **2019**, *41*, 1476–1486. [CrossRef] [PubMed]
73. Qiang, F.; Shin, H.-J.; Lee, B.-J.; Han, H.-K. Enhanced systemic exposure of fexofenadine via the intranasal administration of chitosan-coated liposome. *Int. J. Pharm.* **2012**, *430*, 161–166. [CrossRef] [PubMed]
74. Chen, M.-X.; Li, B.-K.; Yin, D.-K.; Liang, J.; Li, S.-S.; Peng, D.-Y. Layer-by-layer assembly of chitosan stabilized multilayered liposomes for paclitaxel delivery. *Carbohydr. Polym.* **2014**, *111*, 298–304. [CrossRef] [PubMed]
75. Salva, E.; Turan, S.O.; Eren, F.; Akbuğa, J. The enhancement of gene silencing efficiency with chitosan-coated liposome formulations of siRNAs targeting HIF-1α and VEGF. *Int. J. Pharm.* **2015**, *478*, 147–154. [CrossRef]
76. Otake, K.; Shimomura, T.; Goto, T.; Imura, T.; Furuya, T.; Yoda, S.; Takebayashi, Y.; Sakai, H.; Abe, M. One-Step Preparation of Chitosan-Coated Cationic Liposomes by an Improved Supercritical Reverse-Phase Evaporation Method. *Langmuir* **2006**, *22*, 4054–4059. [CrossRef]
77. Mozuraityte, R.; Rustad, T.; Storrø, I. The Role of Iron in Peroxidation of Polyunsaturated Fatty Acids in Liposomes. *J. Agric. Food Chem.* **2008**, *56*, 537–543. [CrossRef]
78. Lin, L.; Gu, Y.; Sun, Y.; Cui, H. Characterization of chrysanthemum essential oil triple-layer liposomes and its application against Campylobacter jejuni on chicken. *LWT* **2019**, *107*, 16–24. [CrossRef]
79. Li, N.; Zhuang, C.-Y.; Wang, M.; Sui, C.-G.; Pan, W.-S. Low molecular weight chitosan-coated liposomes for ocular drug delivery: In vitro and in vivo studies. *Drug Deliv.* **2012**, *19*, 28–35. [CrossRef]
80. Jeon, S.; Yoo, C.Y.; Park, S.N. Improved stability and skin permeability of sodium hyaluronate-chitosan multilayered liposomes by Layer-by-Layer electrostatic deposition for quercetin delivery. *Colloids Surf. B Biointerfaces* **2015**, *129*, 7–14. [CrossRef]
81. Takeuchi, H.; Matsui, Y.; Yamamoto, H.; Kawashima, Y. Mucoadhesive properties of carbopol or chitosan-coated liposomes and their effectiveness in the oral administration of calcitonin to rats. *J. Control. Release* **2003**, *86*, 235–242. [CrossRef]
82. Takeuchi, H.; Matsui, Y.; Sugihara, H.; Yamamoto, H.; Kawashima, Y. Effectiveness of submicron-sized, chitosan-coated liposomes in oral administration of peptide drugs. *Int. J. Pharm.* **2005**, *303*, 160–170. [CrossRef] [PubMed]
83. Jøraholmen, M.W.; Bhargava, A.; Julin, K.; Johannessen, M.; Škalko-Basnet, N. The Antimicrobial Properties of Chitosan Can Be Tailored by Formulation. *Mar. Drugs* **2020**, *18*, 96. [CrossRef] [PubMed]

84. Andersen, T.; Mishchenko, E.; Flaten, G.E.; Sollid, J.U.E.; Mattsson, S.; Tho, I.; Škalko-Basnet, N. Chitosan-Based Nanomedicine to Fight Genital Candida Infections: Chitosomes. *Mar. Drugs* **2017**, *15*, 64. [CrossRef] [PubMed]
85. Niaz, T.; Shabbir, S.; Noor, T.; Rahman, A.; Bokhari, H.; Imran, M. Potential of polymer stabilized nano-liposomes to enhance antimicrobial activity of nisin Z against foodborne pathogens. *LWT* **2018**, *96*, 98–110. [CrossRef]
86. Serra, L.; Doménech, J.; Peppas, N. Engineering design and molecular dynamics of mucoadhesive drug delivery systems as targeting agents. *Eur. J. Pharm. Biopharm.* **2009**, *71*, 519–528. [CrossRef]
87. Dünnhaupt, S.; Barthelmes, J.; Thurner, C.C.; Waldner, C.; Sakloetsakun, D.; Bernkop-Schnürch, A. S-protected thiolated chitosan: Synthesis and in vitro characterization. *Carbohydr. Polym.* **2012**, *90*, 765–772. [CrossRef]
88. Sugihara, H.; Yamamoto, H.; Kawashima, Y.; Takeuchi, H. Effects of food intake on the mucoadhesive and gastroretentive properties of submicron-sized chitosan-coated liposomes. *Chem. Pharm. Bull.* **2012**, *60*, 1320–1323. [CrossRef]
89. Haidar, Z.S.; Hamdy, R.C.; Tabrizian, M. Protein release kinetics for core-shell hybrid nanoparticles based on the layer-by-layer assembly of alginate and chitosan on liposomes. *Biomaterials* **2008**, *29*, 1207–1215. [CrossRef]
90. Liu, W.; Liu, J.; Liu, W.; Li, T.; Liu, C. Improved Physical and in Vitro Digestion Stability of a Polyelectrolyte Delivery System Based on Layer-by-Layer Self-Assembly Alginate–Chitosan-Coated Nanoliposomes. *J. Agric. Food Chem.* **2013**, *61*, 4133–4144. [CrossRef]
91. Gibis, M.; Zeeb, B.; Weiss, J. Formation, characterization, and stability of encapsulated hibiscus extract in multilayered liposomes. *Food Hydrocoll.* **2014**, *38*, 28–39. [CrossRef]
92. Dajic Stevanovic, Z.; Sieniawska, E.; Glowniak, K.; Obradovic, N.; Pajic-Lijakovic, I. Natural Macromolecules as Carriers for Essential Oils: From Extraction to Biomedical Application. *Front. Bioeng. Biotechnol.* **2020**, *8*, 563. [CrossRef] [PubMed]
93. Bakkali, F.; Averbeck, S.; Averbeck, D.; Idaomar, M. Biological effects of essential oils—A review. *Food Chem. Toxicol.* **2008**, *46*, 446–475. [CrossRef] [PubMed]
94. Swamy, M.K.; Akhtar, M.S.; Sinniah, U.R. Antimicrobial Properties of Plant Essential Oils against Human Pathogens and Their Mode of Action: An Updated Review. *Evid. Based Complement. Altern. Med.* **2016**, *2016*, 1–21. [CrossRef] [PubMed]
95. Dilworth, L.L.; Riley, C.K.; Stennett, D.K. Plant Constituents: Carbohydrates, Oils, Resins, Balsams, and Plant Hormones. In *Pharmacognosy. Fundamentals, Applications and Strategy*; Badal, S., Delgoda, R., Eds.; Academic Press: London, UK, 2017; pp. 61–80.
96. Schmidt, E. Production of Essential Oils. In *Handbook of Essential Oils: Science, Technology, and Applications*; Can Baser, K.H., Buchbauer, G., Eds.; CRC Press: Boca Raton, FL, USA, 2010; pp. 83–120.
97. Bucar, F.; Wube, A.; Schmid, M. Natural product isolation: How to get from biological material to pure compounds. *Nat. Prod. Rep.* **2013**, *30*, 525–545. [CrossRef]
98. Simona, J.; Dani, D.; Petr, S.; Marcela, N.; Jakub, T.; Bohuslava, T. Edible Films from Carrageenan/Orange Essential Oil/Trehalose—Structure, Optical Properties, and Antimicrobial Activity. *Polymers* **2021**, *13*, 332. [CrossRef] [PubMed]
99. Hyldgaard, M.; Mygind, T.; Meyer, R.L. Essential Oils in Food Preservation: Mode of Action, Synergies, and Interactions with Food Matrix Components. *Front. Microbiol.* **2012**, *3*, 12. [CrossRef] [PubMed]
100. Raut, J.S.; Karuppayil, S.M. A status review on the medicinal properties of essential oils. *Ind. Crop. Prod.* **2014**, *62*, 250–264. [CrossRef]
101. Sarkic, A.; Stappen, I. Essential Oils and Their Single Compounds in Cosmetics—A Critical Review. *Cosmetics* **2018**, *5*, 11. [CrossRef]
102. Hammer, K.A.; Carson, C.F. Antibacterial and antifungal activities of essential oils. In *Lipids and Essential Oils as Antimicrobial Agents*; Thormar, H., Ed.; John Wiley & Sons, Ltd.: Chichester, UK, 2011; pp. 255–295.
103. Bassolé, I.H.N.; Juliani, H.R. Essential Oils in Combination and Their Antimicrobial Properties. *Molecules* **2012**, *17*, 3989–4006. [CrossRef] [PubMed]
104. Nazzaro, F.; Fratianni, F.; De Martino, L.; Coppola, R.; De Feo, V. Effect of Essential Oils on Pathogenic Bacteria. *Pharmaceuticals* **2013**, *6*, 1451–1474. [CrossRef] [PubMed]
105. Langeveld, W.T.; Veldhuizen, E.J.A.; Burt, S.A. Synergy between essential oil components and antibiotics: A review. *Crit. Rev. Microbiol.* **2014**, *40*, 76–94. [CrossRef] [PubMed]
106. Tariq, S.; Wani, S.; Rasool, W.; Shafi, K.; Bhat, M.A.; Prabhakar, A.; Shalla, A.H.; Rather, M.A. A comprehensive review of the antibacterial, antifungal and antiviral potential of essential oils and their chemical constituents against drug-resistant microbial pathogens. *Microb. Pathog.* **2019**, *134*, 103580. [CrossRef]
107. Trifan, A.; Luca, S.V.; Greige-Gerges, H.; Miron, A.; Gille, E.; Aprotosoaie, A.C. Recent advances in tackling microbial multidrug resistance with essential oils: Combinatorial and nano-based strategies. *Crit. Rev. Microbiol.* **2020**, *46*, 1–20. [CrossRef] [PubMed]
108. Kon, K.V.; Rai, M.K. Plant essential oils and their constituents in coping with multidrug-resistant bacteria. *Expert Rev. Anti Infect. Ther.* **2012**, *10*, 775–790. [CrossRef] [PubMed]
109. Subramani, R.; Narayanasamy, M.; Feussner, K.-D. Plant-derived antimicrobials to fight against multi-drug-resistant human pathogens. *3 Biotech* **2017**, *7*, 172. [CrossRef]
110. Kfoury, M.; Auezova, L.; Greige-Gerges, H.; Fourmentin, S. Promising applications of cyclodextrins in food: Improvement of essential oils retention, controlled release and antiradical activity. *Carbohydr. Polym.* **2015**, *131*, 264–272. [CrossRef]
111. Doost, A.S.; Nasrabadi, M.N.; Kassozi, V.; Nakisozi, H.; Van Der Meeren, P. Recent advances in food colloidal delivery systems for essential oils and their main components. *Trends Food Sci. Technol.* **2020**, *99*, 474–486. [CrossRef]

112. Sherry, M.; Charcosset, C.; Fessi, H.; Greige-Gerges, H. Essential oils encapsulated in liposomes: A review. *J. Liposome Res.* **2013**, *23*, 268–275. [CrossRef] [PubMed]
113. Majeed, H.; Bian, Y.-Y.; Ali, B.; Jamil, A.; Majeed, U.; Khan, Q.F.; Iqbal, K.J.; Shoemaker, C.F.; Fang, Z. Essential oil encapsulations: Uses, procedures, and trends. *RSC Adv.* **2015**, *5*, 58449–58463. [CrossRef]
114. Ahmad, R.; Srivastava, S.; Ghosh, S.; Khare, S.K. Phytochemical delivery through nanocarriers: A review. *Colloids Surf. B Biointerfaces* **2021**, *197*, 111389. [CrossRef]

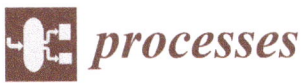

Review

Contribution of Essential Oils to the Fight against Microbial Biofilms—A Review

Diana Camelia Nuță [1,*], Carmen Limban [1], Cornel Chiriță [2], Mariana Carmen Chifiriuc [3], Teodora Costea [4], Petre Ioniță [5], Ioana Nicolau [5] and Irina Zarafu [5]

1. Department of Pharmaceutical Chemistry, Faculty of Pharmacy, "Carol Davila" University of Medicine and Pharmacy, TraianVuia no.6, 020956 Bucharest, Romania; carmen.limban@umfcd.ro
2. Department of Pharmacology and Clinical Pharmacy, Faculty of Pharmacy, "Carol Davila" University of Medicine and Pharmacy, TraianVuia no.6, 020956 Bucharest, Romania; cornel.chirita@umfcd.ro
3. Department of Microbiology, Faculty of Biology, Universtity of Bucharest, AleeaPortocalelor no.1-3, 060101 Bucharest, Romania; carmen_balotescu@yahoo.com
4. Department of Pharmacognosy, Phytochemistry, Phytotherapy, Faculty of Pharmacy, "Carol Davila" University of Medicine and Pharmacy, TraianVuia no.6, 020956 Bucharest, Romania; teodora.costea@umfcd.ro
5. Department of Organic Chemistry, Biochemistry and Catalysis, Faculty of Chemistry, University of Bucharest, Regina Elisabeta no.4-12, 030018 Bucharest, Romania; petre.ionita@chimie.unibuc.ro (P.I.); ioana.nicolau@chimie.unibuc.ro (I.N.); irina.zarafu@chimie.unibuc.ro (I.Z.)
* Correspondence: diana.nuta@umfcd.ro

Abstract: The increasing clinical use of artificial medical devices raises the issue of microbial contamination, which is a risk factor for the occurrence of biofilm-associated infections. A huge amount of scientific data highlights the promising potential of essential oils (EOs) to be used for the development of novel antibiofilm strategies. We aimed to review the relevant literature indexed in PubMed and Embase and to identify the recent directions in the field of EOs, as a new modality to eradicate microbial biofilms. We paid special attention to studies that explain the mechanisms of the microbicidal and antibiofilm activity of EOs, as well as their synergism with other antimicrobials. The EOs are difficult to test for their antimicrobial activity due to lipophilicity and volatility, so we have presented recent methods that facilitate these tests. There are presented the applications of EOs in chronic wounds and biofilm-mediated infection treatment, in the food industry and as air disinfectants. This analysis concludes that EOs are a source of antimicrobial agents that should not be neglected and that will probably provide new anti-infective therapeutic agents.

Keywords: essential oils; bacterial biofilm; antimicrobial; medical devices

Citation: Nuță, D.C.; Limban, C.; Chiriță, C.; Chifiriuc, M.C.; Costea, T.; Ioniță, P.; Nicolau, I.; Zarafu, I. Contribution of Essential Oils to the Fight against Microbial Biofilms—A Review. *Processes* **2021**, *9*, 537. https://doi.org/10.3390/pr9030537

Academic Editors: Elwira Sieniawska, Greige-Gerges Helene and Adriana Trifan

Received: 12 February 2021
Accepted: 15 March 2021
Published: 18 March 2021

Publisher's Note: MDPI stays neutral with regard to jurisdictional claims in published maps and institutional affiliations.

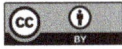

Copyright: © 2021 by the authors. Licensee MDPI, Basel, Switzerland. This article is an open access article distributed under the terms and conditions of the Creative Commons Attribution (CC BY) license (https://creativecommons.org/licenses/by/4.0/).

1. Introduction

In the past decade, essential oils (EOs) use for the prophylaxis and therapy of biofilm-associated infections (BAIs) have become very popular. The universally accepted definition of a biofilm refers to a sessile multicellular community of microbial cells with a modified transcriptome and phenotype (exhibiting increased resistance to both therapeutic doses of current antimicrobials and immune effectors) that adhere to a surface and, among them, being protected by an auto-secreted extracellular polymeric matrix [1,2]. It is considered that BAIs represent up to 85% of the total microbial infections, occurring after microbial colonization of either viable tissues or medical devices and having serious consequences [3], because they are persistent and hard or impossible to treat, even in immunocompetent individuals.

On the other hand, the food manufacturing industry is facing the formation of microbial biofilms that can affect industrial processes, and researchers are in constant search of new ways to eradicate this phenomenon. The protective mechanisms of microbial cells within biofilms are multifactorial and differ from those that occurred in planktonic cells and include matrix impermeability, modified transcription rate, selection of persister cells, accumulation of antibiotic inactivating enzymes, increased horizontal transfer rate of resistance genes, etc. [4]. Therefore, biofilm cells can become up to100–1000 times more resistant to antimicrobial substances than planktonic cells [5]. This high phenotypic resistance, also called tolerance, interferes not only with the BAI treatment but also with the efficacy of surface disinfection processes [6,7]. The discovery of natural products with antimicrobial activity represents a direction of current research trying to limit microbial diseases.

Therefore, the purpose of this paper was to review the recent literature on EOs antibiofilm activities.

2. Methods

For this purpose, the PubMed (National Library of Medicine, Washington, DC) and Embase (Elsevier) databases were searched for all relevant articles written in English, using the following keywords: "essential oils", and "biofilm", and then "dentistry", "chronic wound infections", "medical devices", "food industry". We also reviewed additional relevant articles identified from the referenced citations. We limited our investigation to English-language journals.

EOs (also called volatile or ethereal oils) are natural aromatic oily liquids with complex compositions obtained from different plant organs by various methods, including expression, fermentation, enfleurage and extraction. The most used technique is steam distillation [8]. From the 20–60 low molecular weight components, which can be found in the composition of EOs in different amounts, at least one, such as terpenes and terpenoids or other aromatic compounds, exhibit antimicrobial activity [9] (Figure 1).

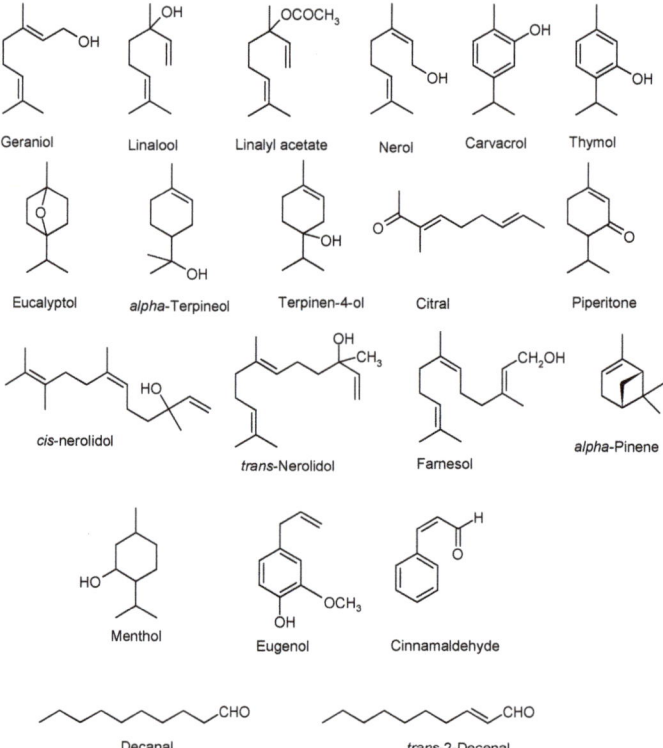

Figure 1. The main components of essential oils (EOs).

EOs of vegetal origin have been used for millennia in ethnomedicine as a natural antimicrobial and antiviral agents. Their antimicrobial activity is due to the alteration of microbial cell envelope leading to cellular lysis with cell contents leakage and proton motive force inhibition. Their benefits result from the fact that microbial resistance is less probably to be installed, as compared to chemical substances, the facile preparation, high biocompatibility and biodegradability [6]. Besides their antimicrobial activity, EOs also exhibit anti-inflammatory effects. In addition, their antibiofilm activity came to researchers' attention in the last ten years [4].

3. Discussion
3.1. EOs Mechanism of Action as Antibiofilm Agents

The complex composition of EOs suggests that multiple mechanisms, probably acting synergically, are involved in their biological effects [3]. From the studied articles, we identified several types of mechanisms of action that we describe below.

In the review of Saviuc et al., it is shown that EOs are potent antibiofilm agents, acting by inhibition of the intercellular communication systems and by inducing changes in the substrate (referring to changing of redox potential, resistivity or pH) [10]. EOs could also kill the biofilm embedded cells by the alteration of the cytoplasmic membrane due to their hydrophobic constituents [11]. The research performed by Selim and Burt groups revealed that the absence of the outer membrane in Gram-positive bacteria favors the direct interaction of the EOs with the cellular membrane, either affecting its permeability and causing the leakage of intracellular content or inactivating the bacterial enzymes [8,12].

As presented by Melo et al. in terms of action on the biofilm produced by *S. aureus*, the action of EOs depends on the hydrophobicity, reactivity and diffusion rate of EOs in the matrix, as well as to the composition and structure of the biofilm. The EOs can stop the formation of biofilm by blocking the quorum-sense system, inhibiting the transcription of flagellar genes or by interfering with bacterial motility [13].

Tang et al. analyzed the EOs from *Amomum villosum* Lour against methicillin-resistant *S. aureus* (MRSA) and established that the mechanism of action consists in reducing the bacterial adherence to inert surfaces. They realized the first proteomic study of the mechanism of action of *A. villosum* Lour EO against MRSA and showed that the inhibitory effect is dose—and temperature-dependent [14].

EOs could also increase the oxidative stress in microbial cells, causing damages of intracellular macromolecules, leading to cellular apoptosis., e.g., Das et al. found that Chamomile EO induced the accumulation of reactive oxygen species (superoxide and peroxide) that could be responsible for the antimicrobial activity of this EO [15].

In their article from 2015, Fde et al. showed that geraniol, the main constituent of some EOs, such as *Cymbopogon martini* EO, inhibits the ergosterol synthesis, a major constituent of the fungal plasma membrane [16]. *Cymbopogon citratus* EO has an effect of inhibiting glucosyltransferase activity in addition to the mechanism of degrading membrane proteins and cell permeability. This enzyme is involved in glucans synthesis, which is important for the stabilization of *E. coli* O157: H7 biofilms. The study carried out by Ortega-Ramirez in 2020 presented a type of enzymatic mechanism that essential oils can have, which can overcome the resistance to disinfection processes of microorganisms that affect the food industry, such as *E. coli* O157: H7, which can form a very resistant biofilm [17].

3.2. Disadvantages EOs Administration

However, the EOs disadvantages should not be neglected, as Glinel et al. have shown. The chemical composition of EOs varies, depending on the ripeness, the harvesting season and the geographical origin. The EOs have low stability when exposed to temperature or UV radiation. Some EOs are toxic after internal administration or could cause hypersensitivity reactions, dizziness, headache, nausea, or lightheadedness, mostly after skin or mucosal administration [4].

3.3. EOs Formulation

Particular importance presents the research on obtaining different formulations and appropriate to the use of EOs, following at the same time an accurate determination of their mode of action.

In their article from 2019, Das et al. highlighted the disadvantages of EOs, due to their increased lipophilicity and volatility, which makes it difficult the evaluate the antimicrobial effect. That's why they proposed Pickering nanoemulsion of *Chamomile* EO as a new and promising formulation, which proved to be more effective and assuring the EO intracellular delivery when tested on a wide range of bacterial and yeast strains [15].

The Pickering oil-in-water (AEP) nanoemulsion of *Artemisia annua* EO, stabilized using silica nanoparticles, was very efficient against mature *Candida* biofilms, as compared to the emulsions stabilized with Tween-80 and with the *A. annua* EO ethanolic solution, the possible mechanism of action being through the generation of the oxidative stress and superior penetration of lipid membranes, as demonstrated using the unilamellar liposomes model [18]. For the same purpose, ethanol, methanol and dimethylsulfoxide (DMSO) solvents and Tween-80 or 20 surfactant-based formulations have been used to stabilize the hydrophobic EOs, reduce the volatility and improve the penetration of cellular envelope [19–22]. However, the need to obtain new formulations that increase the solubility of EO or the emulsification capacity in an aqueous medium for a more advanced release of the components still exists [22].

In the attempt to characterize the antimicrobial activity as precisely as possible, the aim was to incorporate the essential oils in modified cyclodextrins or silica nanoparticles [23–25].

Recently, inert and biocompatible solid particles have been used as stabilizing agents instead of surfactants to stabilize EO emulsions. This approach involves the adsorption of solid particles at the oil–water interface reducing the interfacial tension and thus, increasing the stability [19,26].

3.4. EOs as Antibiofilm Agents

At present, there are only a few compounds with demonstrated activity agents have on fungal biofilms. For this reason, new anti-biofilm molecules are needed, and some essential oils have proven effective in combating antibacterial and antifungal biofilms. The chemical composition of commonly used EOs and the biofilm-producing microbial species used in antibiofilm tests are presented in Table 1. Table 2 shows the most tested EOs in terms of the antibiofilm effect on medical devices or different surfaces.

As it is presented in Table 2, much attention has been paid lately to *Melaleuca alternifolia* (tea tree oil) (TTO EO) [27], which exhibits antibacterial and antifungal activity, preventing the formation of biofilms on different surfaces having a high-risk of contamination.

A study from 2011 performed by Budzyńska et al. presents the activity of TTO EO, *Lavandula angustifolia* (lavender essential oil) (LEO), *Melissa officinalis* (*Melissa* essential oilor lemon balm) (MEO) and linalool, linalyl acetate, α-terpineol, terpinen-4-ol on biofilms formed by *S. aureus* and *E. coli* reference strains. MEO, α-terpineol and terpinen-4-ol, showed a higher antibiofilm effect than LEO and its major components, i.e., linalool and linalyl acetate. The tests demonstrated that *E. coli* biofilm was more susceptible than the *S. aureus* biofilms to the action of EOs, especially to TTO, that destroyed it after 1 h exposure to a 0.78% concentration, contrary to the opinion stating that Gram-negative microorganisms are more resistant to EOs. In comparison with LEO and TTO, the MEO effect is more dependent on the action time. The in vivo tests on biomedical surfaces of urinary catheters and tracheal tubes showed that TTO and terpinen-4-ol used at 2 × MIC (minimal inhibitory concentration) caused visible biofilm eradication, while increased concentrations were required to eradicate the microbial biofilm on surgical mesh [5].

Karpanen and coworkers studied the antimicrobial effect of chlorhexidine digluconate, either alone or combined with TTO eucalyptus oil and thymol on planktonic and adherent *S. epidermidis*. Thymol exhibited a higher activity on biofilm cells. This was the first study in that EOs demonstrated the best potential of inhibiting the biofilm produced by *S. epidermidis* TK1 and RP62A when they were combined with chlorhexidine digluconate. This synergistic activity is particularly valuable for skin antisepsis and for removing *S. epidermidis* from hard disinfection surfaces [28].

The study was deepened by Kwiecinski et al., who also studied the antimicrobial action of TTO; this research demonstrated the TTO effectiveness against *S. aureus* clinical strains in different growth phases, including stationary phase and biofilms. The minimum biofilm eradication concentration was usually 2x CMI, lower than 1% v/v. The inhibition of biofilm took place in 15 min at a TTO concentration >1% v/v [29].

The TTO was also tested on clinical and reference *C. albicans* strains in biofilm growth state on both biotic (human epithelial cells) and abiotic (polystyrene) surfaces, but inhibition at 0.008% concentration occurred only for one *C. albicans* reference strain [30].

In another experiment, the *Boswellia papyrifera* resin EO (BEO) proved antibiofilm activity against *S. epidermidis* and *S. aureus* preformed biofilms of 24 h, at concentrations close to the MICs. Sub-MIC concentrations of BEO exhibited a good inhibitory effect against *C. albicans* growth, adhesion, biofilm development, mature biofilm eradication (at 44 µg/mL concentration) and germ tube formation [31].

The sub-MIC concentrations of EO from *T. vulgaris* reduced the *S. aureus* biofilm development rate, inducing some cellular adaptation to this EO. This suggests that EOs treatments should envisage their rotation and combination with other biocides to prevent the emergence of resistant isolates [32].

A very recently published research on clove and thyme oils efficiency against *Fusarium* spp. development on soft contact lenses indicated that at concentrations lower than 50 µL/L that can be used without affecting the device material, the fungal cell adherence and formation were inhibited [33].

The *Mentha piperita* EO inhibits *C. albicans* and *C. dubliniensis* biofilm formation at a concentration of a maximum of 2 µL/mL in a dose-dependent manner. The effect is due to the increased concentration in menthol of this EO, which can be incorporated into the fungal cell membrane; the phenolic monoterpene, bearing a hydroxyl group on the phenolic ring, also exhibits antimicrobial effect due to the cytoplasmic membrane disruption. This mechanism of action results in the antifungal efficacy of EO of *Mentha piperita* on those strains resistant to azoles [34].

Table 1 indicates that much research has been devoted to identifying the EOs that can be used in biofilm eradication produced by *S. aureus* strains. In the study of Lee et al. (2014), from 83 EOs, nine of them (bay (*Pimenta racemosa*), cade (*Juniperus oxycedrus*), cedarwood (*Calocedrus decurrens*), frankincense (*Boswellia carterii*), lovage root (*Levisticum officinale*), oregano (*Origanum vulgare*), sandalwood (*Santalum album*), thyme red (*Thymus vulgaris*), and Vetiver Haiti (*Cymbopogon martini*) oils) inhibited the *S. aureus* biofilm at 0.01% (v/v) concentration. Three of them (black pepper (*Piper nigrum*), cananga (*Cananga odorata*), and myrrh (*Commiphora myrrha*) oils) at a sub-MIC exhibited a strong antibiofilm activity. One of the active compounds was cis-nerolidol (0.01% (v/v)), which proved to be more efficient than trans-nerolidol contained by the three EOs, inhibiting by more than 80% versus 45% the *S. aureus* biofilm growth. The black pepper EOs inhibited the expression of nuc1 and nuc2 (nucleases) and sarA (staphylococcal accessory regulator A), showing promise, together with cis-nerolidol for fighting MRSA and vancomycin–methicillin-resistant *S. aureus* infections [35].

The antimicrobial effect of carvacrol is often described in the literatureand the EOs rich in this compound, such as *Satureja hortensis* one (even in sub-MIC concentrations), proved to inhibit *Candida*, *Staphylococcus* and periodontal bacteria biofilms [36].

Gomes et al. demonstrated the efficiency of farnesol on *S. epidermidis* (one of the main nosocomial agents of indwelling medical devices BAIs) biofilm, producing significant destruction of biofilm structure and a significative reduction of biofilm thickness [37].

Gursoy et al. studied the antibiofilm activity of *Satureja hortensis* essential oil, tested on *Candida* and *Staphylococcus* biofilms, at and 0.03% and 0.06% concentrations. The growth inhibitory effect against periodontal bacteria and the anti-biofilm effect in subinhibitory concentration was registered [36].

The EOs from two plants from the *Apiaceae* family, *Ferula asafetida* and *Dorema aucheri*, were also tested for their antibiofilm activity against *P. aeruginosa* using 25 µg/mL concentration. *Ferula* EO decreased pigmentogenesis, protease and biofilm development, while *Dorema* EO affected only pyoverdine and elastase production [38].

The EOs of *Cinnamomum burmannii* and *Massoia aromatic* are another source of antibiofilm agents, proving to inhibit both *P. aeruginosa* and *S. aureus* biofilms. The effectiveness of these EOs can be due to their main components, highlighted by GC–MS analysis, which are cinnamic aldehyde and massoia lactone, respectively [39].

Kavanaugh and Ribbeck demonstrated that the EOs of cassia, Peru balsam, and red thyme oils are very efficient against MRSA biofilms. In addition, the three EOs at MIC values have also inhibited *P. aeruginosa* biofilm cells; for cassia EO (0.2%), the effect is more intensive than that of colistin (3 µg mL^{-1}) [7].

The *Eucalyptus smithii* and *Juniperus communis* EOs inhibited both initial phases as well as the maturation of biofilms formed by *S. aureus* and *P. aeruginosa* respiratory isolates and reference strains [40].

A study of antibiofilm effect from 2014 used EOs from *Lamiaceae* and *Apiaceae* families (*Ammi visnaga*, *Ammoides verticillata*, *Artemisia arborescens*, *Dittrichia graveolens*, *Lavandula dentate*, *Lavandula multifida*, *Mentha piperita*, *Origanum vulgare*, *Rosmarinus eriocalyx*, *Thymbra capitata*), rich in oxygenated monoterpenes (mostly alcohols, such as thymol, carvacrol, linalool).The EOs from *T. capitata* and *O. glandulosum* (0.75–1.5%) inhibited *E. faecalis* biofilms, similar to those extracted from *A. verticillata* and *L. multifida* (1.50–3.00%). The study also confirmed that the administration of EOs is more efficient than the administration of the main component itself [41]. The *Baccharis psiadioides* (*Asteraceae*) EO, known for their antipyretic and anti-inflammatory properties, as well as a snake bites antidote, has been proved to exhibit antimicrobial and antibiofilm action on 13 *E. faecalis* resistant strains [42].

Many studies have focused on the research of eugenol, found as a major compound in clove (*S. aromaticum*) EO, and of citral, containing geranial (trans-citral, citral A) and neral (cis-citral, citral B), found in the citrus plants leaves and fruits. Eugenol acts by disrupting cellular membrane permeability, while citral affects both the cytoplasmic/outer membrane as well as the stress response mediated by the sigma factor RpoSin *E. coli* [43].

The *Thymbra capitata* EO inhibited the preformed biofilms of different *Candida* spp. at 2xMIC, excepting *C. glabrata*, probably due to the increased content in phenols (carvacrol) [44]. Starting from these observations on antifungal activity of EOs, Dalleau et al. (2008) have tried to deepen this study by testing ten terpenes, the main components of EOs (carvacrol, citral, eucalyptol, eugenol, farnesol, geraniol, linalool, menthol, γ-terpinene, and thymol), on different *Candida* strains (*C. albicans*, *C. parapsilosis*, *C. glabrata*). The best activity was recorded using carvacrol against *C. albicans*, *C. glabrata* and *C.parapsilosis* biofilms, the effect being biofilm age and concentration-independent. They also obtained good results for geraniol and thymol [45]. In another study [46], the antibiofilm effect of *Citrus limon* and *Zingiber officinale* EOs were investigated, and it has been shown that they can be used against biofilms of *Klebsiella ornithinolytica*, *K. oxytoca* and *K. terrigena*.

In an interesting article from 2019, Kerekeset al. described the antibiotic effect of *Cinnamomum zeylanicum*, *Origanum majorana*, and *Thymus vulgaris* EOs on dual-species biofilms.

Studying the effect on the biofilm produced by *L. monocytogenes* SZMC 21307 and *E. coli* SZMC 0582, they found that treatment with cinnamon EO at concentrations of 1 mg/mL eradicated the dual biofilm. In the case of marjoram EO, the biofilm elimination started from 0.5 mg/mL concentration, and in the case of thyme EO, the inhibitory effect was detected starting with 1 mg/mL concentrations. These values were surprisingly much lower than those recorded in the eradication of monoculture biofilms. All studied

EOs decreased biofilm formation but at concentrations higher than those required for monospecific biofilms eradication.

These polymicrobial biofilms can be found in the food industry, and the recorded results suggest the possible use of EOs as food preservatives, but however, their use is limited by the strong odor and taste, requiring further study to mitigate these effects [47].

The promising results on the antibiofilm effect of EOs have outlined a new challenge for researchers to study whether the association of EOs with antibiotics is beneficial. In this regard, Rosato et al. published in 2020 a series of research that is intended to be just the beginning of a comprehensive study on the synergistic effect of EO antibiotics. They studied the activity of *Cinnamomum zeylanicum*, *Mentha piperita*, *Origanum vulgare* and *Thymus vulgaris* EOs associated with norfloxacin, oxacillin, and gentamicin on bacterial biofilm produced by *S. aureus*, *S. epidermidis* IG4, and *E. faecalis*. The synergistic effects were tested through the checkerboard microdilution method. The study showed that all EOs have a synergistic effect, the best being in combination with norfloxacin, leading, for example, in the case of *Cinnamomum zeylanicum* EO to a decrease from 128 µg/mL to 3.99 g/mL of gentamicin MIC50.The advantages of combined therapy are obvious: the decrease of antibiotic doses and implicitly reducing the resistance to antimicrobial drugs [48].

3.5. EOs Used in Dentistry

Many studies were devoted to finding new irrigants or interappointment to remove the microbial biofilms formed in the mouth, which prevent endodontic treatments [49]. Therefore, there is a need for chemical substances as medications that have both antibacterial and antibiofilm activities. *E. faecalis* is commonly recovered from teeth with persistent endodontic infections, creating biofilms attached to the canal walls or located in isthmuses and ramifications from where are difficult to eliminate by current substances, such as sodium hypochlorite and chlorhexidine [41,50]. Microbial biofilms and smear layer must be eradicated during endodontic treatment. Because the substances used as chemical irrigants are not bio-friendly with the dental and peri-radicular tissues, different natural substances have been studied as disinfectantsof root canals [51]. Chloroformic solutions of eucalyptus and orange EOs associated with cetrimide at concentrations varying from 0.05% to 0.3% reduced the biofilm by 70–85%. The two EOs enhanced the efficiency of cetrimide, which effectively eradicated the biofilms in lower doses, the synergic effect being probably due to lipophilic compounds (e.g., terpenoids or phenolics) [50].

The *Melaleuca alternifolia* EO used as a gel with antibacterial effect was very effective against oral *S. mutans* biofilm, decreasing the gingival bleeding index. Mouthwashes with this EO have also decreased not only *S. mutans* but also the total oral bacteria counts. The EO was used in 5% concentration, which was well accepted, without side effects [52,53].

Testing several oral disinfectants, including those containing a mixture of *Aloe vera* and TTO, Smith et al. (2013) demonstrated that none of the mouthwashes effectively eradicated biofilms formed from oral and bloodstream isolates MRSA.The antibiofilm effect can be improved by increasing the concentration and exposure time [54]. Carvacrol and oregano oil were also the subjects of the research study undertaken by Nostro in 2007. Both of them are known for their effect on *Staphylococcus* strains; they showed in vitro effects on staphylococcal biofilms, the biofilm inhibitory concentrations values have registered at 2–4xCMI values. Dental plaque biofilm plays an essential role in oral pathology, the etiology of dental caries, but also in contamination of dental materials surfaces, such as those used in the implant–prosthetic rehabilitation (implants, impression materials, alloys for prosthetic use, etc.) [55]. Due to the biofilm matrix destabilizing effect, thymol is used in the mouthwash with anti-plaque effects [56].

Cortelli et al. (2014) noted how important could be the use of EOs (menthol, thymol, and eucalyptol) for oral health by preventing the biofilm formation in patients with prostheses [57]. In several cases, the EOs can be more efficient than cetylpyridinium chloride [58]. Haas et al. suggested that EOs can be used daily, in the long-term, for reducing the supragingival plaque and, thus, gingivitis [59]. Quintas et al. have shown that EOs prevented de novo plaque-like biofilm development for 7 h after mouthwash, representing a possible alternative to chlorhexidine for the pre-surgical rinse or after periodontitis treatments [60,61]. In a study from 2013, Erriu et al. demonstrated that the mouthwash containing EOs compounds, such as eucalyptol, methyl salicylate, menthol and thymol, combined with ethanol, exhibits an improved antibiofilm activity at high dilution. The nonalcoholic mixture of EOs tested on *Aggregatibacter actinomycetemcomitans* strains had better anti-planktonic behavior [62]. It was also demonstrated the benefit of association of these EOs with xylitol in mouthrinse against *S. mutans*-derived biofilms, independent of the type of treatment or age of biofilm. This is a very promising treatment for the treatment and prevention of caries [63].The *Mentha piperita* and *Rosmarinus officinalis* EOs proved to be effective against *S. mutans*, one of the main agents of dental caries. Of the *Mentha piperita* EO, having a menthol concentration below 3.6% was more effectivethan rosemary oil(containing piperitone as the main component) and chlorhexidine (at 4000 and 8000 ppm). The use of toothpaste blended with EOsindicated that lower concentrations of the EOs were more effective than chlorhexidine [64]. The association of chlorhexidine with EO is indicated for better antibiofilm activity in oral treatment [65].

Eugenol and citral could represent better alternatives to chlorhexidine because, at subinhibitory concentrations, they are affecting biofilm formation and virulence of methicillin-susceptible *S. aureus*, MRSA and *L. monocytogenes* strains, having a low-risk for selecting resistance [66].

Bersan et al. studied the EOs (1 mg/mL) from twenty medicinal and aromatic species on biofilms produced in vitro by different microbial strains and compared the results with nystatin and chlorhexidine digluconate. The *Aloysia gratissima* and *Coriandrum* spp. EOs have strongly inhibited *C. albicans*, *Fusobacterium nucleatum*, *P. gingivalis*, *S. mitis* and *S. sanguis*. The *C. articulates* EO inhibited *F. nucleatum* and *P. gingivalis* biofilms. *A. gratissima* (1 mg/mL or 9% concentration) inhibited the *S. mitis* biofilm more intensively than chlorhexidine [67]. EOs, stannous fluoride and hexetidine associated with methylparaben and propylparaben decreased the in vitro peri-implant biofilm mass and activity by 39% to 56% and decreased gingivitis by 59% after continuous application. These EOs have also been shown to reduce the release of bacterial endotoxins and pathogenicity [68].

In a recent study, Marinković et al. studied the antibiofilm efficacy of *Cymbopogon martini* and *Thymus zygis* EOs on the multispecific biofilms of *S. mitis*, *S. sanguinis* and *E. faecalis* in the root canals of extracted teeth. They found that the addition of an oil-based irrigant to 1.5% sodium hypochlorite proved to be more efficient against biofilm development [69]. On the other side, exposure to biocides (e.g., triclosan) can increase the *S. mutans* hydrophobicity, increasing its susceptibility to EOs. Therefore, a combination of triclosan-containing toothpaste with EOS-based mouthrinse could reduce the acidic bacteria [70]. A good antibiofilm and anti-caries effect, comparable to that of chlorhexidine (0.12%), was observed for a mouth rinse containing *Matricaria chamomilla* L. EO (PerioGard®–Palmolive). The antibiofilm effect has been evaluated as a decrease in Colony-forming units (CFUs) for total *S. mutans*, *S. sobrinus* and *Lactobacillus* sp., and the anti-caries effect has been studied as the effect on enamel demineralization compared to phosphate-buffered saline (PBS) solution. The authors found a mineral loss reduction by 39.4% in the case of mouthwash containing EO from *Matricaria chamomilla* L., very close to that of chlorhexidine (47.4%). The authors considered that the experimental product having Chamomile EO significantly reduced enamel demineralization [71]. The *Mentha spicata* essential oil was tested for in vitro and in vivo antimicrobial and biofilm activities on *S. mutans* [72].

These results suggest that rosemary EO is efficient against cariogenic oral streptococci. Due to its major compound, eugenol, clove oil is a potent fungicidal, bactericidal and natural anesthetic compound. The *Eucalyptus* EO, reach in eucalyptol, showed antibiofilm activity against *C. albicans* biofilms [73]. The EOs from *A. gratissima*, *Baccharis dracunculifolia*, *C. sativum*, and *Lippia sidoides* demonstrated a potent inhibitory activity on *S. mutans* biofilm, probably due to the presence of thymol, carvacrol, and trans-nerolidol [74]. Mouthwashes containing *Citrus hystrix* leaf EO alone or in combination with chlorhexidine inhibited the periodontopathogenic bacteria and *S. sanguinis* and *S. mutans* biofilms [75]. The EO of *B. dracunculifolia* has been studied for use in dental care because it is known that this EO inhibits the growth of *S. mutans*. This EO reduced the rate of biofilm after one week of use, at the same level as triclosan, being a good candidate to be implemented in new material for dental care [76]. *Curcuma longa* EO (0.5 to 4 mg/mL) inhibited the growth, acid production and *S. mutans* adherence to saliva-coated hydroxyapatite beads and biofilm development [77]. The EO extracted from seeds of the *Butia capitata* tree was tested on biofilms produced by aciduric bacteria, lactobacilli, and *S. mutans*, comparing with three commercial self-etching adhesives, and it was demonstrated that they were equally effective against tested microorganisms [78].

The *Coriandrum sativum* EOs exhibited an inhibitory activity against *C. albicans* oral isolates from patients with a periodontal disease, similar to nystatin, suggesting its promising potential for the prophylaxis and treatment of oral candidiasis [79]. The *Citrus limonum* and *C. aurantium* EOs exhibited an antibiofilm effect comparable to 0.2% chlorhexidine but lower than 1% sodium hypochlorite on multispecific biofilms formed by *C. albicans*, *E. faecalis* and *E. coli* [80]. *C. sativum* EO isprobably active through its major compounds (decanal and trans-2-decenal) that could bind membrane ergosterol, acting similarly to nystatin and amphotericin B. *C. articulatus* contains α-pinene that could interfere with cellular envelopes integrity, respiratory chain and ion transport *A. gratissima* and *L. sidoides* EOs were bactericidal and inhibited the production extracellular polysaccharides in *S. mutans* [81]. The *C. sativum* EO also inhibited the proteolytic activity of *C. albicans* and affected the normal morphology of yeast cells (at 156.0 to 312.50 mg/mL concentration), probably by affecting the membrane permeability, due to the presence of mono- and sesquiterpene hydrocarbons [82].

3.6. EOs in Chronic Wound Infection Treatment

Wounds chronicity is often associated with biofilm development. Farnesol and xylitol exhibited a significant inhibitory effect against *E. faecalis* biofilms, being, therefore, proposed as adjuvants for the treatment of chronic wound infections or caries [83]. Notably, Anghel et al. demonstrated the benefit of using a modified wound dressing nanofunctionalized with magnetite nanoparticles with sustained release of *S. hortensis* EO (rich in phenolic compounds, such as thymol, carvacrol, and para-cymene) against *C. albicans* biofilm [84].

3.7. EOs in the BAIs Treatment

BAIs are a major cause of morbidity and mortality in hospitalized patients. The treatment of biofilm-mediated infections requires the development of new antibiofilm strategies, which represent new scientific challenges.

When Park et al. (2007) tested the antibacterial effect of TTO on silicone tympanostomy tubes, they found that all tested concentration of EO (100%, 50%, 10% in tween) produced a reduced bacterial adherence of all MRSA strains, which may be explained by the alteration of adherence factors present on the bacterial cell surface. The bacterial cultures were obtained from otorrhea in patients with chronic suppurative otitis media, and the antibiofilm effect of TTO was evaluated in comparison to vancomycin. The MRSA exhibited a similar susceptibility to 50% TTO and vancomycin. The authors proposed TTO as an alternative for pediatric MRSA otorrhea treatment with tympanostomy tubes [85]. Brady et al. studied the *S. aureus* biofilm, formed on a cochlear implant resistant to all conventional antimicrobials, but 5% TTO completely eradicated it in one hour [86]. Recently, Malic et al. studied the antimicrobial activities of TTO, comparatively to terpinene, eucalyptol (1,8-cineole) and eugenol against *p. mirabilis* involved in catheter-associated urinary tract infections, for further use to obtain modified catheter biomaterials, but they found a reduced antibiofilm activity [87]. Previously, a study from 2010 showed that the pomelo EO inhibited the *S. epidermidis* and *P. aeruginosa* biofilms development on soft contact lenses in a time and temperature-dependent manner [88]. In their study, Selim et al. presented the *Cupressus sempervirens* EO inhibitory effect on *K. pneumoniae* cells adherence capacity to intravenous infusion tubes made of polyvinyl chloride (PVC) at 500 μg concentration. It was observed that biomaterial surface pretreatment with EO rendered it repellent the microbial cells, thereby reducing surface adhesion [12]. *C. citratus* (at 0.5× and 0.25× MIC) and *Syzygium aromaticum* EOs inhibited the *C. albicans* clinical and reference strains biofilms formed under static conditions in polystyrene tubes [89,90], proposing them as an alternative to amphotericin B and fluconazole [91]. Cinnamon bark EO (containing as major components cinnamaldehyde and eugenol) has been shown to exhibit a potent antibiofilm on *P. aeruginosa*, reducing it by up to 96%. When mixed with 2% poly(D,L-lactide-co-glycolide) (PLGA) (a biodegradable polymer), it prevented *p* biofilm formation [92]. In their paper, Chmit et al. reported that they could not determine a notable antibiofilm effect of the EO from *Laurus nobilis* using a *S. epidermidis* strain. Despite these results, the *L. nobilis* EO remains in attention due to its large spectrum of activity against pathogenic bacteria [93,94]. The medical industry is in a constant search for new materials, but also of biocidal products, the potential applications of EOs and polymer systems attracting the attention of researchers. Nostro et al. incorporated eugenol, citronellol and linalool in poly(ethylene-co-vinyl acetate) copolymer (EVA) and tested against *E. coli*, *P. aeruginosa*, *L. monocytogenes*, *S. epidermidis*, and *S. aureus*. The EO diffused through the polymeric matrix, and the combinations EVA + citronellol and EVA + eugenol at 7% concentration induced a 40–90% biofilm decrease [95].

3.8. EOs Used in Food Industry

In the food industry, bacteria adhere to vats, tanks and tubes, impairing food safety and quality. Therefore, strategies are needed to inhibit biofilm formation or the elimination of mature biofilms. Current strategies used in the food industry, such as disinfection, surface preconditioning, ultrasonication, etc., although effective, cannot control microbial biofilms. The quorum-sensing systems that assure a coordinate gene expression depending on cellular density also regulating biofilm formation represent a promising lead for the development of novel antibiofilm strategies [96]. The food-contact surfaces rise many problems to the meat industry because of the risk of contamination with pathogenic (e.g., *Salmonella enterica*, *L. monocytogenes*, *E. coli*) ormeat spoilage bacteria (e.g., *Pseudomonas* spp., *Brochothrix thermosphacta* and *Lactobacillus* spp.) bacteria, predominantly growing in biofilms. Disinfection of the food contact surfaces is a difficult and challenging problem that can be solved by finding new disinfectants, such as EOs [6,97,98]. To find new food preservatives, detergents and sanitizers, which can be used in the food industry, Chorianopoulos et al. tested the *S. thymbra* EO (1% *v/v*) against monospecific or polyspecific biofilms formed by Gram-positive (*S. simulans*, *L. fermentum*, *L. monocytogenes*) or Gram-negative (*P. putida*, *S. enterica*) bacteria. The strong inhibitory effect of EO on microorganisms was associated with carvacrol and thymol compounds, acting as membrane permeabilizing agents [99]. *Mentha piperita*, *C. citratus* and *Cinnamomum zeylanicum* EOs inhibited *S. enterica*-serotype *Enteritidis* biofilm development on stainless steel surfaces, for the first two EOs, after 10–40 min [100]. Sub-MIC concentrations of cinnamon EO and cinnamaldehyde reduced the biofilm counts at 156–234 μg/mL. Cinnamaldehyde is probably acting by inhibiting the macromolecules synthesis and damaging the cell membrane [101]. The *C. citratus* EO was also tested comparing with the *T. vulgaris* EO against *A. hydrophila* biofilm development on stainless steel coupons in UHT skimmed milk [11]. The *Thymbra capitata* EO was evaluated against both planktonic and biofilm cells of *S. enterica* serovar *Typhimurium* and proved very efficient in comparison with benzalkonium chloride [102]. One of the proposed alternatives to overcome the bacterial contamination of the food, both in suspension and in the biofilm, can be the use of a mixture of essential components of volatile oils (thymol, eugenol, berberine and cinnamaldehyde), to create a synergistic effect with streptomycin, useful in controlling foodborne pathogens [103]. The antimicrobial activity of 19 EOs was evaluated to determine their effectiveness in eliminating the pathogenic agent *S. aureus* from the food processing plants. Thus, planktonic cells of *S. aureus* strains have shown increased sensitivity to volatile thyme, lemon and vetiver oils. The 48 h old biofilms of the same strains, formed on stainless steel installations in the food industry, could not be eliminated by the volatile oils tested, with increased efficiency of oils of thyme and patchouli. The efficiency of thyme oil was increased by the use of benzalkonium chloride. To prevent the emergence of resistant strains, it is necessary to combine different types of essential oils, as well as their use in combination with various biocides [32].

3.9. EOs as Air Disinfectants

Laird et al. examined how Citri-V, a mixture of citrus EOs (orange: bergamot, 1:1 v/v), removes *Enterococcus* spp. and *S. aureus* biofilms from then stainless steel and plastic surfaces after aerial release in a concentration of 15 mg/L. The citrus vapors may be used for additional decontamination if they are also used with routine cleaning, as they are less toxic than ozone or hydrogen peroxide used for air decontamination treatments [104].

3.10. Nanoparticles with EOs Used in Controlling and Preventing Infections

Nanoparticles used in antibiofilm therapy have been intensively studied lately due to their unique properties, helping to fight resistant infections because they can easily penetrate the biofilm matrix and can also functionalize biomedical surfaces by coating, impregnating or embedding, thus preventing biofilm formation [105].

The use of functionalized nanoparticles with EOs can be a method for controlling and preventing infections associated with microbial biofilms, limiting at the same time the consumption of synthetic antimicrobial drugs and thus, reducing microbial resistance.

Nanoparticles can be used as controlled and local delivery systems for EOs and also for enhancing their activity. The development of combinations between nanoparticles and EOs is a new research direction approached also by Chifiriuc et al., who used *Rosmarinus officinalis* EO to obtain a nanobiosystem used for coating catheter surface that successfully inhibited the adherence of *C. tropicalis* and *C. albicans* clinical strains. After 48–72 h, the biofilm was almost absent on the surface of the coated materials [106].

As we also presented in this paper, many studies have shown the beneficial effect of carvacrol in inhibiting microbial biofilms, attracting the attention of researchers in the field of nanotechnology, which have tried to encapsulate this EO in PLGA nanocapsules to obtain a new drug delivery system, that altered the architecture of the *S. epidermidis* biofilm when added in the initial phases of biofilm formation [107].

The aim of a study performed by Bilcu and coworkers figured out the characteristics resulted from combining the antimicrobial activity of three EOs obtained from *Pogostemon cablin*, *Vanilla planifolia* and *Cananga odorata* subsp. with that of iron oxide@C14 nanoparticles for obtaining coatings for the surfaces of medical devices. These hybrid coatings inhibited the *S. aureus* and *K. pneumoniae* adherence and biofilm formation in both initial and maturation (in the case of vanilla EO) phases [108].

Polylactic acid (PLA) nanoparticles with EOs can be used to design new ecological strategies based on natural alternatives efficiently in the treatment of severe infections with biofilms formed by pathogenic and/or resistant bacteria. PLA was combined with lemon EO to obtain functional nanocapsules that exhibited better antimicrobial activity than PLA alone [109]. Using a solvent evaporation method and coated with matrix-assisted pulsed laser evaporation (MAPLE), a hybrid nanocoating composed of magnetite nanoparticles functionalized with *Melissa officinalis* EO, PLA and chitosan, was obtained and characterized. In vitro experiments revealed significant inhibitory activity of prokaryotic cell adhesion properties [110]. New research has been effectuated on the development of nanoemulsions containing geranium oil that demonstrated inhibitory effect against *C. albicans*, *C. tropicalis*, *C. glabrata* and *C. krusei* biofilms, quantified by measuring the total protein and bioluminescence. The results showed a better activity on *C. albicans* and *C. tropicalis* biofilms. Both geranium oil and nanoemulsions containing this oil significantly inhibited biofilm formation in all species tested on polyethylene surfaces, with nanoemulsions having a better activity, proving that they can become an effective alternative for reducing the microbial adhesion on the surface of the medical devices and preventing consecutive infections [111]. For increasing its thermal stability, carvacrol is incorporated into polymers of the type of halloysite nanotubes, which then allow subsequent mixing with the low-density polyethylene melt. The nanocomposites exhibited antimicrobial activity against *E. coli*, *L. innocua* and *Alternaria alternate* biofilms. They have proven effective and can be excellent candidates for a wide range of applications, such as controlling microbial contamination of food [112].

Table 1. The EOs studied in terms of microbial antibiofilm action.

Latin Name of Plant Source of EO	Main Components of EO	Microbial Strain That Produces Biofilms on Which the EO Has Been Tested	Reference
Boswellia papyrifera *Boswellia rivae*	n-octyl acetate, octanol, limonene, a-pinene, verticilla-4 (20), 7,11-triene, acetate, incensole	*Staphylococcus epidermidis* *S. aureus* *C. albicans*	[31]
Butia capitata	capric, caprylic, lauric, linoleic, myristic, oleic, palmitic, stearic acids	Aciduric bacteria Lactobacilli *Streptococcus mutans*	[78]
Cananga odorata subsp. *Genuine* (ylang-ylang oil)	*p*-cresyl methyl ether, linalool, geranyl acetate, geraniol, eucalyptol	*S. aureus* *Klebsiella pneumoniae*	[109]
Cinnamomum aromaticum (Cassia oil)	cinnamaldehyde, eugenol, linalool	*P. aeruginosa* *P. putida* *S. aureus*	[7]
Cinnamomum zeylanicum	e-cinnamaldehyde	*Salmonella* Saintpaul	[102]
Citrus hystrix	citronellal	*S. sanguinis* *S. mutans*	[75]
Coriandrum sativum	decanal, trans-2-decenal, 2-decen-1-ol, cyclodecane	*C. albicans* *C. tropicalis* *C. krusei* *C. dubliniensis* *C. rugosa*	[82]
Cupressus sempervirens	α-pinene, α-terpinolene, δ-3-carene, limonene	*K. pneumoniae*	[12]
Curcuma longa	curlone, *trans*-β-elemenone, germacrone, β-sesquiphellandrene, α-turmerone, α*r*-turmerone, α-zingiberene	*S. mutans*	[77]
Cymbopogon citratus (lemongrass oil)	geranial, neral, myrcene	*C. albicans* *C. tropicalis* *C. glabrata* *C. krusei* *P. gingivalis* *P. intermedia* *Aeromonas hydrophila*	[89–91] [73] [11]
Eucalyptus camaldulensis	eucalyptol	*Porphyromonas gingivalis* *Actinobacillus actinomycetemcomitans* *Fusobacterium nucleatum* *S. mutans* *S. sobrinus* *C. albicans*	[73]

Table 1. Cont.

Latin Name of Plant Source of EO	Main Components of EO	Microbial Strain That Produces Biofilms on Which the EO Has Been Tested	Reference
Eugenia caryophyllata (*Syzygium aromaticum*) (clove oil)	biflorin, caryophyllene oxide, eugenol, eugenyl acetate, ellagic acid, gallic acid, kaempferol, myricetin, oleanolic acid, rhamnocitrin	C. albicans C. tropicalis C. glabrata C. krusei P. gingivalis P. intermedia	[73,89–91]
Laurus nobilis	acetate, eucalyptol, linalool, methyleugenol, α-terpinyl	S. epidermidis	[93,94]
Lavandula angustifolia (lavender essential oil, LEO)	camphor, caryophyllene, eucalyptol, lavendulyl acetate, limonene, linalool, linalyl acetate, *cis*-ocimene, 3-octanone, a-pinene, transocimene, terpinen-4-ol	S. aureus E. coli	[5]
Matricaria chamomilla (Chamomile EO)	(E)-β-farnesene α-bisabolol oxide A	S. mutans S. sobrinus Lactobacillus sp.	[71]
Melaleuca alternifolia (tea tree oil, TTO)	α-pinene, *p*-cymene, eucalyptol, terpinen-4-ol, γ-terpinene, α-terpinene, terpinolene	S. mutans Proteus mirabilis	[52] [87]
Melissa officinalis (Melissa essential oil, MEO or lemon balm)	citrals (geranial + neral, citronellal, limonene, geraniol, β-caryophyllene, β-caryophyllene oxide, and germacrene D	S. aureus E. coli	[5]
Mentha piperita	menthofuran, menthol, menthyl acetate, eucalyptol, menthone, α-pinene, sabinene, β-pinene	C. albicans C. dubliniensis	[34]
Mentha spicata	carvone, trans-carveol, myrcenecarvyl-acetate-Z	S. mutans	[73,98]
Ocimum gratissimum	eugenol, 1,8-cineole	S. aureus E. coli	[13]
Origanum vulgare (oregano oil)	carvacrol, thymol, γ-terpinene, *p*-cymene	S. aureus S. epidermidis	[55]
Pogostemon cablin (patchouli essential oil)	α-guaiene, β-caryophyllene, δ-cadinene, pogostol, (-)-patchoulol, seychellene, α- and β-patchoulene	S. aureus K. pneumoniae	[109]
Rosmarinus officinalis (rosemary oil)	eucalyptol, alpha-pinene, camphor, verbenone, borneol	S. sobrinus	[73]
Satureja thymbra	carvacrol, thymol, *p*-cymene	S. simulans Lactobacillus fermentum P. putida Salmonella enterica Listeria monocytogenes	[6]
Thymbra capitata	carvacrol, γ-terpinene, *p*-cymene	Candida albicans C. glabrata C. tropicalis C. parapsilosis C. guilliermondii	[44]
Thymus vulgaris (thyme oil)	eucalyptol, camphor	A. hydrophila	[11]
Vanilla planifolia (vanilla oil)	ethylvanillin, 4-hydroxybenzaldehyde, methyl anisate, 4-hydroxybenzyl methyl ether, piperonal, vanillic acid, vanillin	S. aureus K. pneumoniae	[109]

Table 2. The EOs studied in terms of microbial antibiofilm action formed on a medical device or live surface.

Latin Name of Plant Source of EO	The Support (Medical Device) on Which the Biofilm Was Studied	Reference
Baccharis dracunculifolia *Mentha spicata* *Melaleuca alternifolia*	Dental biofilm	[76] [73] [52]
Cananga odorata subsp. *genuine* *Pogostemoncablin* *Vanilla planifolia*	Catheter	[109]
Cupressus sempervirens	Intravenous infusion tube	[12]
Cymbopogon citratus *Thymus vulgaris* *Saturejathymbra*	Stainless steel coupons	[11] [11] [6]
Eugenia caryophyllata *(Syzygiumaromaticum)* *Thymus vulgaris*	Soft contact lenses	[33]
Lavandula angustifolia *Melissa officinalis* *Melaleuca alternifolia*	Urological catheter, infusion tube, surgical mesh	[5]
Melaleuca alternifolia	Catheter-associated urinary tract infections	[87]
	Cochlear implant	[86]
	Silicone tympanostomy tubes	[85]

4. Conclusions

Essential oils represent safe and efficient alternatives for the development of novel antibiofilm agents that could find a potential role in the medical and food industries for infection control, especially BAIs associated with artificial medical devices, susceptible to the formation of microbial films resistant to conventional antibiotic treatment. The great advantage of EOs is that their usage is not likely to select for microbial resistance because they have a complex composition and, therefore, multiple targets in the microbial cells.

An increasing idea to combat microbial biofilms is to combine the conventional antimicrobials with EOs, based on studies already conducted, which have shown promising results.

Our review shows that most studies were performed in vitro, thus further in vivo studies are necessary, as well as the elucidation of many additional therapeutic aspects, such as EOs formulation, frequency and duration of therapy, safety issues; these aspects need to be optimized to ensure the best possible clinical outcomes.

It cannot be neglected the potential advantage of using EOs prophylactically, and in this context, a promising lead is to obtain bioactive nanobiocoatings containing EOs for inhibiting bacterial and fungal adhesion and further biofilm development on the different surface from the medical, industrial and natural environment.

Author Contributions: Conceptualization, D.C.N. and C.L.; methodology, I.Z.; software, C.C. and I.N.; investigation, T.C. and P.I.; data curation, D.C.N., C.L., M.C.C. and I.Z.; writing—original draft preparation, D.C.N., C.L., C.C., M.C.C., T.C., P.I., I.N. and I.Z.; writing—review and editing, D.C.N., M.C.C. and P.I.; visualization, T.C.; supervision, D.C.N., C.L. and I.Z. All authors have read and agreed to the published version of the manuscript.

Funding: This research was funded by UEFISCDI, PN-III-P1-1.1-TE-2019-1506, project number 147TE/2020.

Institutional Review Board Statement: Not applicable.

Informed Consent Statement: Not applicable.

Data Availability Statement: Not applicable.

Conflicts of Interest: The authors declare no conflict of interest.

References

1. Rodney, M.D.; Costerton, J.W. Biofilms: Survival Mechanisms of Clinically Relevant Microorganisms. *Clin. Microbiol. Rev.* **2002**, *15*, 167–193.
2. Mohammadi, Z.; Palazzi, F.; Giardino, L.; Shalavi, S. Microbial biofilms in endodontic infections: An update review. *Biomed. J.* **2013**, *36*, 59–70. [CrossRef] [PubMed]
3. Lazăr, V.; Chifiriuc, M.C. Medical significance and new therapeutical strategies for biofilm associated infections. *Roum. Arch. Microbiol. Immunol.* **2010**, *69*, 125–138. [PubMed]
4. Glinel, K.; Thebault, P.; Humblot, V.; Pradier, C.M.; Jouenne, T. Antibacterial surfaces developed from bio-inspired approaches. *Acta Biomater.* **2012**, *8*, 1670–1684. [CrossRef]
5. Budzyñska, A.; Wiêckowska-Szakiel, M.; Sadowska, B.; Kalemba, D.; Rózalska, B. Antibiofilm Activity of Selected Plant Essential Oils and their Major Components. *Pol. J. Microbiol.* **2011**, *60*, 35–41. [CrossRef] [PubMed]
6. Chorianopoulos, N.G.; Giaouris, E.D.; Skandamis, P.N.; Haroutounian, S.A.; Nychas, G.J.E. Disinfectant test against monoculture and mixed-culture biofilms composed of technological, spoilage and pathogenic bacteria: Bactericidal effect of essential oil and hydrosol of *Satureja thymbra* and comparison with standard acid–base sanitizers. *J. Appl. Microbiol.* **2008**, *104*, 1586–1596. [CrossRef]
7. Kavanaugh, N.L.; Ribbeck, K. Selected Antimicrobial Essential Oils Eradicate *Pseudomonas* spp. and *Staphylococcus aureus* Biofilms. *Appl. Environ. Microbiol.* **2012**, *78*, 4057–4061. [CrossRef] [PubMed]
8. Burt, S. Essential oils: Their antibacterial properties and potential applications in foods—A review. *Int. J. Food Microbiol.* **2004**, *94*, 223–253. [CrossRef] [PubMed]
9. Bakkali, F.; Averbeck, S.; Averbeck, D.; Idaomar, M. Biological effects of essential oils—A review. *Food Chem. Toxicol.* **2008**, *46*, 446–475. [CrossRef]
10. Saviuc, C.M.; Drumea, V.; Olariu, L.; Chifiriuc, M.C.; Bezirtzoglou, E.; Lazăr, V. Essential Oils with Microbicidal and Antibiofilm Activity. *Curr. Pharm. Biotechnol.* **2015**, *16*, 137–151. [CrossRef]
11. Millezi, A.F.; das Graças Cardoso, M.; Alves, E.; Piccoli, R.H. Reduction of *Aeromonas hidrophyla* biofilm on stainless stell surface by essential oils. *Braz. J. Microbiol.* **2013**, *44*, 73–80. [CrossRef] [PubMed]
12. Selim, S.A.; Adam, M.E.; Hassan, S.M.; Albalawi, A.R. Chemical composition, antimicrobial and antibiofilm activity of the essential oil and methanol extract of the Mediterranean cypress (*Cupressus sempervirens* L.). *BMC Complement. Altern. Med.* **2014**, *14*, 179. [CrossRef]
13. Melo, R.S.; Albuquerque Azevedo, Á.M.; Gomes Pereira, A.M.; Rocha, R.R.; Bastos Cavalcante, R.M.; Carneiro Matos, M.N.; Ribeiro Lopes, P.H.; Gomes, G.A.; Soares Rodrigues, T.H.; Santos, H.S.d.; et al. Chemical Composition and Antimicrobial Effectiveness of *Ocimum gratissimum* L. Essential Oil Against Multidrug-Resistant Isolates of *Staphylococcus aureus* and *Escherichia coli*. *Molecules* **2019**, *24*, 3864. [CrossRef] [PubMed]
14. Tang, C.; Chen, J.; Zhang, L.; Zhang, R.; Zhang, S.; Ye, S.; Zhao, Z.; Yang, D. Exploring the antibacterial mechanism of essential oils by membrane permeability, apoptosis and biofilm formation combination with proteomics analysis against methicillin-resistant *Staphylococcus aureus*. *Int. J. Med. Microbiol.* **2020**, *5*, 151435. [CrossRef] [PubMed]
15. Das, S.; Horváth, B.; Šafranko, S.; Jokić, S.; Széchenyi, A.; Kőszegi, T. Antimicrobial Activity of Chamomile Essential Oil: Effect of Different Formulations. *Molecules* **2019**, *24*, 4321. [CrossRef] [PubMed]
16. Fde, O.P.; Mendes, J.M.; Lima, I.O.; Mota, K.S.; Oliveira, W.A.; Ede, O.L. Antifungal activity of geraniol and citronellol, two monoterpenes alcohols, against Trichophyton rubrum involves inhibition of ergosterol biosynthesis. *Pharm. Biol.* **2015**, *53*, 228–234.
17. Ortega-Ramirez, L.A.; Gutiérrez-Pacheco, M.M.; Vargas-Arispuro, I.; González-Aguilar, G.A.; Martínez-Téllez, M.A.; Ayala-Zavala, J.F. Inhibition of Glucosyltransferase Activity and Glucan Production as an Antibiofilm Mechanism of Lemongrass Essential Oil against Escherichia coli O157:H7. *Antibiotics* **2020**, *9*, 102. [CrossRef] [PubMed]
18. Das, S.; Vörös-Horváth, B.; Bencsik, T.; Micalizzi, G.; Mondello, L.; Horváth, G.; Kőszegi, T.; Széchenyi, A. Antimicrobial Activity of Different Artemisia Essential Oil Formulations. *Molecules* **2020**, *25*, 2390. [CrossRef]
19. Pina-Barrera, A.M.; Alvarez-Roman, R.; Baez-Gonzalez, J.G.; Amaya-Guerra, C.A.; Rivas-Morales, C.; Gallardo-Rivera, C.T.; Galindo-Rodriguez, S.A. Application of a multisystem coating based on polymeric nanocapsule containing essential oil of *Thymus vulgaris* L. to increase the shelf life of table grapes (*Vitis vinifera* L.). *IEEE Trans. NanoBioscience* **2019**, *18*, 549–557. [CrossRef]
20. Alizadeh Behbahani, B.; Tabatabaei Yazdi, F.; Vasiee, A.; Mortazavi, S.A. Oliveria decumbens essential oil: Chemical compositions and antimicrobial activity against the growth of some clinical and standard strains causing infection. *Microb. Pathog.* **2018**, *114*, 449–452. [CrossRef] [PubMed]
21. Tang, X.; Shao, Y.-L.; Tang, Y.-J.; Zhou, W.-W. Antifungal Activity of Essential Oil Compounds (Geraniol and Citral) and Inhibitory Mechanisms on Grain Pathogens (*Aspergillus flavus* and *Aspergillus ochraceus*). *Mol. J. Synth. Chem. Nat. Prod. Chem.* **2018**, *23*, 2108. [CrossRef]

22. Inouye, S.; Tsuruoka, T.; Uchida, K.; Yamaguchi, H. Effect of Sealing and Tween 80 on the Antifungal Susceptibility Testing of Essential Oils. *Microbiol. Immunol.* **2001**, *45*, 201–208. [CrossRef] [PubMed]
23. Abarca, R.L.; Rodríguez, F.J.; Guarda, A.; Galotto, M.J.; Bruna, J.E. Characterization of beta-cyclodextrin inclusion complexes containing an essential oil component. *Food Chem.* **2016**, *196*, 968–975. [CrossRef] [PubMed]
24. Wang, T.; Li, B.; Si, H.; Lin, L.; Chen, L. Release characteristics and antibacterial activity of solid state eugenol/β-cyclodextrin inclusion complex. *J. Incl. Phenom. Macrocycl. Chem.* **2011**, *71*, 207–213. [CrossRef]
25. Astray, G.; Gonzalez-Barreiro, C.; Mejuto, J.C.; Rial-Otero, R.; Simal-Gándara, J. A review on the use of cyclodextrins in foods. *Food Hydrocoll.* **2009**, *23*, 1631–1640. [CrossRef]
26. Zhou, Y.; Sun, S.; Bei, W.; Zahi, M.R.; Yuan, Q.; Liang, H. Preparation and antimicrobial activity of oreganoessential oil Pickering emulsion stabilized by cellulose nanocrystals. *Int. J. Biol. Macromol.* **2018**, *112*, 7–13. [CrossRef]
27. Halcón, L.; Milkus, K. Staphylococcus aureus and wounds: A review of tea tree oil as a promising antimicrobial. *Am. J. Infect. Control.* **2004**, *32*, 4002–4008. [CrossRef]
28. Karpanen, T.J.; Worthington, T.; Hendry, E.R.; Conway, B.R.; Lambert, P.A. Antimicrobial efficacy of chlorhexidine digluconate alone and in combination with eucalyptus oil, tea tree oil and thymol against planktonic and biofilm cultures of *Staphylococcus epidermidis*. *J. Antimicrob. Chemother.* **2008**, *62*, 1031–1036. [CrossRef]
29. Kwiecinski, J.; Eick, S.; Wojcik, K. Effects of tea tree (*Melaleuca alternifolia*) oil on *Staphylococcus aureus* in biofilms and stationary growth phase. *Int. J. Antimicrob. Agents* **2009**, *33*, 343–347. [CrossRef]
30. Sudjana, A.N.; Carson, C.F.; Carson, K.C.; Riley, T.V.; Hammer, K.A. *Candida albicans* adhesion to human epithelial cells and polystyrene and formation of biofilm is reduced by sub-inhibitory *Melaleuca alternifolia* (tea tree) essential oil. *Med. Mycol.* **2012**, *50*, 863–870. [CrossRef]
31. Schillaci, D.; Arizza, V.; Dayton, T.; Camarda, L.; Di Stefano, V. In vitro anti-biofilm activity of *Boswellia spp. oleogum* resin essential oils. *Lett. Appl. Microbiol.* **2008**, *47*, 433–438. [CrossRef] [PubMed]
32. Vázquez-Sánchez, D.; Cabo, M.L.; Rodríguez-Herrera, J.J. Antimicrobial activity of essential oils against *Staphylococcus aureus* biofilms. *Food Sci. Technol. Int.* **2014**, *21*, 559–570. [CrossRef] [PubMed]
33. Olivier, E.I. Antimicrobial activities of selected essential oils against *Fusarium oxysporum* isolates and their biofilms. *S. Afr. J. Bot.* **2015**, *99*, 115–121.
34. Saharkhiz, M.J.; Motamedi, M.; Zomorodian, K.; Pakshir, K.; Miri, R.; Hemyari, K. Chemical Composition, Antifungal and Antibiofilm Activities of the Essential Oil of *Mentha piperita* L. *ISRN Pharm.* **2012**, *2012*, 718645. [CrossRef] [PubMed]
35. Lee, K.; Lee, J.H.; Kim, S.I.; Cho, M.H.; Lee, J. Anti-biofilm, anti-hemolysis, and anti-virulence activities of black pepper, cananga, myrth oils, and nerolidol against *Staphylococcus aureus*. *Appl. Microbiol. Biotechnol.* **2014**, *98*, 9447–9457. [CrossRef] [PubMed]
36. Gursoy, U.K.; Gursoy, M.; Gursoy, O.V.; Cakmakci, L.; Könönen, E.; Uitto, V.J. Anti-biofilm properties of *Satureja hortensis* L. essential oil against periodontal pathogens. *Anaerobe* **2009**, *15*, 164–167. [CrossRef] [PubMed]
37. Gomes, F.; Teixeira, P.; Cerca, N.; Azeredo, J.; Oliveira, R. Effect of Farnesol on Structure and Composition of *Staphylococcus epidermidis* Biofilm Matrix. *Curr. Microbiol.* **2011**, *63*, 354–359. [CrossRef] [PubMed]
38. Sepahi, E.; Tarighi, S.; Ahmadi, F.S.; Bagheri, A. Inhibition of quorum sensing in *Pseudomonas aeruginosa* by two herbal essential oils from Apiaceae family. *J. Microbiol.* **2015**, *53*, 176–180. [CrossRef]
39. Pratiwi, S.U.T.; Lagendijk, E.L.; de Weert, S.; Idroes, R.; Hertiani, T.; Van den Hondel, C. Effect of Cinnamomum burmannii Nees ex Bl. and Massoiaaromatica Becc. Essential oils on planktonic growth and biofilm formation of *Pseudomonas aeruginosa* and *Staphylococcus aureus* In Vitro. *Int. J. Appl. Res. Nat. Prod.* **2015**, *8*, 1–13.
40. Camporese, A. In vitro activity of *Eucalyptus smithii* and *Juniperus communis* essential oils against bacterial biofilms and efficacy perspectives of complementary inhalation therapy in chronic and recurrent upper respiratory tract infections. *Infez Med.* **2013**, *2*, 117–124.
41. Benbelaïd, F.; Khadir, A.; Abdoune, M.A.; Bendahou, M.; Muselli, A.; Costa, J. Antimicrobial activity of some essential oils against oral multidrugresistant *Enterococcus faecalis* in both planktonic and biofilm state. *Asian Pac. J. Trop. Biomed.* **2014**, *4*, 463–472. [CrossRef]
42. Negreiros, M.; Pawlowski, Â.; Zini, C.A.; Soares, G.L.G.; Motta, A.; Frazzon, A.P.G. Antimicrobial and antibiofilm activity of *Baccharis psiadioides* essential oil against antibiotic-resistant *Enterococcus faecalis* strains. *Pharm. Biol.* **2016**, *54*, 3272–3279. [CrossRef]
43. Zhou, L.; Zheng, H.; Tang, Y.; Yu, W.; Gong, Q. Eugenol inhibits quorum sensing at sub-inhibitory concentrations. *Biotechnol. Lett.* **2013**, *35*, 631–637. [CrossRef]
44. Palmeira-de-Oliveira, A.; Gaspar, C.; Palmeira-de-Oliveira, R.; Silva-Dias, A.; Salgueiro, L.; Cavaleiro, C.; Pina-Vaz, C.; Martinez-de-Oliveira, J.; Queiroz, J.A.; Rodrigues, A.G. The anti-Candida activity of *Thymbra capitata* essential oil: Effect upon pre-formed biofilm. *J. Ethnopharmacol.* **2012**, *140*, 379–383. [CrossRef]
45. Dalleau, S.; Cateau, E.; Berges, T.; Berjeaud, J.M.; Imbert, C. In vitro activity of terpenes against Candida biofilms. *Int. J. Antimicrob. Agents* **2008**, *31*, 572–576. [CrossRef] [PubMed]
46. Avcioglu, N.H.; Sahal, G.; Bilkay, I.S. Antibiofilm effects of citrus limonum and zingiber officinale oils on biofilm formation of Klebsiella ornithinolytica, Klebsiella oxytoca and klebsiella terrigena species. *Afr. J. Tradit. Complement. Altern. Med.* **2016**, *13*, 61–67. [CrossRef] [PubMed]

47. Kerekes, E.B.; Vidács, A.; Takó, M.; Petkovits, T.; Vágvölgyi, C.; Horváth, G.; Balázs, V.L.; Krisch, J. Anti-Biofilm Effect of Selected Essential Oils and Main Components on Mono- and Polymicrobic Bacterial Cultures. *Microorganisms* **2015**, *7*, 345. [CrossRef] [PubMed]
48. Rosato, A.; Sblano, S.; Salvagno, L.; Carocci, A.; Clodoveo, M.L.; Corbo, F.; Fracchiolla, G. Anti-Biofilm Inhibitory Synergistic Effects of Combinations of Essential Oils and Antibiotics. *Antibiotics* **2020**, *9*, 637. [CrossRef] [PubMed]
49. Teles, R.P.; Teles, F.R.F. Antimicrobial agents used in the control of periodontal biofilms: Effective adjuncts to mechanical plaque control. *Braz. Oral. Res.* **2009**, *23*, 39–48. [CrossRef]
50. Martos, J.; Ferrer Luque, C.M.; González-Rodríguez, M.P.; Arias-Moliz, M.T.; Baca, P. Antimicrobial activity of essential oils and chloroform alone and combinated with cetrimide against *Enterococcus faecalis* biofilm. *Eur. J. Microbiol. Immunol.* **2013**, *3*, 44–48. [CrossRef]
51. Venkateshbabu, N.; Anand, S.; Abarajithan, M.; Sheriff, S.O.; Jacob, P.S.; Sonia, N. Natural therapeutic options in endodontics—A review. *Open Dent. J.* **2016**, *10*, 214–226. [CrossRef] [PubMed]
52. Santamaria, M., Jr.; Petermann, K.D.; Vedovello, A.S.; Degan, V.; Lucato, A.; Franzinic, C.M. Antimicrobial effect of *Melaleuca alternifolia* dental gel in orthodontic patients. *Am. J. Orthod. Dentofac. Orthop.* **2014**, *145*, 198–202. [CrossRef] [PubMed]
53. Carson, C.F.; Hammer, K.A.; Riley, T.V. *Melaleuca alternifolia* (Tea Tree) Oil: A Review of Antimicrobial and Other Medicinal Properties. *Clin. Microbiol. Rev.* **2006**, *19*, 50–62. [CrossRef] [PubMed]
54. Smith, K.; Robertson, D.P.; Lappin, D.F.; Ramage, G. Commercial mouth washes are ineffective against oral MRSA biofilms. *Oral Med.* **2013**, *115*, 624–629.
55. Stanecu, F.; Bancescu, G.; Constantinescu, M.V.; Defta, C. Microbial biofilm as a form of bacteria high organization and communication. *Rom. J. Stomatol.* **2012**, *58*, 284–290.
56. Nostro, A.; SudanoRoccaro, A.; Bisignano, G.; Marino, A.; Cannatelli, M.A.; Pizzimenti, F.C.; Cioni, P.L.; Procopio, F.; Blanco, A.R. Effects of oregano, carvacrol and thymol on *Staphylococcus aureus* and *Staphylococcus epidermidis* biofilms. *J. Med. Microbiol.* **2007**, *56*, 519–523. [CrossRef]
57. Cortelli, S.C.; Costa, F.O.; Rode, S.; Haas, A.N.; Pintode Andrade, A.K.; Pannuti, C.M.; Escobar, E.C.; de Almeida, E.R.; Cortelli, J.R.; Pedrazzi, V.; et al. Mouthrinserecommendation for prosthodontic patients. *Braz. Oral Res.* **2014**, *28*, 1–9. [CrossRef]
58. Marsh, P.D. Controlling the oral biofilm with antimicrobials. *J. Dent.* **2010**, *38*, S11–S15. [CrossRef]
59. Haas, A.N.; Pannuti, C.M.; Andrade, A.K.P.; Escobar, E.C.; Almeida, E.R.; Costa, F.O.; Cortelli, J.R.; Cortelli, S.C.; Rode, S.; Pedrazzi, V.; et al. Mouthwashes for the control of supragingival biofilm and gingivitis in orthodontic patients: Evidence-based recommendations for clinicians. *Braz. Oral. Res.* **2014**, *28*, 1–8. [CrossRef]
60. Quintas, V.; Prada-López, I.; Prados-Frutos, J.C.; Tomás, I. In situ antimicrobial activity on oral biofilm: Essential oils vs. 0.2% chlorhexidine. *Clin. Oral Investig.* **2015**, *19*, 97–107. [CrossRef] [PubMed]
61. Quintas, V.; Prada-López, I.; Donos, N.; Suárez-Quintanilla, D.; Tomás, I. Antiplaque Effect of Essential Oils and 0.2% Chlorhexidine on an In Situ Model of Oral Biofilm Growth: A Randomised Clinical Trial. *PLoS ONE* **2015**, *10*, e0117177. [CrossRef] [PubMed]
62. Erriu, M.; Pili, F.M.G.; Tuveri, E.; Pigliacampo, D.; Scano, A.; Montaldo, C.; Piras, V.; Denotti, G.; Pilloni, A.; Garau, V.; et al. Oil Essential Mouthwashes Antibacterial Activity against Aggregati bacteractinomycetemcomitans: A Comparison between Antibiofilm and Antiplanktonic Effects. *Int. J. Dent.* **2013**, *164267*. [CrossRef]
63. Sun, F.C.; Engelman, E.E.; McGuire, J.A. Impact of an Anticaries Mouthrinse on In Vitro Remineralization and Microbial Control. *Int. J. Dent.* **2014**, *2014*, 982071. [CrossRef] [PubMed]
64. Rasooli, I.; Shayegh, S.; Taghizadeh, M.; Astaneh, S.D.A. Phytotherapeutic Prevention of Dental Biofilm Formation. *Phytother. Res.* **2008**, *22*, 1162–1167. [CrossRef]
65. Hofer, D.; Meier, A.; Sener, B.; Guggenheim, B.; Attin, T.; Schmidlin, P.R. Biofilm reduction and staining potential of a 0.05% chlorhexidine rinse containing essential oils. *Int. J. Dent. Hyg.* **2011**, *9*, 60–67. [CrossRef] [PubMed]
66. Apolonio, J.; Faleiro, M.L.; Miguel, M.G.; Neto, L. No induction of antimicrobial resistance in *Staphylococcus aureus* and *Listeria monocytogenes* during continuous exposure to eugenol and citral. *FEMS Microbiol. Lett.* **2014**, *354*, 92–101.
67. Bersan, S.M.F.; Galvão, L.C.C.; Goes, V.F.F. Action of essential oils from Brazilian native and exotic medicinal species on oral biofilms. *BMC Complement. Altern. Med.* **2014**, *14*, 1–12. [CrossRef] [PubMed]
68. Pedrazzi, V.; Escobar, E.C.; Cortelli, J.R.; Haas, A.N.; Pintode Andrade, A.K.; Pannuti, C.M.; Rodriguesde Almeida, E.; Costa, F.O.; Cortelli, S.C.; de Mello Rode, S. Antimicrobial mouth rinse use as an adjunct method in peri-implant biofilmcontrol. *Braz. Oral Res.* **2014**, *28*, 1–9. [CrossRef] [PubMed]
69. Marinković, J.; Ćulafić, D.M.; Nikolić, B.; Đukanović, S.; Marković, T.; Tasić, G.; Ćirić, A.; Marković, D. Antimicrobial potential of irrigants based on essential oils of *Cymbopogon martinii* and *Thymus zygis* towards in vitro multispecies biofilm cultured in ex vivo root canals. *Arch. Oral Biol.* **2020**, *117*, 104842. [CrossRef]
70. Jongsma, M.A.; van der Mei, H.C.; Atema-Smit, J.; Busscher, H.J.; Ren, Y. In vivo biofilm formation on stainless steel bonded retainers during different oral health-care regimens. *Int. J. Oral Sci.* **2015**, *7*, 42–48. [CrossRef]
71. Braga, A.S.; de Melo Simas, L.L.; Pires, J.G.; Martines Souza, B.; de Souza Rosa de Melo, F.P.; Saldanha, L.L.; Dokkedal, A.L.; Magalhães, A.C. Antibiofilm and anti-caries effects of an experimental mouth rinse containing *Matricaria chamomilla* L. extract under microcosm biofilm on enamel. *J. Dent.* **2020**, *99*, 103415. [CrossRef] [PubMed]

72. Rasooli, I.; Shayegh, S.; Astaneh, S. The effect of *Mentha spicata* and *Eucalyptus camaldulensis* essential oils on dental biofilm. *Int. J. Dent. Hyg.* **2009**, *7*, 196–203. [CrossRef] [PubMed]
73. Kouidhi, B.; Mohammed, Y.A.; Qurashi, A.L.; Chaieb, K. Drug resistance of bacterial dental biofilm and the potential use of natural compounds as alternative for prevention and treatment. *Microb. Pathog.* **2015**, *80*, 39–49. [CrossRef] [PubMed]
74. de Carvalho Galváo, L.C.; Furletti, V.F.; Bersan, S.M.F.; da Cunha, M.G.; Ruiz, A.L.T.G.; Ernesto de Carvalho, J.; Sartoratto, A.; Rehder, V.L.G.; Figueira, G.M.; Duarte, M.C.T.; et al. Antimicrobial activity of essential oils against *Streptococcus mutans* and their antiproliferative effects. *Evid. Based Complement. Altern. Med.* **2012**. [CrossRef]
75. Wongsariya, K.; Phanthong, P.; Bunyapraphatsara, N.; Srisukh, V.; Chomnawang, M.T. Synergistic interaction and mode of action of *Citrus hystrix* essential oil against bacteria causing periodontal diseases. *Pharm. Biol.* **2014**, *52*, 273–280. [CrossRef]
76. Pedrazzi, V.; Leite, M.F.; Tavares, C.R.; Sato, S.; do Nascimento, G.C.; Issa, J.P.M. Herbal mouthwash containing extracts of *Baccharis dracunculifoliaas* agent for the control of biofilm: Clinical evaluation in humans. *Sci. World J.* **2015**. [CrossRef]
77. Lee, K.H.; Kim, B.S.; Keum, K.S.; Yu, H.H.; Kim, Y.-H.; Chang, B.-S.; Ra, J.-Y.; Moon, H.-D.; Seo, B.-R.; Choi, N.-Y.; et al. Essential oil of Curcuma longa inhibits Streptococcus mutans biofilm formation. *J. Food Sci.* **2011**, *76*. [CrossRef] [PubMed]
78. Peraltaa, S.L.; Carvalhob, P.H.A.; van de Sandea, F.H.; Pereirac, C.M.P.; Pivaa, E.; Lund, R.G. Self-etching dental adhesive containing a natural essential oil: Anti-biofouling performance and mechanical properties. *Biofouling* **2013**, *29*, 345–355. [CrossRef] [PubMed]
79. Furletti, V.F.; Teixeira, L.P.; Obando-Pereda, G. Action of *Coriandrum sativum* L. essential oil upon oral *Candida albicans* biofilm formation. *Evid. Based Complement. Altern. Med.* **2011**. [CrossRef]
80. Oliveira, S.A.; Zambrana, J.R.; Iorio, F.B.; Pereira, C.A.; Jorge, A.O. The antimicrobial effects of *Citrus limonum* and *Citrus aurantium* essential oils on multi-species biofilms. *Braz. Oral. Res.* **2014**, *28*, 22–27. [CrossRef]
81. Freires, I.A.; Bueno-Silva, B.; Câmara de Carvalho Galvão, L.; Duarte, M.C.T.; Sartoratto, A.; Figueira, G.M.; de Alencar, S.M.; Rosalen, P.L. The effect of essential oils and bioactive fractions on *Streptococcus mutans* and *Candida albicans* biofilms: A confocal analysis. *Evid. Based Complement. Altern. Med.* **2015**. [CrossRef]
82. de Almeida Freires, I.; Murata, R.M.; Furletti, V.F. *Coriandrum sativum* L. (Coriander) essential oil: Antifungal activity and mode of action on *Candida* spp., and molecular targets affected in human whole-genome expression. *PLoS ONE* **2014**, *9*, e099086. [CrossRef]
83. Alves, F.R.F.; Neves, M.A.S.; Silva, M.G.; Rôcas, I.N.; Siqueira, J.F., Jr. Antibiofilm and antibacterial activities of farnesol and xylitol as potential endodontic irrigants. *Braz. Dent. J.* **2013**, *24*, 224–229. [CrossRef] [PubMed]
84. Anghel, I.; Grumezescu, A.M.; Holban, A.M.; Ficai, A.; Anghel, A.G.; Chifiriuc, M.C. Biohybrid nanostructured iron oxide nanoparticles and *Satureja hortensis* to prevent fungal biofilm development. *Int. J. Mol. Sci.* **2013**, *14*, 18110–18123. [CrossRef] [PubMed]
85. Park, H.; Jang, C.H.; Cho, Y.B.; Choi, C.H. Antibacterial effect of Tea-tree oil on methicillin-resistant *Staphylococcus aureus* biofilm formation of the tympanostomy tube: An in vitro study. *In Vivo* **2007**, *21*, 1027–1030.
86. Brady, A.J.; Farnan, T.B.; Toner, J.G.; Gilpin, D.F.; Tunney, M.M. Treatment of a cochlear implant biofilm infection: A potential role for alternative antimicrobial agents. *Ann. Otol. Rhinol. Laryngol.* **2010**, *124*, 729–738. [CrossRef]
87. Malic, S.; Jordan, R.P.C.; Waters, M.G.J.; Stickler, D.J.; Williamsa, D.W. Biocide activity against urinary catheter pathogen. *Antim. Agents Chemother.* **2014**, *58*, 1192–1194. [CrossRef]
88. Saviuc, C.; Dascălu, L.; Chifiriuc, M.C.; Rădulescu, V.; Oprea, E.; Popa, M.; Hristu, R.; Stanciu, G.; Lazăr, V. The inhibitory activity of pomelo essential oil on the bacterial biofilms development on soft contact lenses. *Roum. Arch. Microbiol. Immunol.* **2010**, *69*, 145–152.
89. Gbenou, J.D.; Ahounou, J.F.; Akakpo, H.B.; Laleye, A.; Yayi, E.; Gbaguidi, F.; Baba-Moussa, L.; Darboux, R.; Dansou, P.; Moudachirou, M.; et al. Phytochemical composition of *Cymbopogon citratus* and *Eucalyptus citriodora* essential oils and their anti-inflammatory and analgesic properties on Wistar rats. *Mol. Biol. Rep.* **2013**, *40*, 1127–1134. [CrossRef]
90. Nassar, M.I.; Gaara, A.H.; El-Ghorab, A.H.; Farrag, A.-R.H.; Shen, H.; Huq, E.; Mabry, T. Chemical constituents of Clove (*Syzygium aromaticum*, Fam. Myrtaceae) and their antioxidant activity. *Rev Latinoamer. Quím.* **2007**, *35*, 47–57.
91. Khan, M.S.A.; Ahmad, I. Biofilm inhibition by *Cymbopogon citratus* and *Syzygium aromaticum* essential oils in the strains of Candida albicans. *J. Ethnopharmacol.* **2012**, *140*, 416–423. [CrossRef]
92. Kim, Y.G.; Lee, J.H.; Kim, S.I.; Baek, K.H.; Lee, J. Cinnamon bark oil and its components inhibit biofilm formation and toxin production. *Int. J. Food Microbiol.* **2015**, *195*, 30–39. [CrossRef]
93. Chmit, M.; Kanaan, H.; Habib, J.; Abbass, M.; Mcheik, A.; Chokr, A. Antibacterial and antibiofilm activities of polysaccharides, essential oil, and fatty oil extracted from *Laurus nobilis* growing in Lebanon. *Asian Pac. J. Trop. Med.* **2014**, *7*, S546–S552. [CrossRef]
94. Caredda, A.; Marongiu, B.; Porcedda, S.; Soro, C. Supercritical carbon dioxide extraction and characterization of *Laurus nobilis* essential oil. *J. Agric. Food Chem.* **2002**, *50*, 1492–1496. [CrossRef]
95. Nostro, A.; Scaffaro, R.; D'Arrigo, M.; Botta, L.; Filocamo, A.; Marino, A.; Bisignano, G. Development and characterization of essential oil component-based polymer films: A potential approach to reduce bacterial biofilm. *Appl. Microbiol. Biotechnol.* **2013**, *97*, 9515–9523. [CrossRef]
96. Coughlan, L.M.; Cotter, P.D.; Hill, C.; Alvarez-Ordóñez, A. New weapons to fight old enemies: Novel strategies for the (bio)control of bacterial biofilms in the food industry. *Front. Microbiol.* **2016**. [CrossRef]

97. Giaouris, E.; Heir, E.; Hébraud, M.; Chorianopoulos, N.; Langsrud, S.; Møretrø, T.; Habimana, O.; Desvaux, M.; Renier, S.; Nychas, G.J. Attachment and biofilm formation by foodborne bacteria in meat processing environments: Causes, implications, role of bacterial interactions and control by alternative novel methods. *Meat Sci.* **2014**, *97*, 298–309. [CrossRef] [PubMed]
98. Znini, M.; Bouklah, M.; Majidi, L.; Kharchouf, S.; Aouniti, A.; Bouyanzer, A.; Hammouti, B.; Costa, J.; Al-Deyab, S.S. Chemical composition and inhibitory effect of *Mentha spicata* essential oil on the corrosion of steel in molar hydrochloric acid. *Int. J. Electrochem. Sci.* **2011**, *6*, 691–704.
99. Gachkar, L.; Yadegari, D.; Rezaei, M.B.; Taghizadeh, M.; Astaneh, S.A.; Rasooli, I. Chemical and biological characteristics of *Cuminum cyminum* and *Rosmarinus officinalis* essential oils. *Food Chem.* **2007**, *102*, 898–904. [CrossRef]
100. Valeriano, C.; de Oliveira, T.L.C.; de Carvalhoa, S.M.; das Graças Cardoso, M.; Alves, E.; Piccoli, R.H. The sanitizing action of essential oil-based solutions against *Salmonella enterica* serotype *Enteritidis* S64 biofilm formation on AISI 304 stainless steel. *Food Control* **2012**, *25*, 673–677. [CrossRef]
101. Piovezan, M.; Uchida, N.S.; da Silva, A.F.; Grespan, R.; Santos, P.R.; Silva, E.L.; Cuman, R.K.N.; Machinski Junior, M.; Mikcha, J.M.G. Effect of cinnamon essential oil and cinnamaldehyde on *Salmonella* Saintpaul biofilm on a stainless steel surface. *J. Gen. Appl. Microbiol.* **2014**, *60*, 119–121. [CrossRef]
102. Karampoula, F.; Giaouris, E.; Deschamps, J.; Doulgeraki, A.I.; Nychas, G.-J.E.; Dubois-Brissonnet, F. Hydrosol of *Thymbra capitata* is a highly efficient biocide against *Salmonella enterica* serovar *Typhimurium* biofilms. *Appl. Environ. Microbiol.* **2016**, *82*, 5309–5319. [CrossRef]
103. Liu, Q.; Niu, H.; Zhang, W.; Mu, H.; Sun, C.; Duan, J. Synergy among thymol, eugenol, berberine, cinnamaldehyde and streptomycin against planktonic and biofilm-associated food-borne pathogens. *Lett. Appl. Microbiol.* **2015**, *60*, 421–430. [CrossRef]
104. Laird, K.; Armitage, D.; Phillips, C. Reduction of surface contamination and biofilms of *Enterococcus* sp. and *Staphylococcus aureus* using a citrus-based vapour. *J. Hosp. Infect.* **2012**, *80*, 61–66. [CrossRef] [PubMed]
105. Qayyum, S.; Khan, A.U. Nanoparticles vs. biofilms: A battle against another paradigm of antibiotic resistance. *Med. Chem. Commun.* **2016**, *7*, 1479–1498. [CrossRef]
106. Chifiriuc, M.C.; Grumezescu, V.; Grumezescu, A.M.; Saviuc, C.; Lazăr, V.; Andronescu, E. Hybrid magnetite nanoparticles/*Rosmarinus officinalis* essential oil nanobiosystem with antibiofilm activity. *Nanoscale Res. Lett.* **2012**, *7*, 209. [CrossRef] [PubMed]
107. Iannitelli, A.; Grande, R.; Di Stefano, A.; Di Giulio, M.; Sozio, P.; Bessa, L.J.; Laserra, S.; Paolini, C.; Protasi, F.; Cellini, L. Potential antibacterial activity of carvacrol-loaded poly(DL-lactide-co-glycolide) (PLGA) nanoparticles against microbial biofilm. *Int. J. Mol. Sci.* **2011**, *12*, 5039–5051. [CrossRef]
108. Bilcu, M.; Grumezescu, A.M.; Oprea, A.E.; Popescu, R.C.; Mogoșanu, G.D.; Hristu, R.; Stanciu, G.A.; Mihailescu, D.F.; Lazar, V.; Bezirtzoglou, E.; et al. Efficiency of vanilla, patchouli and ylang ylang essential oils stabilized by iron oxide@C14 nanostructures against bacterial adherence and biofilms formed by *Staphylococcus aureus* and *Klebsiella pneumoniae* clinical strains. *Molecules* **2014**, *19*, 17943–17956. [CrossRef]
109. Liakos, I.L.; Grumezescu, A.M.; Holban, A.M.; Florin, I.; D'Autilia, F.; Carzino, R.; Bianchini, P.; Athanassiou, A. Polylacticacid-lemongrass essential oil nanocapsules with antimicrobial properties. *Pharmaceuticals* **2016**, *9*, 42. [CrossRef]
110. Grumezescu, A.M.; Andronescu, E.; Oprea, A.E.; Holban, A.M.; Socol, G.; Grumezescu, V.; Chifiriuc, M.C.; Iordache, F.; Maniu, H. MAPLE fabricated magnetite@ *Melissa officinalis* and polylactic acid: Chitosan coated surfaces with anti-staphylococcal properties. *J. Sol-Gel Sci. Technol.* **2015**, *73*, 612–619. [CrossRef]
111. Giongo, J.L.; de Almeida Vaucher, R.; Fausto, V.P.; Quatrin, P.M.; Lopes, L.Q.S.; Santos, R.C.V.; Gündel, A.; Gomes, P.; Steppe, M. Anti-*Candida* activity assessment of *Pelargonium graveolens* oil free and nanoemulsion in biofilm formation in hospital medical supplies. *Microb. Pathog.* **2016**, *100*, 170–178. [CrossRef] [PubMed]
112. Shemesh, R.; Krepker, M.; Natan, M.; Danin-Poleg, Y.; Banin, E.; Kashi, Y.; Nitzan, N.; Vaxman, A.; Segal, E. Novel LDPE/halloysite nanotube films with sustained carvacrol release for broad-spectrum antimicrobial activity. *RSC Adv.* **2015**, *5*, 87108–87117. [CrossRef]

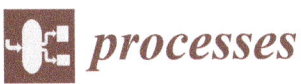

Review

Combination Therapy Involving *Lavandula angustifolia* and Its Derivatives in Exhibiting Antimicrobial Properties and Combatting Antimicrobial Resistance: Current Challenges and Future Prospects

Wye-Hong Leong [1], Kok-Song Lai [2] and Swee-Hua Erin Lim [2,*]

[1] School of Medicine, Perdana University-Royal College of Surgeons in Ireland, Kuala Lumpur 50490, Malaysia; kennethleong9607@gmail.com
[2] Health Sciences Division, Abu Dhabi Women's College, Higher Colleges of Technology, Abu Dhabi 41012, United Arab Emirates; lkoksong@hct.ac.ae
* Correspondence: erinlimsh@gmail.com

Citation: Leong, W.-H.; Lai, K.-S.; Lim, S.E. Combination Therapy Involving *Lavandula angustifolia* and Its Derivatives in Exhibiting Antimicrobial Properties and Combatting Antimicrobial Resistance: Current Challenges and Future Prospects. *Processes* **2021**, *9*, 609. https://doi.org/10.3390/pr9040609

Academic Editor: Elwira Sieniawska

Received: 13 December 2020
Accepted: 29 December 2020
Published: 30 March 2021

Publisher's Note: MDPI stays neutral with regard to jurisdictional claims in published maps and institutional affiliations.

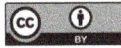

Copyright: © 2021 by the authors. Licensee MDPI, Basel, Switzerland. This article is an open access article distributed under the terms and conditions of the Creative Commons Attribution (CC BY) license (https://creativecommons.org/licenses/by/4.0/).

Abstract: Antimicrobial resistance (AMR) has been identified as one of the biggest health threats in the world. Current therapeutic options for common infections are markedly limited due to the emergence of multidrug resistant pathogens in the community and the hospitals. The role of different essential oils (EOs) and their derivatives in exhibiting antimicrobial properties has been widely elucidated with their respective mechanisms of action. Recently, there has been a heightened emphasis on lavender essential oil (LEO)'s antimicrobial properties and wound healing effects. However, to date, there has been no review published examining the antimicrobial benefits of lavender essential oil, specifically. Previous literature has shown that LEO and its constituents act synergistically with different antimicrobial agents to potentiate the antimicrobial activity. For the past decade, encapsulation of EOs with nanoparticles has been widely practiced due to increased antimicrobial effects and greater bioavailability as compared to non-encapsulated oils. Therefore, this review intends to provide an insight into the different aspects of antimicrobial activity exhibited by LEO and its constituents, discuss the synergistic effects displayed by combinatory therapy involving LEO, as well as to explore the significance of nano-encapsulation in boosting the antimicrobial effects of LEO; it is aimed that from the integration of these knowledge areas, combating AMR will be more than just a possibility.

Keywords: antimicrobial resistance; combination therapy; lavender essential oil; nanoencapsulation; synergy

1. Introduction

The phenomenon of antimicrobial resistance (AMR) has escalated substantially over the past few decades and it has been ascertained to be one of the greatest global health crisis at present [1]. AMR can be broadly categorized into three different patterns of resistance exhibited in AMR-organisms: multi-drug resistant (MDR) is defined as acquired non-susceptibility to one agent in at least three or more different antimicrobial categories, extensively-drug resistant (XDR) means non-susceptibility to at least one agent in all but two or fewer antimicrobial categories (where bacterial isolates are susceptible to agents from only one or two antimicrobial categories), and pan-drug resistant (PDR) refers to non-susceptibility to all agents in all available antimicrobial categories [2]. Emergence of different strains of drug-resistant pathogens, especially in a significant proportion of hospital-acquired infections has rendered the use of conventional antimicrobial agents ineffective worldwide [3,4]. A specific group of MDR-organisms known as the "ESKAPEE" pathogens which encompasses seven different bacteria: *Enterococcus faecium*, *Staphylococcus aureus*, *Klebsiella pneumoniae*, *Acinetobacter baumannii*, *Pseudomonas aeruginosa*, *Enterobacter* spp., and

Escherichia coli, are the leading causes of hospital-acquired or nosocomial infections [5,6]. These pathogens are also associated with a significant risk of mortality and morbidity in hospitalized patients as a consequence of therapeutic failure, resulting in considerable healthcare and economic repercussions [7]. In the United Kingdom, incidences of bloodstream infection caused by MDR-pathogens, particularly Enterobacteriaceae like *K. pneumoniae*, *E. coli*, and Gram-positive bacteria like *Enterococcus* spp. in the hospitals have steadily increased by 32% between year 2015 and 2019 [8]. Similarly, in Malaysia, the most recent National Surveillance of Antibiotic Resistance report in 2016 has noted significant increase in prevalence of meropenem-resistant *Acinetobacter baumannii* and vancomycin-resistant *Enterococcus faecium* in various hospitals, resulting in poorer patient prognosis [9]. It has been postulated that the incessant dissemination of AMR is accelerated by many extrinsic and intrinsic factors. Inappropriate and indiscriminate prescribing of antibiotics in clinical settings due to non-adherence to proper antibiotic stewardship remains as the leading extrinsic cause of the emergence of AMR [10,11]. Other extrinsic factors such as widespread and unregulated use of antibiotics in veterinary and agricultural sectors, patient's non-adherence to prescribed antibiotics and unauthorized self-prescribing of easily-available antibiotics which are over-the-counter tended to speed up the trajectory of AMR [12,13].

On the other hand, intrinsic resistance in bacteria to antibiotics is acquired through inherent or mutational changes in functional or structural attributes of both the pathogens or molecular targets. These adaptations obtained by resistant strains of pathogens are mediated by genetic mutations in the bacteria themselves or through horizontal gene transfer. Certain bacteria possess the ability to employ certain hydrolytic enzymes to inhibit the intracellular binding between the drug and the target pathogen [14]. One such example would be the production of *K. pneumoniae* carbapenemase (KPC) seen in *K. pneumoniae* which degrades antibiotics, such as the β-lactam antibiotics (including carbapenems), aminoglycosides, and fluoroquinolones, before reaching the drug-binding protein targets, eventually nullifying their antimicrobial effects [15,16]. Another essential mechanism utilized by MDR-pathogens is via the presence of active drug efflux pumps, which promotes the active transport of the antibiotics out of the bacterial cell, eventually decreasing the intracellular concentration of the drug significantly [17,18]. Efflux pump up-regulation is more commonly seen in Gram-negative organisms, particularly in biofilm-producing *P. aeruginosa*, whereby the presence of different efflux pumps confers additional biofilm resistance to different forms of antibiotics [19].

Therefore, due to the rapid spread and acceleration of life-threatening MDR-strains of pathogens, there is a dire need in researching for novel yet effective antimicrobial agents and possible alternatives involving natural products to mitigate the development of AMR. Various natural compounds with medicinal properties have been proposed as antimicrobial agents against MDR pathogens, especially when used in association with conventional antibiotics [20,21]. Plant-derived metabolites such as essential oils (EOs) have been investigated extensively for their tremendous use as antimicrobial agents [22,23]. EOs are naturally-occurring compounds which are extracted from plants and they consist of different small complexes which are lipophilic and highly volatile [24,25]. In recent years, there has been a heightened emphasis on the therapeutic benefits of lavender essential oils (LEOs) and their derivatives especially on their antimicrobial effects. LEOs (primarily *Lavandula angustifolia*) have been shown to possess an extensive array of biological properties such as analgesic, antimutagenic, anti-inflammatory, anxiolytic, and a range of antimicrobial benefits [26–30]. Furthermore, combinatorial therapies incorporating the use of EOs has been shown by numerous in vitro studies to drastically potentiate the bactericidal effects against the MDR pathogens, which can be potential approaches in mitigating AMR [31,32]. Such strategies can be adopted via a few different combinations: (i) combination of different natural adjuvants (i.e., combining LEO with one or more types of EOs), (ii) incorporation of LEO into conventional antibiotics, (iii) optimization of LEO with inclusion of nanoparticles [33]. EOs (including LEOs) have poor oral bioavailability and are chemically unstable to oxygen and humidity, which may limit their application as potential novel antimicrobial agents [34]. However, incorporation of LEOs into different types of nanoparticle delivery systems enables a more sustained and controlled release of the EOs, which enhances their antimicrobial benefits [35].

To date, there are limited reviews focusing on the antimicrobial benefits of LEOs and none elucidating the antimicrobial benefits of combinatorial therapies involving LEOs. This review aims to highlight the main antimicrobial properties that are exhibited by LEOs and their derivatives. In addition, application of different combinatorial therapies involving LEOs in augmenting their antimicrobial effects will be outlined, including the advantages of nano-based approaches in potentiating the therapeutic benefits of LEOs.

2. Components of LEO with Their Respective Antimicrobial Properties

Numerous qualitative and quantitative studies, done via different methods such as the gas chromatography, high-performance liquid chromatography and gas chromatography/mass spectrometry analyses have been conducted extensively in the past to identify the different constituents of LEOs [36,37]. Although there is a considerable amount of variation in terms of the chemical composition of different LEOs due to different areas of plant cultivation, presence of various plant genotypes and different oil extraction methods [38,39], it has been substantiated that it is the synergistic interaction from different components in the LEO that augments its antimicrobial effects.

By and large, LEO is primarily comprised of monoterpenes such as linalool, linalyl acetate, β-ocimene (both cis- and trans-) and lavandulol. Other sesquiterpenes-based compounds like β-caryophyllene and esters, such as lavandulyl acetate, can also be found in LEO [30,40]. Linalool and linalyl acetate constitute the highest proportion of chemical compounds found in extracted LEOs, with percentages ranging from 20 to 40% and 25 to 50%, respectively [41]. Table 1 illustrates the main terpene and terpenoid derivatives found abundantly in LEO that have been proven by previous studies to demonstrate promising antimicrobial properties.

Table 1. Relative abundance of main compounds found in lavender essential oil (LEO) and their antimicrobial effects from different quantitative and qualitative studies.

Chemical Components	Molecular Formula	Percentage (%)	Possible Mechanism of Action in Exhibiting Antimicrobial Effects	References
Linalool	$C_{10}H_{18}O$	20–40	Inhibition of bacterial growth. Disruption of cellular membrane.	[16,42]
Linalyl acetate	$C_{12}H_{20}O_2$	25–50	Disruption of cellular membrane.	[43,44]
β-ocimene	$C_{10}H_{16}$	3–5	Disruption of cellular membrane.	[45]
Terpinen-4-ol	$C_{10}H_{18}O$	3–8	Inhibition of bacterial growth. Disruption of cellular membrane. Inhibition of biofilm formation.	[46,47]
Eucalyptol (1,8-cineole)	$C_{10}H_{18}O$	1–4	Inhibition of bacterial growth. Disruption of cellular membrane. Inhibition of efflux pumps.	[48,49]
Camphor	$C_{10}H_{16}O$	1–10	Disruption of cellular membrane. Inhibition of biofilm formation.	[50,51]
β-caryophyllene	$C_{15}H_{24}$	2–5	Disruption of cellular membrane.	[52]
Geraniol	$C_{10}H_{18}O$	2–5	Disruption of cellular membrane. Inhibition of biofilm formation.	[53,54]
Lavandulyl acetate	$C_{12}H_{20}O_2$	3–8	Inhibition of bacterial growth.	[55]
Linalyl anthranilate	$C_7H_{23}NO_2$	2–12	Disruption of cellular membrane.	[56]

As shown in Table 1, most of the chemical compounds found in LEO exhibits their antimicrobial effects by destroying the lipid cellular membrane of the pathogens, causing increased permeability to these compounds, leakage of intracellular molecules, and eventually irreversible cellular damage. This is possibly due to the fact that LEO and most of its constituents are lipophilic in nature, which promotes the penetration and accumulation of hydrophobic LEO into the phospholipid bilayer of the cellular membrane of the microbes [57].

In previous studies, oxygenated monoterpenes like eucalyptol, linalyl acetate, and linalool are associated with greater antimicrobial effects due to their lipophilic and/or hydrophobic properties [58,59]. Therefore, it is not surprising that LEOs have been proven to possess a broad spectrum of antimicrobial capacity against different Gram-positive and Gram-negative bacteria, a number of fungi such as yeasts and dermatophytes and as well as some parasites like *Schistosoma* spp. and *Trichomonas vaginalis*. The in vitro antimicrobial activities exhibited by LEOs are screened and assessed by measuring the diameters of zones of bacterial growth inhibition, determining the minimum inhibitory concentration (MIC) and minimum bactericidal concentration or minimum fungicidal concentration (MBC/MFC) levels against different pathogens. The MIC of LEO is defined as the lowest concentration of LEO required to inhibit the growth of microbial colonies tested. On the other hand, the MBC value of LEO denotes the minimum concentration needed to kill 99.9% or more of the pathogens, which is an indicator of LEO's bactericidal activity [60,61]. These parameters are evaluated using common bioassays such as the disc-diffusion method, broth macro- and microdilution assays [62]. However, the time-kill test has been found to be the best tool to ascertain the bactericidal or fungicidal effects of LEO due to its ability to establish the presence of any dynamic interaction between LEO and the microbes; which can be concentration-dependent or time-dependent [62,63]. Table 2 shows the MIC values of different clinically relevant pathogens that are obtained from a range of in vitro studies.

Table 2. Minimum inhibitory concentration (MIC) values of LEO against various pathogens obtained from different in vitro studies.

Pathogens	MIC Values (µg/mL)	References
Gram-positive bacteria		
Staphylococcus aureus	5.0	
Listeria monocytogenes	5.5	
Staphylococcus epidermidis	4.0	[33,64–67]
Bacillus cereus	25.0	
Enterococcus faecalis	1.3	
MRSA	100.0	
Gram-negative bacteria		
Escherichia coli	10,000.0	
Klebsiella pneumoniae	10,000.0	
Pseudomonas aeruginosa	5000.0	[68–71]
Proteus mirabilis	1000.0	
Acinetobacter baumannii	2000.0	
Fungi		
Candida albicans	10.0	
Trichophyton rubrum	1.0	
Trichosporon beigelii	2.0	[71–74]
Cryptococcus neoformans	1000.0	
Aspergillus fumigatus	3000.0	

The role of LEO as an alternative antimicrobial agent warrants special attention, particularly in clinical settings against MDR-bacteria as a few studies have reported its therapeutic benefits against different MDR pathogens like *A. baumannii* and *P. aeruginosa*. Sienkiewicz et al. (2014) conducted a study to evaluate the antibacterial properties exhibited by cinnamon, geranium, and LEOs against strains of *A. baumannii* isolated from hospitals which are resistant to most conventional antibiotics, including trimethoprim/sulfamethoxazole, tobramycin, and tigecycline. MIC levels were determined using the broth microdilution method and all the EOs including LEOs have been shown to exhibit inhibitory activity against these resistant strains of *A. baumannii* [75]. In another study, Nikolic et al. (2014) evaluated the cytotoxic and antimicrobial effects of EOs from five different *Lamiaceae* species, including *L. angustifolia* through the microdilution method. Seven bacterial species consisting of *Streptococcus pyogenes*, *Streptococcus mutans*, *Streptococcus sanguis*, *Streptococcus salivarius*, *Lactobacillus acidophilus*, *Enterococcus faecalis*, and *P. aeruginosa*, along with fifty-eight other clinical isolates of oral *Candida* spp. were used in the study. All the EOs, including *L. angustifolia*, have displayed significant bactericidal and fungicidal effects against all tested microbes [76]. On the other hand, Imane et al. (2017) studied the antimicrobial effects of LEOs against three of the most common causes of nosocomial skin and soft tissue infections: *S. aureus*, *P. aeruginosa*, and *E. coli*. From the disc diffusion test, it was reported that LEO exhibited bactericidal effects against both *E. coli* and *P. aeruginosa* with MBC values of 10.67 and 85.33 µL/mL, respectively [77]. Furthermore, the antimicrobial potential and cytotoxic effects of lavender and immortelle EOs against different clinical strains of bacteria and fungi were evaluated by Mesic et al. (2018). LEOs were found to demonstrate significant growth inhibition against all tested Gram-positive and Gram-negative bacteria, including MDR strains of microbes, extended-spectrum β-lactamase (ESBL) producing *E. coli* and MRSA [78].

LEO also has potent antifungal properties against a wide spectrum of different yeasts and dermatophytes [76,78]. Multiple studies have suggested that the antimycotic properties exhibited by LEOs are the results of inhibition of biosynthesis of ergosterol, which is one of the vital components of plasma membrane in most of the fungi. This leads to destruction of the fungi cell membrane and eventually, apoptosis ensues [79,80]. D'Auria et al. (2005) reported the use of LEOs against different clinical strains of *Candida albicans* demonstrated both fungistatic and fungicidal activity in a concentration-dependent manner [81]. *C. albicans*, which is a common opportunistic pathogen found in patients who are usually immunocompromised, is said to exhibit its virulence and pathogenicity via the constant reversible transition between the hyphal and yeast form. This transition process is mediated by the formation of germ tube and the application of LEOs was said to be able to suppress the germ tube formation, hence slowing down the spread and progression of the fungal infection [81,82].

Certain degree of antiparasitic benefits in LEOs were observed in a few studies, where Moon et al. (2006) conducted a study to evaluate the antiprotozoal activities of LEOs against *Trichomonas vaginalis*, the primary cause of non-viral sexually transmitted illnesses and *Giardia duodenalis* or *Giardia lamblia*, an important cause of acute and chronic diarrhoea found usually in contaminated food or water [83–85]. LEOs have been shown to inhibit the growth of both *G. lamblia* and *T. vaginalis* in vitro completely, even at low concentrations [83]. Furthermore, LEOs were shown to possess antileishmanial properties when the use of LEOs in different concentrations were effective in inhibiting the activity of *Leishmania major* promastigotes and significantly reducing the number of amastigotes found in the macrophages [86]. Antischistosomal benefits were noticed in a study conducted by Mantovani et al. (2013), whereby incubation with LEOs exerts considerable effects against adult *Schistosoma mansoni* worms and exponentially decreases the rate of egg development after 120 h [87].

3. Combination Therapy Involving LEO

Many in vitro studies in the past have demonstrated that the combination therapies involving EOs are beneficial in potentiating their antimicrobial properties and has been countlessly recommended as a potential strategy in mitigating the worsening of AMR [88,89]. Combinatory therapy involving LEOs can be classified into three main forms of drug interaction, i.e., additivity, antagonism, and synergism. Additivity or non-interaction is said to occur when two different bioactive compounds used in combination, produces antimicrobial effects that are equal to the sum of the individual drugs [90]. When there is pronounced decline in the efficacy of the combination therapy as compared to its individual compounds, it is termed as antagonism [91]. Previous studies have hypothesized that an antagonistic interaction occurs in combination therapy involving LEOs due to combination of bacteriostatic and bactericidal agents at the same time, use of two compounds with similar mechanisms of action or presence of unfavourable physiochemical properties [92]. On the other hand, synergism, which is most favourable and preferred approach of all three, is when the combined effects of both antimicrobial agents are greater than the sum of the effects of the two individual compounds [93]. Numerous studies involving the combination therapy with LEOs in the past have given special attention to the presence of synergistic interactions due to the utilization of multitargeted antimicrobial activity, which results in marked reduction in toxicity and higher efficacy of LEOs [94,95]. Antimicrobial effects of LEOs can be augmented by employing a few different combinations: (i) between different constituents of LEOs; (ii) LEOs with other EOs; and (iii) LEOs with other antimicrobial agents.

To establish the presence of synergism between LEOs and other agents as mentioned above, different in vitro methods are used to evaluate the antimicrobial interactions in these combinatory therapies. However, the most commonly used techniques for synergy prediction is the checkerboard assay and time-kill curve methods [62,96]. Checkerboard method involves multiple combinations of LEO and other test agents in serial dilutions into different microtiter plates. The LEO combination in which the growth of microbes tested is completely inhibited will be the effective MIC value [97]. Data from the checkerboard assay expresses the antimicrobial interactions of these two compounds on the basis of plotting of isobolograms or determination of fractional inhibitory concentrations (FIC) and FIC index (FICI) [98]. The value of FIC can be expressed and calculated using the following equation:

$$FIC_{LEO} = \frac{\text{MIC of LEO in combination}}{\text{MIC of LEO when used alone}}$$

The value of FICI is obtained by addition of the FIC values of the LEO and the other compound:

$$FICI = FIC_{LEO} + FIC_{\text{other compound}} *, \qquad (1)$$

where $FIC_{\text{other compound}}$ = $MIC_{\text{other compound}}$ in combination/$MIC_{\text{other compound}}$ when used alone.

* other compound denotes substances like EOs other than LEO, constituents of LEO or conventional antibiotics.

Generally, synergistic interaction is said to be achieved when the FICI is equal or less than 0.5, additive or no interaction was seen if the FICI value was between 0.5 and 4.0 and antagonism was portrayed when the FICI is more than 4.0 [99].

The time-kill curve method allows determination of bactericidal effects of each individual compound by measuring the number of viable inoculums in the presence of a certain combination of antibacterial agents at multiple intervals [100]. Although it is time-consuming and labour-intensive, time kill assay is usually deemed as the "gold standard" in synergy prediction due to its good reproducibility and sensitivity [95].

3.1. LEO and Other Essential Oils

One of the biggest studies conducted with regard to combinatory therapy involving LEOs and other EOs was performed by de Rapper et al. (2013), where they evaluated the antimicrobial activity of LEO in combination with 45 other aroma-therapeutic oils against three different microbes: *S. aureus*, *P. aeruginosa*, and *C. albicans*. Upon investigating different ratios of different EOs in combination, FICI analysis revealed favorable interactions, whereby 26.7% of these interactions are synergistic and 48.9% are additive. Only one combination exhibited antagonistic effects (LEO and *Cymbopogon citratus*) with FICI value of 6.7. It was also found that the most optimal synergistic interactions were noted in combinations of LEO with *Cinnamomum zeylanicum* and LEO with *Citrus sinensis* when used against *C. albicans* and *S. aureus* [101]. In another study, Imane et al. (2020) assessed the antimicrobial benefits in a formulation containing the combination of three different EOs, which are LEO, *Artemisia herba alba* and *Rosmarinus officialis* EOs against common wound pathogens. Disc-diffusion assay revealed the combination of these three EOs have bactericidal effects against all the tested microbes. A synergistic effect was also seen in this combination with FICI values ranging from 0.015 to 0.5 [102]. On the other hand, Abboud et al. (2015) conducted a study to ascertain the antimicrobial activities of combined LEO and *Thymus vulgaris* EOs against common *Streptococcus* and *Staphylococcus* strains that cause bovine mastitis. Mixture of LEO and *T. vulgaris* EO has successfully demonstrated a significant decrease in these bacterial colonies in different samples of cow milk [103]. Orchard et al. (2019) conducted an in vitro study to assess the antifungal activity of 128 different combinations of EOs including LEOs against topical fungal pathogens like *C. albicans* and dermatophytes, which commonly cause superficial fungal infection like onychomycosis and ringworms. Broth microdilution methods were utilized and it was found that most of the combinations with LEOs have fungistatic or fungicidal effects against the fungal pathogens. However, from the isobologram studies, most of the interactions resulted in additivity which is slightly different as compared to previous studies [104]. Another similar study done by Cassella et al. (2002) has proven that the combination of tea tree oil (*Melaleuca alternifolia*) and LEO demonstrated significant antifungal activity against tested dermatophytes like *Trichophyton rubrum* and *Trichophyton mentagrophytes*. Isobologram and FICI analysis further revealed that the combination of *M. alternifolia* EO and LEO exhibit a synergistic antimycotic effect against both tested fungal pathogens [105]. Table 3 illustrates the FICI values of the combinatory therapy involving the use of LEOs and other EOs.

Table 3. Synergistic effects exhibited by LEO when used in combination with other EOs from different in vitro studies.

Combination of LEO and Other Essential Oils	Pathogens	MIC of LEO When Used in Combination (mg/mL)	MIC of Tested EO When Used in Combination (mg/mL)	FICI Values	Methods Used to Test for Synergism	Presence of Synergism	References
Cinnamomum zeylanicum (cinnamon)	*C. albicans* *S. aureus* *P. aeruginosa*	1.00 1.00 1.00	1.00 1.00 1.00	0.40 0.50 0.53	Checkerboard assay Isobologram	+ + 0	[101]
Citrus sinensis (sweet orange)	*C. albicans* *S. aureus* *P. aeruginosa*	1.00 1.00 1.00	1.00 1.00 1.00	0.42 0.38 0.51	Checkerboard assay Isobologram	+ + 0	[101]
Artemisia herba alba (desert wormwood)	*S. aureus* *E. coli* *P. aeruginosa*	0.02 0.02 0.02	0.02 0.02 0.02	0.03 0.25 0.50	Checkerboard assay	+ + +	[102]
Rosmarinus officialis (rosemary)	*S. aureus* *E. coli* *P. aeruginosa*	0.02 0.02 0.02	0.02 0.02 0.02	0.13 0.25 0.48	Checkerboard assay	+ + +	[102]
Allium sativum (garlic)	*C. albicans*	0.50	0.50	1.25	Isobologram	0	[104]
	T. mentagrophytes	0.13	0.13	0.23		+	
Syzygium aromaticum (clove)	*C. albicans*	2.00	2.00	1.50	Isobologram	0	[104]
	T. mentagrophytes	0.50	0.50	4.35		-	
Citrus aurantium (bitter orange)	MRSA *E. coli* *P. aeruginosa*	1.00 2.00 0.75	1.00 2.00 0.75	0.50 1.00 0.75	Checkerboard assay Isobologram	+ 0 0	[106]

+ indicates synergy; 0 indicates additivity; - indicates antagonism; MRSA: methicillin-resistant *Staphylococcus aureus*.

3.2. LEO and Antimicrobial Agents

Several studies in the past have demonstrated mostly additive or synergistic activity in combination therapy involving LEOs and conventional antibiotics. The incorporation of natural products (including LEOs) into different antibacterial agents in treating MDR-pathogens has been shown to cause irreversible disruption of bacterial cell membrane [107,108]. These hydrophobic compounds have the propensity to neutralize the lipopolysaccharide (LPS), which is found in the outer membrane of most Gram-negative bacilli. This will subsequently potentiate the bactericidal effects of the combined antimicrobial agent by promoting the influx of these agents into the bacterial cell [109,110]. Yap et al. (2014) reported synergistic interactions between LEOs and piperacillin against MDR-resistant *E. coli* J53 R1 where time-kill analysis revealed complete eradication of the bacteria. The results also indicated the LEO-piperacillin may have a role in reversing the *E. coli* resistance to piperacillin via its anti-quorum sensing effects and ability to alter *E. coli*'s outer membrane permeability [111]. A similar study was conducted involving transcriptomic analysis on the similar strains of MDR-*E. coli* to identify any presence of transcriptional changes to the MDR-*E-coli* genome upon the use of combination of LEO-piperacillin treatment [112]. Pathway enrichment analyses revealed that LEO-piperacillin use causes upregulation of certain genes which affects the biosynthesis of LPS of the bacterial cell wall and the metabolism of *E. coli* in diverse environments, which increases its susceptibility to cellular destruction [112]. In another study conducted by Kwiatkowski et al. (2020), LEO combinations with octenidine dihydrochloride (OCT), an antiseptic agent with broad bactericidal effects were thoroughly investigated. The efficiency of this combination against *S. aureus* ATCC 43300 (reference strains) and other clinical isolates was assessed with checkerboard assays and time-kill curve methods; the FICI was found to be between 0.11 and 0.26, indicating a strong synergistic effect. Further Fourier transform infrared (FTIR) spectroscopy revealed that the combination of LEO/OCT causes modification of cell wall in MRSA, augmenting the penetration of LEO/OCT into the cells [113]. On the other hand, LEO along with the use of chloramphenicol exhibited clear synergism against the Gram-negative *P. aeruginosa*, with the FICI of 0.29. Isobologram analysis further revealed that LEO was able to interact synergistically with many of the conventional antibiotics when combined in ratios with higher proportions of LEO. This is probably the first huge-scaled study focusing on the beneficial effects of LEO when used in combination with other antimicrobial agents [114]. Another study conducted by Yang et al. (2020) detected the presence of synergistic antimicrobial effects when LEOs are used concurrently with meropenem against carbapenemase-producing *K. pneumoniae*, where MIC values of both LEO and meropenem were found to be remarkably decreased. Checkerboard and time-kill assays revealed the FICI to be 0.31 and further proteomic analysis revealed the combination of LEO and meropenem causes disruption of the cellular membrane of *K. pneumoniae* via induction of oxidative stress, resulting in influx of LEO-meropenem and other generated free radicals into the bacterial cell [115]. Other than that, the incorporation of gentamicin into LEO exhibits markedly synergistic interactions when used against different strains of *S. aureus*. In contrast, no interaction was seen when LEO-gentamicin was used against *P. aeruginosa*, which coincides with findings from past studies [116]. Table 4 illustrates the FICI values of the combinatory therapy involving the use of LEOs and other conventional antimicrobial agents.

Table 4. Synergistic effects exhibited by LEO when used in combination with other antibiotics from different in vitro studies.

Combination of LEO and Different Antibiotics	Pathogens	MIC of LEO When Used in Combination (mg/mL)	MIC of Antibiotics When Used in Combination (µg/mL)	FICI Values	Methods Used to Test for Synergism	Presence of Synergism	References
Octenidine dihydrochloride	MRSA	0.12	1.71	0.16	Checkerboard assay Time-kill curve	+	[113]
Chloramphenicol	*C. albicans* *S. aureus* *P. aeruginosa*	3.00 2.00 2.00	0.63 0.31 0.31	1.00 0.75 0.29	Checkerboard assay Isobologram	0 0 +	[114]
Ciprofloxacin	*S. aureus* *P. aeruginosa*	2.00 2.00	0.11 0.04	0.49 0.74	Checkerboard assay Isobologram	+ 0	[114]
Meropenem	Carbapenemase-resistant *K. pneumoniae*	6.30	8.00	0.31	Checkerboard assay Time-kill curve	+	[115]
Gentamicin	MRSA *S. aureus* *P. aeruginosa*	0.13 0.64 2.00	0.13 0.13 0.50	0.14 0.19 0.70	Checkerboard assay	+ + 0	[116]
Piperacillin	*E. coli*	1.30	0.13	0.26	Checkerboard assay	+	[117]
Ceftazidime	*E. coli*	5.00	0.50	1.00	Checkerboard assay	0	[117]
Ketoconazole	*C. albicans*	0.16	0.06	0.53	Checkerboard assay	0	[118]

+ indicates synergy; 0 indicates additivity; MRSA: methicillin-resistant *Staphylococcus aureus*.

4. Significance of Nanotechnology in LEO Use

Nanotechnology refers to the emerging field of molecular studies, dealing with the design, production, and application of materials with size ranged between 1 and 100 nm. Previous publications have shown that the incorporation of nanoparticles into bioactive compounds like LEOs is an effective and feasible strategy in enhancing its antimicrobial effects as these materials may facilitate the delivery of LEOs into the cell, resulting in higher intracellular uptake of LEOs [119,120]. Moreover, the use of nanoencapsulation confers the ability to overcome some of the intrinsic drawbacks of LEOs mentioned previously in this review (i.e., poor oral bioavailability, highly hydrophobic and chemically unstable when being exposed to heat, moisture, or oxygen), allowing the utilization as a potential antimicrobial agent to be fully exploited [36,121]. Hence, over the last decade, nano-based approaches are frequently applied in conjunction with the use of EOs in different disciplines, including in food processing and pharmaceutical industries. The use of nanoencapsulation involving EOs encompasses a wide variety of different nanocarriers designs and materials; however, polymeric nanoparticles (i.e., chitosan and sodium alginate), lipid-based nanoparticles (i.e., liposomes, solid lipid nanoparticles, and micro- and nanoemulsions), and formation of inclusion complexes are some of the common nanosystem platforms employed for the encapsulation of EOs [122,123]. To the best of our knowledge, only a limited range of antimicrobial nanodelivery systems have been utilized into studies involving LEO-based combinatorial therapies. In fact, there is scarcity of in vitro and clinical studies investigating the antimicrobial properties of these LEOs-based nanoparticles against clinically relevant MDR-bacteria, such as *K. pneumoniae*, *P. aeruginosa*, MRSA, and *E. coli* and none reported against strains like *E. faecium* or *A. baumannii*.

One of the common nanoencapsulation strategies used in delivering LEO into the target sites effectively and augmenting its antimicrobial effects is via the formation of molecular complexes like cyclodextrins (CDs) and their derivatives. CDs are macrocyclic oligosaccharide compounds with a central hydrophobic core and outer hydrophilic surface, which plays a role in increasing the chemical stability of LEO [124]. Previous studies with other EOs have shown that complexation with cyclodextrins allows a more sustained and controlled release of the EOs and may potentiate their antimicrobial effects [125,126]. Yuan et al. (2019) investigated the biochemical properties and antimicrobial capacity of LEO when encapsulated in hydroxypropyl-β-cyclodextrin (HPCD) in comparison with non-encapsulated LEO against strains of *E. coli*, *S. aureus*, and *C. albicans*. Disc diffusion assay revealed both high bactericidal and fungicidal effects exhibited by the combination of LEO and HPCD composite against all three tested pathogens. The MIC levels of LEO/HPCD composite against those tested microbes were considerably lower when compared to the values obtained when using LEO or the composite extract alone. This marked growth in biocidal activity may be attributed to the increased LEO aqueous solubility after HPCD encapsulation, which facilitates the access of LEO into the bacterial cytoplasm and cell membrane [127]. Similar study was done by Das et al. (2019) whereby four different essential oils including LEO were encapsulated with randomly methylated β-cyclodextrin (RAMEB). The findings from this in vitro study are in accordance with the results obtained from Yuan et al., as the LEO-RAMEB inclusion complexes demonstrated remarkable antibacterial properties against *E. coli* and *S. aureus*; the antimicrobial activities were found to be elevated by at least two to four folds as compared with LEOs only [128].

Over the past decade, there has been a steady increase in publications focusing on the use of various types of polymeric nanofibres as a medium for the delivery of EOs because they demonstrated promising wound healing and antibacterial benefits [129,130]. The fabrication of these nanofibres via the electrospinning technology is considered the most versatile and feasible process where this technique is frequently adopted by fellow scientists [131]. Balasubramanian and Kodam (2014) incorporated LEOs into electrospun polyacrylonitrile (PAN) nanofibrous mats where the process of electrospinning was further facilitated by the addition of an electrolytic solution of sodium chloride with various concentrations, ranging from 0.1% to 0.3%. The antibacterial efficacy of these LEO/PAN nanofibres against different strains of *S. aureus* and *K. pneumoniae* were evaluated via disc diffusion assays and unsurprisingly, the combination of LEO/PAN exhibited clear zones of inhibition against both bacteria with MIC value of 0.1 mg/mL, which signifies excellent antibacterial activity. Cytotoxicity tests via MTT assay also revealed that the use of LEO/PAN nanofibres results in 100% cellular viability, even at a high concentration of 200μg/mL, which may suggest that PAN are suitable nanocarriers for medical applications with a low risk for cellular damage [132]. On the other hand, the biosynthesis of silver nanoparticles (AgNP) as an alternative disinfectant and antimicrobial agent has been widely described in many studies, due to its potent bactericidal properties against both Gram-positive and Gram-negative pathogens [133,134]. Sofi et al. (2019) engineered nanofibre-based wound dressings where AgNP and LEOs are simultaneously incorporated into polyurethane nanofibres. These nanofibrous wound dressings fabricated with LEOs and AgNP exhibited significant bactericidal activity against different isolates of both *S. aureus* and *E. coli*. From the in vitro tests as well, gradual increase in concentrations of both LEOs and AgNP demonstrated larger zones of inhibition for both microbes, which may be attributed to the presence of synergistic effects when these two components are combined together. From studies done on other nanoparticles, the addition of AgNP to LEOs is also said to be able to overcome the problems encountered when using polymers such as PAN and sodium alginate nanofibres, such as the presence of narrow spectrum antibacterial properties or low tensile strength [135]. Therefore, these LEOs-AgNP-polyurethrane nanofibres wound dressings have a great potential in promoting wound healing and possessing remarkable bactericidal effects against commonly seen skin pathogens.

Other forms of nanoformulations like rhamnolipid-based emulsions and inclusion of hydroxyapatite nanoparticles are becoming increasingly popular when used in combination with LEOs as these nanocarrier systems have been indicated to enhance the antimicrobial potentials of LEOs [136,137]. For the purpose of this review, studies pertaining to the antimicrobial benefits of LEOs when incorporated into different types of nanoparticles against clinically relevant pathogens are summarized in Table 5.

Table 5. The use of LEOs in combination with different nanocarrier systems in boosting their antimicrobial activities.

Encapsulation Method	Encapsulating Agent	Target Pathogens	Antimicrobial Activity	References
Inclusion complexes formation	Cyclodextrin (HPCD, RAMEB)	S. aureus E. coli C. albicans	Increases LEOs aqueous solubility, which promotes penetration into cells.	[127,128]
Nanofibres electrospinning	Polyacrylonitrile (PAN)	S. aureus K. pneumoniae	Causes membrane disruption. Inhibition of bacterial growth.	[132]
	AgNP + polyurethane	E. coli S. aureus	Causes membrane disruption. Inhibition of bacterial growth. Exhibits synergistic antimicrobial effects.	[135]
Nanoemulsion	Rhamnolipids	MRSA C. albicans	Increases LEOs aqueous solubility, which promotes penetration into cells. Causes membrane disruption.	[136]
	Refined, bleached and deodorized sunflower oil (RBDSFo)	S. aureus B. subtilis E. coli S. enterica	Causes membrane disruption. Inhibition of bacterial growth. Exhibits synergistic antimicrobial effects.	[138]
Nanoencapsulation	Hydroxyapatite	E. coli ESBL E. coli ATCC 25922 S. aureus MRSA	Causes depolarization of bacterial cell membrane. Inhibition of bacterial growth.	[137,139]
Nanoprecipitation	Starch nanoparticles	E. coli S. aureus	Causes membrane disruption. Inhibition of bacterial growth.	[140]

5. Current Challenges and Future Prospects

It is without a doubt that different strategies or approaches have to be adopted in order to slow down or mitigate the acceleration of AMR. One of the main challenges in coming up with an effective solution is that there is no "one-size-fits-all" approach in circumventing this issue. A multitude of strategies and therapies have to be applied concurrently in order to have the maximum therapeutic benefits due to the presence of a multifaceted antimicrobial mechanism. LEO and its derivatives have been shown to exhibit a broad spectrum of antimicrobial activities against many different Gram-positive and Gram-negative bacteria, fungal pathogens, and parasites. Studies in the past have also demonstrated the therapeutic benefits of combinatorial therapies involving LEO. However, there is a scarcity of information regarding the pharmacokinetics and pharmacodynamics of these combinatorial therapies involving LEO. More clinical and in vitro studies should be done to reinforce the presence of promising synergistic interactions between LEO and other essential oils or antimicrobial agents. Different clinical trials, including cytotoxicity studies on these combinatory therapies should be conducted to explore the safety and efficacy of these LEO-based formulations, with hope that these can lead to the development of formulations which will be a safe and prospective alternative for the common antibiotics when used in the clinical practice in treating infections caused by MDR-pathogens. Formulation enhancement will also enable the revival of previously sidelined antibiotics due to growing resistance.

Furthermore, there is a heightened interest in developing novel strategies involving nano-encapsulation of LEOs as these nanomolecules are able to compensate for the suboptimal physicochemical characteristics of using LEOs only. By increasing its chemical stability and solubility in water, encapsulated LEOs have more reliable and potent antimicrobial effects as compared to non-encapsulated ones due to a more sustained and controlled release of these bioactive compounds into the bacterial cells. However, there is paucity in knowledge about the detailed mechanism on how these nanoparticles have the capacity to potentiate the bactericidal and fungicidal effects of these LEOs. Moreover, only a limited array of nanodelivery systems have been explored in combination with the use of LEOs. Hence, future studies should explore the specific mechanisms of action of these nanomolecules in augmenting the antimicrobial potentials of LEOs and possibly, demonstrating any presence of synergism or additivity when LEOs are incorporated into them. More emphasis should also be placed into employing a broader range of different nanocarriers when using LEOs as a therapeutic approach in combatting AMR.

6. Conclusions

In summary, the present review has managed to highlight the importance of LEO and its derivatives as novel antimicrobial agents due to its efficacious bactericidal effects against many drug-resistant pathogens, which are the predominant causes of life-threatening hospital-acquired infections. A range of different combinatory therapies involving LEOs which are proven to exhibit potent antimicrobial benefits have been outlined, where some of these formulations may even have the potential to reverse the resistance to common antibiotics in certain bacteria. In addition, this review discussed the different forms of nanodelivery system that are employed in previous research involving LEO, where these nanocarriers have the capacity to potentiate the therapeutic benefits of LEOs. The integration of these diverse approaches may provide knowledge areas which are imperative in mitigating the threats of AMR.

Author Contributions: Conceptualization, S.-H.E.L.; resources, data curation, and writing—original draft preparation, W.-H.L.; writing—review and editing, W.-H.L. and K.-S.L.; visualization, S.-H.E.L. and K.-S.L.; supervision, project administration, and funding acquisition, S.-H.E.L. All authors have read and agreed to the published version of the manuscript.

Funding: This research was funded by the Research Excellence and Innovation Grant (REIG_2020_043) from UCSI University, Malaysia.

Institutional Review Board Statement: Not applicable.

Informed Consent Statement: Not applicable.

Data Availability Statement: No new data were created or analyzed in this study. Data sharing is not applicable to this article.

Acknowledgments: The authors would like to thank the Higher Colleges of Technology and Perdana University for making this work possible.

Conflicts of Interest: The authors declare no conflict of interest.

References

1. Shriram, V.; Khare, T.; Bhagwat, R.; Shukla, R.; Kumar, V. Inhibiting bacterial drug efflux pumps via phyto-therapeutics to combat threatening antimicrobial resistance. *Front. Microbiol.* **2018**, *9*, 2990. [CrossRef]
2. Magiorakos, A.P.; Srinivasan, A.; Carey, R.; Carmeli, Y.; Falagas, M.; Giske, C.; Harbarth, S.; Hindler, J.; Kahlmeter, G.; Olsson-Liljequist, B.; et al. Multidrug-resistant, extensively drug-resistant and pandrug-resistant bacteria: An international expert proposal for interim standard definitions for acquired resistance. *Clin. Microbiol. Infect.* **2012**, *18*, 268–281. [CrossRef]
3. Esposito, S.; De Simone, G. Update on the main MDR pathogens: Prevalence and treatment options. *Infez. Med.* **2017**, *25*, 301–310.
4. Pendleton, J.N.; Gorman, S.P.; Gilmore, B.F. Clinical relevance of the ESKAPE pathogens. *Expert Rev. Anti Infect. Ther.* **2013**, *11*, 297–308. [CrossRef] [PubMed]
5. Subramani, R.; Narayanasamy, M.; Feussner, K.D. Plant-derived antimicrobials to fight against multi-drug-resistant human pathogens. *3 Biotech* **2017**, *7*, 172. [CrossRef] [PubMed]
6. Ma, Y.X.; Wang, C.Y.; Li, Y.Y.; Li, J.; Wan, Q.Q.; Chen, J.H.; Tay, F.R.; Niu, L.N. Considerations and caveats in combating ESKAPE pathogens against nosocomial infections. *Adv. Sci.* **2020**, *7*, 1901872. [CrossRef]
7. Founou, R.C.; Founou, L.L.; Essack, S.Y. Clinical and economic impact of antibiotic resistance in developing countries: A systematic review and meta-analysis. *PLoS ONE* **2017**, *12*, e0189621. [CrossRef] [PubMed]
8. Public Health England. *English Surveillance Programme for Antimicrobial Utilisation and Resistance (ESPAUR)*; PHE: London, UK, 2020. Available online: https://www.gov.uk/government/publications/english-surveillance-programme-antimicrobial-utilisation-and-resistance-espaur-report (accessed on 26 November 2020).
9. Gerald, N.M.J. Malaysian Action Plan on Antimicrobial Resistance (MyAP-AMR) 2017-2021. Available online: https://www.moh.gov.my/moh/resources/Penerbitan/Garis%20Panduan/Garis%20panduan%20Umum%20(Awam)/National_Action_Plan_-_FINAL_29_june.pdf (accessed on 26 November 2020).
10. Laxminarayan, R.; Duse, A.; Wattal, C.; Zaidi, A.K.; Wertheim, H.F.; Sumpradit, N.; Vlieghe, E.; Hara, G.L.; Gould, I.M.; Goossens, H. Antibiotic resistance—the need for global solutions. *Lancet Infect. Dis.* **2013**, *13*, 1057–1098. [CrossRef]
11. Srivastava, J.; Chandra, H.; Nautiyal, A.R.; Kalra, S.J. Antimicrobial resistance (AMR) and plant-derived antimicrobials (PDA ms) as an alternative drug line to control infections. *3 Biotech* **2014**, *4*, 451–460. [CrossRef]
12. Ayukekbong, J.A.; Ntemgwa, M.; Atabe, A.N. The threat of antimicrobial resistance in developing countries: Causes and control strategies. *Antimicrob. Resist Infect. Control* **2017**, *6*, 47. [CrossRef]
13. Yang, S.K.; Yusoff, K.; Mai, C.W.; Lim, W.M.; Yap, W.S.; Lim, S.H.E.; Lai, K.S. Additivity vs synergism: Investigation of the additive interaction of cinnamon bark oil and meropenem in combinatory therapy. *Molecules* **2017**, *22*, 1733. [CrossRef] [PubMed]
14. Ali, J.; Rafiq, Q.A.; Ratcliffe, E. Antimicrobial resistance mechanisms and potential synthetic treatments. *Future Sci. OA* **2018**, *4*, FSO290. [CrossRef] [PubMed]
15. Sidjabat, H.; Nimmo, G.R.; Walsh, T.R.; Binotto, E.; Htin, A.; Hayashi, Y.; Li, J.; Nation, R.L.; George, N.; Paterson, D.L. Carbapenem resistance in Klebsiella pneumoniae due to the New Delhi metallo-β-lactamase. *Clin. Infect. Dis.* **2011**, *52*, 481. [CrossRef] [PubMed]
16. Yang, S.K.; Yusoff, K.; Ajat, M.; Thomas, W.; Abushelaibi, A.; Akseer, R.; Lim, S.H.E.; Lai, K.S. Disruption of KPC-producing Klebsiella pneumoniae membrane via induction of oxidative stress by cinnamon bark (*Cinnamomum verum* J. Presl) essential oil. *PLoS ONE* **2019**, *14*, e0214326. [CrossRef] [PubMed]
17. Masi, M.; Réfregiers, M.; Pos, K.M.; Pagès, J.M. Mechanisms of envelope permeability and antibiotic influx and efflux in Gram-negative bacteria. *Nat. Microbiol.* **2017**, *2*, 1–7. [CrossRef]
18. Moo, C.L.; Yang, S.K.; Yusoff, K.; Ajat, M.; Thomas, W.; Abushelaibi, A.; Lim, S.H.E.; Lai, K.S. Mechanisms of antimicrobial resistance (AMR) and alternative approaches to overcome AMR. *Curr. Drug Discov. Technol.* **2020**, *17*, 430–447. [CrossRef]
19. Soto, S.M. Role of efflux pumps in the antibiotic resistance of bacteria embedded in a biofilm. *Virulence* **2013**, *4*, 223–229. [CrossRef]
20. Gavarić, N.; Kovač, J.; Kretschmer, N.; Kladar, N.; Možina, S.S.; Bucar, F.; Bauer, R.; Božin, B.J. *Concepts, Compounds and the Alternatives of Antibacterials*; InTech: London, UK, 2015; pp. 123–152.
21. Gargano, M.L.; Zervakis, G.I.; Isikhuemhen, O.S.; Venturella, G.; Calvo, R.; Giammanco, A.; Fasciana, T.; Ferraro, V. Ecology, phylogeny, and potential nutritional and medicinal value of a rare white maitake collected in a Mediterranean forest. *Diversity* **2020**, *12*, 230. [CrossRef]
22. Solórzano-Santos, F.; Miranda-Novales, M.G. Essential oils from aromatic herbs as antimicrobial agents. *Curr. Opin. Biotechnol.* **2012**, *23*, 136–141. [CrossRef]

23. Bhavaniramya, S.; Vishnupriya, S.; Al-Aboody, M.S.; Vijayakumar, R.; Baskaran, D. Role of essential oils in food safety: Antimicrobial and antioxidant applications. *Grain Oil Sci. Technol.* **2019**, *2*, 49–55. [CrossRef]
24. Yang, S.K.; Low, L.Y.; Yap, P.S.X.; Yusoff, K.; Mai, C.W.; Lai, K.S.; Lim, S.H.E. Plant-derived antimicrobials: Insights into mitigation of antimicrobial resistance. *Rec. Nat. Prod.* **2018**, *12*, 295–316. [CrossRef]
25. Bakkali, F.; Averbeck, S.; Averbeck, D.; Idaomar, M. Biological effects of essential oils–a review. *Food Chem. Toxicol.* **2008**, *46*, 446–475. [CrossRef] [PubMed]
26. Karadag, E.; Samancioglu, S.; Ozden, D.; Bakir, E. Effects of aromatherapy on sleep quality and anxiety of patients. *Nurs. Crit. Care* **2017**, *22*, 105–112. [CrossRef] [PubMed]
27. Vakilian, K.; Atarha, M.; Bekhradi, R.; Chaman, R. Healing advantages of lavender essential oil during episiotomy recovery: A clinical trial. *Complementary Ther. Clin. Pract.* **2011**, *17*, 50–53. [CrossRef] [PubMed]
28. Evandri, M.; Battinelli, L.; Daniele, C.; Mastrangelo, S.; Bolle, P.; Mazzanti, G. The antimutagenic activity of Lavandula angustifolia (lavender) essential oil in the bacterial reverse mutation assay. *Food Chem. Toxicol.* **2005**, *43*, 1381–1387. [CrossRef] [PubMed]
29. Cardia, G.F.E.; Silva-Filho, S.E.; Silva, E.L.; Uchida, N.S.; Cavalcante, H.A.O.; Cassarotti, L.L.; Salvadego, V.E.C.; Spirinello, R.A.; Bersani-Amado, C.A.; Cuman, R.K.N. Effect of lavender (*Lavandula angustifolia*) essential oil on acute inflammatory response. *Evid. Based Complementary Altern. Med.* **2018**, *2018*, 1–10. [CrossRef] [PubMed]
30. Woronuk, G.; Demissie, Z.; Rheault, M.; Mahmoud, S. Biosynthesis and therapeutic properties of *Lavandula* essential oil constituents. *Planta Med.* **2011**, *77*, 7–15. [CrossRef]
31. Yang, S.K.; Yap, P.S.X.; Krishnan, T.; Yusoff, K.; Gan, K.C.; Yap, W.S.; Lai, K.S.; Lim, S.H.E. Mode of action: Synergistic interaction of peppermint (*Mentha x piperita* L. Carl) essential oil and meropenem against plasmid-mediated resistant *E. Coli*. *Rec. Nat. Prod.* **2018**, *12*, 582.
32. Van Vuuren, S.; Suliman, S.; Viljoen, A. The antimicrobial activity of four commercial essential oils in combination with conventional antimicrobials. *Lett. Appl. Microbiol.* **2009**, *48*, 440–446. [CrossRef]
33. Miladinović, D.L.; Ilić, B.S.; Mihajilov-Krstev, T.M.; Nikolić, N.D.; Miladinović, L.C.; Cvetković, O.G. Investigation of the chemical composition–antibacterial activity relationship of essential oils by chemometric methods. *Anal. Bioanal. Chem.* **2012**, *403*, 1007–1018. [CrossRef]
34. Trifan, A.; Luca, S.V.; Greige-Gerges, H.; Miron, A.; Gille, E.; Aprotosoaie, A.C. Recent advances in tackling microbial multidrug resistance with essential oils: Combinatorial and nano-based strategies. *Crit. Rev. Microbiol.* **2020**, *46*, 338–357. [CrossRef] [PubMed]
35. Turek, C.; Stintzing, F.C. Stability of essential oils: A review. *Compr. Rev. Food Sci. Food Saf.* **2013**, *12*, 40–53. [CrossRef]
36. Prakash, B.; Kujur, A.; Yadav, A.; Kumar, A.; Singh, P.P.; Dubey, N. Nanoencapsulation: An efficient technology to boost the antimicrobial potential of plant essential oils in food system. *Food Control* **2018**, *89*, 1–11. [CrossRef]
37. Dong, G.; Bai, X.; Aimila, A.; Aisa, H.A.; Maiwulanjiang, M. Study on lavender essential oil chemical compositions by GC-MS and improved pGC. *Molecules* **2020**, *25*, 3166. [CrossRef]
38. Cavanagh, H.M.; Wilkinson, J.M. Lavender essential oil: A review. *Aust. Infect. Control* **2005**, *10*, 35–37. [CrossRef]
39. Maietti, S.; Rossi, D.; Guerrini, A.; Useli, C.; Romagnoli, C.; Poli, F.; Bruni, R.; Sacchetti, G. A multivariate analysis approach to the study of chemical and functional properties of chemo-diverse plant derivatives: Lavender essential oils. *Flavour Frag. J.* **2013**, *28*, 144–154. [CrossRef]
40. Danh, L.T.; Triet, N.D.A.; Zhao, J.; Mammucari, R.; Foster, N. Antioxidant activity, yield and chemical composition of lavender essential oil extracted by supercritical CO_2. *J. Supercrit. Fluids* **2012**, *70*, 27–34. [CrossRef]
41. Beale, D.J.; Morrison, P.D.; Karpe, A.V.; Dunn, M.S. Chemometric analysis of lavender essential oils using targeted and untargeted GC-MS acquired data for the rapid identification and characterization of oil quality. *Molecules* **2017**, *22*, 1339. [CrossRef]
42. Liu, X.; Cai, J.; Chen, H.; Zhong, Q.; Hou, Y.; Chen, W.; Chen, W. Antibacterial activity and mechanism of linalool against *Pseudomonas aeruginosa*. *Microb. Pathog.* **2020**, *141*, 103980. [CrossRef]
43. Khayyat, S. Thermal, photo-oxidation and antimicrobial studies of linalyl acetate as a major ingredient of lavender essential oil. *Arab. J. Chem.* **2020**, *13*, 1575–1581. [CrossRef]
44. Trombetta, D.; Castelli, F.; Sarpietro, M.G.; Venuti, V.; Cristani, M.; Daniele, C.; Saija, A.; Mazzanti, G.; Bisignano, G. Mechanisms of antibacterial action of three monoterpenes. *Antimicrob. Agents Chemother.* **2005**, *49*, 2474–2478. [CrossRef] [PubMed]
45. Mighri, H.; Sabri, K.; Eljeni, H.; Neffati, M.; Akrout, A. Chemical composition and antimicrobial activity of *Pituranthos chloranthus* (Benth.) hook and *Pituranthos tortu-osus* (Coss.) maire essential oils from southern Tunisia. *Adv. Biol. Chem.* **2015**, *5*, 273. [CrossRef]
46. Li, W.R.; Li, H.L.; Shi, Q.S.; Sun, T.L.; Xie, X.B.; Song, B.; Huang, X.M. The dynamics and mechanism of the antimicrobial activity of tea tree oil against bacteria and fungi. *Appl. Microbiol. Biotechnol.* **2016**, *100*, 8865–8875. [CrossRef] [PubMed]
47. Bordini, E.A.F.; Tonon, C.C.; Francisconi, R.S.; Magalhães, F.A.C.; Huacho, P.M.M.; Bedran, T.L.; Pratavieira, S.; Spolidorio, L.C.; Spolidorio, D.P. Antimicrobial effects of terpinen-4-ol against oral pathogens and its capacity for the modulation of gene expression. *Biofouling* **2018**, *34*, 815–825. [CrossRef]
48. Saviuc, C.; Gheorghe, I.; Coban, S.; Drumea, V.; Chifiriuc, M.C.; Banu, O.; Bezirtzoglou, E.; Lazar, V. *Rosmarinus officinalis* essential oil and eucalyptol act as efflux pumps inhibitors and increase ciprofloxacin efficiency against *Pseudomonas aeruginosa* and *Acinetobacter baumannii* MDR strains. *Rom. Biotechnol. Lett.* **2016**, *21*, 11783.
49. Taha, A.M.; Eldahshan, O.A. Chemical characteristics, antimicrobial, and cytotoxic activities of the essential oil of Egyptian *Cinnamomum glanduliferum* bark. *Chem. Biodivers.* **2017**, *14*, e1600443. [CrossRef]

50. Bouazama, S.; Harhar, H.; Costa, J.; Desjobert, J.; Talbaoui, A.; Tabyaoui, M. Chemical composition and antibacterial activity of the essential oils of *Lavandula pedunculata* and *Lavandula dentate*. *J. Mater. Environ. Sci.* **2017**, *8*, 2154–2160.
51. Manoharan, R.K.; Lee, J.H.; Lee, J. Antibiofilm and antihyphal activities of cedar leaf essential oil, camphor, and fenchone derivatives against *Candida albicans*. *Front. Microbiol.* **2017**, *8*, 1476. [CrossRef]
52. Moo, C.L.; Yang, S.K.; Osman, M.A.; Yuswan, M.H.; Loh, J.Y.; Lim, W.M.; Lim, S.H.E.; Lai, K.S. Antibacterial activity and mode of action of β-caryophyllene on *Bacillus cereus*. *Pol. J. Microbiol.* **2020**, *69*, 49. [CrossRef]
53. Coutinho, H.D.M.; de Freitas, M.A.; Gondim, C.N.F.L.; de Albuquerque, R.S.; de Alencar Ferreira, J.V.; Andrade, J.C. *In vitro* antimicrobial activity of geraniol and cariophyllene against *Staphylococcus aureus*. *Rev. Cuba. Plantas Med.* **2015**, *20*, 98–105.
54. De Lira, M.H.P.; de Andrade Júnior, F.P.; Moraes, G.F.Q.; da Silva Macena, G.; de Oliveira Pereira, F.; Lima, I.O. Antimicrobial activity of geraniol: An integrative review. *J. Essent. Oil Res.* **2020**, *32*, 187–197. [CrossRef]
55. Bamoniri, A.; Ebrahimabadi, A.H.; Mazoochi, A.; Behpour, M.; Kashi, F.J.; Batooli, H. Antioxidant and antimicrobial activity evaluation and essential oil analysis of *Semenovia tragioides* Boiss. from Iran. *Food Chem.* **2010**, *122*, 553–558. [CrossRef]
56. Yang, S.K.; Yusoff, K.; Ajat, M.; Yap, W.S.; Lai, K.S. Antimicrobial activity and mode of action of terpene linalyl anthranilate against carbapenemase-producing *Klebsiella pneumoniae*. *J. Pharm. Anal.* **2020**. [CrossRef]
57. Białoń, M.; Krzyśko-Łupicka, T.; Nowakowska-Bogdan, E.; Wieczorek, P.P. Chemical composition of two different lavender essential oils and their effect on facial skin microbiota. *Molecules* **2019**, *24*, 3270. [CrossRef]
58. Zengin, H.; Baysal, A.H. Antibacterial and antioxidant activity of essential oil terpenes against pathogenic and spoilage-forming bacteria and cell structure-activity relationships evaluated by SEM microscopy. *Molecules* **2014**, *19*, 17773–17798. [CrossRef]
59. Mahizan, N.A.; Yang, S.K.; Moo, C.L.; Song, A.A.L.; Chong, C.M.; Chong, C.W.; Abushelaibi, A.; Lim, S.H.E.; Lai, K.S. Terpene derivatives as a potential agent against antimicrobial resistance (AMR) pathogens. *Molecules* **2019**, *24*, 2631. [CrossRef]
60. Yilmaz, M.T. Minimum inhibitory and minimum bactericidal concentrations of boron compounds against several bacterial strains. *Turk. J. Med Sci.* **2012**, *42*, 1423–1429.
61. Miller, R.; Walker, R.; Carson, J.; Coles, M.; Coyne, R.; Dalsgaard, I.; Gieseker, C.; Hsu, H.; Mathers, J.; Papapetropoulou, M. Standardization of a broth microdilution susceptibility testing method to determine minimum inhibitory concentrations of aquatic bacteria. *Dis. Aquat. Org.* **2005**, *64*, 211–222. [CrossRef]
62. Balouiri, M.; Sadiki, M.; Ibnsouda, S.K. Methods for in vitro evaluating antimicrobial activity: A review. *J. Pharm. Anal.* **2016**, *6*, 71–79. [CrossRef]
63. Chouhan, S.; Sharma, K.; Guleria, S. Antimicrobial activity of some essential oils—present status and future perspectives. *Medicines* **2017**, *4*, 58. [CrossRef]
64. Soković, M.; Glamočlija, J.; Marin, P.D.; Brkić, D.; Van Griensven, L.J. Antibacterial effects of the essential oils of commonly consumed medicinal herbs using an in vitro model. *Molecules* **2010**, *15*, 7532–7546. [CrossRef] [PubMed]
65. Blažeković, B.; Yang, W.; Wang, Y.; Li, C.; Kindl, M.; Pepeljnjak, S.; Vladimir-Knežević, S. Chemical composition, antimicrobial and antioxidant activities of essential oils of *Lavandula*× intermedia 'Budrovka'and *L. angustifolia* cultivated in Croatia. *Ind. Crops Prod.* **2018**, *123*, 173–182. [CrossRef]
66. Zenão, S.; Aires, A.; Dias, C.; Saavedra, M.J.; Fernandes, C. Antibacterial potential of *Urtica dioica* and *Lavandula angustifolia* extracts against methicillin resistant *Staphylococcus aureus* isolated from diabetic foot ulcers. *J. Herb. Med.* **2017**, *10*, 53–58. [CrossRef]
67. Danh, L.T.; Triet, N.D.A.; Zhao, J.; Mammucari, R.; Foster, N. Comparison of chemical composition, antioxidant and antimicrobial activity of lavender (*Lavandula angustifolia* L.) essential oils extracted by supercritical CO_2, hexane and hydrodistillation. *Food Bioprocess Technol.* **2013**, *6*, 3481–3489. [CrossRef]
68. Mayaud, L.; Carricajo, A.; Zhiri, A.; Aubert, G. Comparison of bacteriostatic and bactericidal activity of 13 essential oils against strains with varying sensitivity to antibiotics. *Lett. Appl. Microbiol.* **2008**, *47*, 167–173. [CrossRef]
69. Javed, H.; Tabassum, S.; Erum, S.; Murtaza, I.; Muhammad, A.; Amin, F.; Nisar, M.F. Screening and characterization of selected drugs having antibacterial potential. *Pak. J. Pharm. Sci.* **2018**, *31*, 933–939.
70. Hossain, S.; Heo, H.; De Silva, B.; Wimalasena, S.; Pathirana, H.; Heo, G.J. Antibacterial activity of essential oil from lavender (*Lavandula angustifolia*) against pet turtle-borne pathogenic bacteria. *Lab. Anim. Res.* **2017**, *33*, 195–201. [CrossRef]
71. Moon, T.; Wilkinson, J.; Cavanagh, H. Antibacterial activity of essential oils, hydrosols and plant extracts from Australian grown *Lavandula* spp. *Int. J. Aromather.* **2006**, *16*, 9–14. [CrossRef]
72. Adam, K.; Sivropoulou, A.; Kokkini, S.; Lanaras, T.; Arsenakis, M. Antifungal activities of *Origanum vulgare* subsp. *hirtum*, *Mentha spicata*, *Lavandula angustifolia*, and *Salvia fruticosa* essential oils against human pathogenic fungi. *J. Agric. Food Chem.* **1998**, *46*, 1739–1745.
73. Khoury, M.; Stien, D.; Eparvier, V.; Ouaini, N.; El Beyrouthy, M. Report on the medicinal use of eleven Lamiaceae species in Lebanon and rationalization of their antimicrobial potential by examination of the chemical composition and antimicrobial activity of their essential oils. *Evid. Based Complementary Altern. Med.* **2016**, *2016*, 1–17. [CrossRef]
74. Shin, S. Anti-*Aspergillus* activities of plant essential oils and their combination effects with ketoconazole or amphotericin B. *Arch. Pharmacal. Res.* **2003**, *26*, 389. [CrossRef] [PubMed]
75. Sienkiewicz, M.; Głowacka, A.; Kowalczyk, E.; Wiktorowska-Owczarek, A.; Jóźwiak-Bębenista, M.; Łysakowska, M. The biological activities of cinnamon, geranium and lavender essential oils. *Molecules* **2014**, *19*, 20929–20940. [CrossRef] [PubMed]
76. Nikolić, M.; Jovanović, K.K.; Marković, T.; Marković, D.; Gligorijević, N.; Radulović, S.; Soković, M. Chemical composition, antimicrobial, and cytotoxic properties of five Lamiaceae essential oils. *Ind. Crops Prod.* **2014**, *61*, 225–232. [CrossRef]

77. Moussi Imane, M.; Houda, F.; Said Amal, A.H.; Kaotar, N.; Mohammed, T.; Imane, R.; Farid, H. Phytochemical composition and antibacterial activity of Moroccan *Lavandula angustifolia* Mill. *J. Essent. Oil Bear. Plants* **2017**, *20*, 1074–1082. [CrossRef]
78. Mesic, A.; Mahmutović-Dizdarević, I.; Tahirović, E.; Durmišević, I.; Eminovic, I.; Jerković-Mujkić, A.; Bešta-Gajević, R. Evaluation of toxicological and antimicrobial activity of lavender and immortelle essential oils. *Drug Chem. Toxicol.* **2018**, *4*, 1–8. [CrossRef]
79. Sharifi-Rad, J.; Sureda, A.; Tenore, G.C.; Daglia, M.; Sharifi-Rad, M.; Valussi, M.; Tundis, R.; Sharifi-Rad, M.; Loizzo, M.R.; Ademiluyi, A.O. Biological activities of essential oils: From plant chemoecology to traditional healing systems. *Molecules* **2017**, *22*, 70. [CrossRef]
80. da Cruz Cabral, L.; Pinto, V.F.; Patriarca, A. Application of plant derived compounds to control fungal spoilage and mycotoxin production in foods. *Int. J. Food Microbiol.* **2013**, *166*, 1–14. [CrossRef]
81. D'auria, F.; Tecca, M.; Strippoli, V.; Salvatore, G.; Battinelli, L.; Mazzanti, G. Antifungal activity of *Lavandula angustifolia* essential oil against *Candida albicans* yeast and mycelial form. *Med. Mycol.* **2005**, *43*, 391–396. [CrossRef]
82. McKenzie, C.; Koser, U.; Lewis, L.; Bain, J.; Mora-Montes, H.; Barker, R.; Gow, N.; Erwig, L. Contribution of *Candida albicans* cell wall components to recognition by and escape from murine macrophages. *Infect. Immun.* **2010**, *78*, 1650–1658. [CrossRef]
83. Moon, T.; Wilkinson, J.M.; Cavanagh, H.M. Antiparasitic activity of two *Lavandula* essential oils against *Giardia duodenalis*, *Trichomonas vaginalis* and *Hexamita inflata*. *Parasitol. Res.* **2006**, *99*, 722–728. [CrossRef]
84. Johnston, V.J.; Mabey, D.C. Global epidemiology and control of *Trichomonas vaginalis*. *Curr. Opin. Infect. Dis.* **2008**, *21*, 56–64. [CrossRef] [PubMed]
85. Adam, R.D. Biology of *Giardia lamblia*. *Clin. Microbiol. Rev.* **2001**, *14*, 447–475. [CrossRef] [PubMed]
86. Shokri, A.; Saeedi, M.; Fakhar, M.; Morteza-Semnani, K.; Keighobadi, M.; Teshnizi, S.H.; Kelidari, H.R.; Sadjadi, S. Antileishmanial activity of *Lavandula angustifolia* and *Rosmarinus officinalis* essential oils and nano-emulsions on Leishmania major (MRHO/IR/75/ER). *Iran. J. Parasitol.* **2017**, *12*, 622. [PubMed]
87. Mantovani, A.L.; Vieira, G.P.; Cunha, W.R.; Groppo, M.; Santos, R.A.; Rodrigues, V.; Magalhães, L.G.; Crotti, A.E. Chemical composition, antischistosomal and cytotoxic effects of the essential oil of *Lavandula angustifolia* grown in Southeastern Brazil. *Rev. Bras. Farmacogn.* **2013**, *23*, 877–884. [CrossRef]
88. Aljaafari, M.; Alhosani, M.S.; Abushelaibi, A.; Lai, K.S.; Lim, S.H.E. *Essential Oils-Oils of Nature*; IntechOpen: London, UK, 2019.
89. Yu, Z.; Tang, J.; Khare, T.; Kumar, V. The alarming antimicrobial resistance in ESKAPEE pathogens: Can essential oils come to the rescue? *Fitoterapia* **2020**, *140*, 104433. [CrossRef]
90. Bush, K.; Courvalin, P.; Dantas, G.; Davies, J.; Eisenstein, B.; Huovinen, P.; Jacoby, G.A.; Kishony, R.; Kreiswirth, B.N.; Kutter, E. Tackling antibiotic resistance. *Nat. Rev. Microbiol.* **2011**, *9*, 894–896. [CrossRef]
91. Bhat, A.S.; Ahangar, A.A. Methods for detecting chemical–chemical interaction in toxicology. *Toxicol. Mech. Methods* **2007**, *17*, 441–450. [CrossRef]
92. Hyldgaard, M.; Mygind, T.; Meyer, R.L. Essential oils in food preservation: Mode of action, synergies, and interactions with food matrix components. *Front. Microbiol.* **2012**, *3*, 12. [CrossRef]
93. Efferth, T.; Koch, E. Complex interactions between phytochemicals. The multi-target therapeutic concept of phytotherapy. *Curr. Drug Targets* **2011**, *12*, 122–132. [CrossRef]
94. Jugreet, B.S.; Mahomoodally, M.F. Essential oils from 9 exotic and endemic medicinal plants from Mauritius shows in vitro antibacterial and antibiotic potentiating activities. *S. Afr. J. Bot.* **2020**, *132*, 355–362. [CrossRef]
95. Owen, L.; Laird, K. Synchronous application of antibiotics and essential oils: Dual mechanisms of action as a potential solution to antibiotic resistance. *Crit. Rev. Microbiol.* **2018**, *44*, 414–435. [CrossRef] [PubMed]
96. Hemaiswarya, S.; Kruthiventi, A.K.; Doble, M. Synergism between natural products and antibiotics against infectious diseases. *Phytomedicine* **2008**, *15*, 639–652. [CrossRef] [PubMed]
97. Owen, L.; Grootveld, M.; Arroo, R.; Ruiz-Rodado, V.; Price, P.; Laird, K. A multifactorial comparison of ternary combinations of essential oils in topical preparations to current antibiotic prescription therapies for the control of acne vulgaris-associated bacteria. *Phytother. Res.* **2017**, *31*, 410–417. [CrossRef] [PubMed]
98. van Vuuren, S.; Viljoen, A. Plant-based antimicrobial studies–methods and approaches to study the interaction between natural products. *Planta Med.* **2011**, *77*, 1168–1182. [CrossRef] [PubMed]
99. Odds, F.C. Synergy, antagonism, and what the chequerboard puts between them. *J. Antimicrob. Chemother.* **2003**, *52*, 1–11. [CrossRef]
100. Langeveld, W.T.; Veldhuizen, E.J.; Burt, S.A. Synergy between essential oil components and antibiotics: A review. *Crit. Rev. Microbiol.* **2014**, *40*, 76–94. [CrossRef]
101. de Rapper, S.; Kamatou, G.; Viljoen, A.; van Vuuren, S. The in vitro antimicrobial activity of *Lavandula angustifolia* essential oil in combination with other aroma-therapeutic oils. *Evid. Based Complementary Altern. Med.* **2013**, *2013*, 1–10. [CrossRef]
102. Moussii, I.M.; Nayme, K.; Timinouni, M.; Jamaleddine, J.; Filali, H.; Hakkou, F. Synergistic antibacterial effects of Moroccan *Artemisia herba alba*, *Lavandula angustifolia* and *Rosmarinus officinalis* essential oils. *Synergy* **2020**, *10*, 100057. [CrossRef]
103. Abboud, M.; El Rammouz, R.; Jammal, B.; Sleiman, M. In vitro and in vivo antimicrobial activity of two essential oils *Thymus vulgaris* and *Lavandula angustifolia* against bovine *Staphylococcus* and *Streptococcus* mastitis pathogen. *Middle East J.* **2015**, *4*, 975–983.
104. Orchard, A.; van Vuuren, S.F.; Viljoen, A.M. Commercial essential oil combinations against topical fungal pathogens. *Nat. Prod. Commun.* **2019**, *14*, 1934578X1901400139. [CrossRef]

105. Cassella, S.; Cassella, J.P.; Smith, I. Synergistic antifungal activity of tea tree (*Melaleuca alternifolia*) and lavender (*Lavandula angustifolia*) essential oils against dermatophyte infection. *Int. J. Aromather.* **2002**, *12*, 2–15. [CrossRef]
106. Orchard, A.; Viljoen, A.; van Vuuren, S. Wound pathogens: Investigating antimicrobial activity of commercial essential oil combinations against reference strains. *Chem. Biodivers.* **2018**, *15*, e1800405. [CrossRef] [PubMed]
107. Cho, Y.S.; Oh, J.J.; Oh, K.H. Synergistic anti-bacterial and proteomic effects of epigallocatechin gallate on clinical isolates of imipenem-resistant *Klebsiella pneumoniae*. *Phytomedicine* **2011**, *18*, 941–946. [CrossRef]
108. Aguiar, J.J.; Sousa, C.P.; Araruna, M.K.; Silva, M.K.; Portelo, A.C.; Lopes, J.C.; Carvalho, V.R.; Figueredo, F.G.; Bitu, V.C.; Coutinho, H.D. Antibacterial and modifying-antibiotic activities of the essential oils of *Ocimum gratissimum* L. and *Plectranthus amboinicus* L. *Eur. J. Integr. Med.* **2015**, *7*, 151–156. [CrossRef]
109. Eumkeb, G.; Siriwong, S.; Phitaktim, S.; Rojtinnakorn, N.; Sakdarat, S. Synergistic activity and mode of action of flavonoids isolated from smaller galangal and amoxicillin combinations against amoxicillin-resistant *Escherichia coli*. *J. Appl. Microbiol.* **2012**, *112*, 55–64. [CrossRef]
110. Dra, L.A.; Brahim, M.A.S.; Boualy, B.; Aghraz, A.; Barakate, M.; Oubaassine, S.; Markouk, M.; Larhsini, M. Chemical composition, antioxidant and evidence antimicrobial synergistic effects of *Periploca laevigata* essential oil with conventional antibiotics. *Ind. Crops Prod.* **2017**, *109*, 746–752. [CrossRef]
111. Yap, P.; Krishnan, T.; Yiap, B.; Hu, C.; Chan, K.G.; Lim, S. Membrane disruption and anti-quorum sensing effects of synergistic interaction between *Lavandula angustifolia* (lavender oil) in combination with antibiotic against plasmid-conferred multi-drug-resistant Escherichia coli. *J. Appl. Microbiol.* **2014**, *116*, 1119–1128. [CrossRef]
112. Lai, P.J.; Ng, E.V.; Yang, S.K.; Moo, C.L.; Low, W.Y.; Yap, P.S.X.; Lim, S.H.E.; Lai, K.S. Transcriptomic analysis of multi-drug resistant *Escherichia coli* K-12 strain in response to *Lavandula angustifolia* essential oil. *3 Biotech* **2020**, *10*, 1–9. [CrossRef]
113. Kwiatkowski, P.; Łopusiewicz, Ł.; Kostek, M.; Drozłowska, E.; Pruss, A.; Wojciuk, B.; Sienkiewicz, M.; Zielińska-Bliźniewska, H.; Dołęgowska, B. The antibacterial activity of lavender essential oil alone and in combination with octenidine dihydrochloride against MRSA strains. *Molecules* **2020**, *25*, 95. [CrossRef]
114. de Rapper, S.; Viljoen, A.; van Vuuren, S. The *in vitro* antimicrobial effects of Lavandula angustifolia essential oil in combination with conventional antimicrobial agents. *Evid. Based Complementary Altern. Med.* **2016**, *2016*, 1–9. [CrossRef]
115. Yang, S.K.; Yusoff, K.; Thomas, W.; Akseer, R.; Alhosani, M.S.; Abushelaibi, A.; Lai, K.S. Lavender essential oil induces oxidative stress which modifies the bacterial membrane permeability of carbapenemase producing *Klebsiella pneumoniae*. *Sci. Rep.* **2020**, *10*, 1–14. [CrossRef] [PubMed]
116. Adaszynska-Skwirzynska, M.; Szczerbinska, D.; Zych, S. Antibacterial activity of lavender essential oil and linalool combined with gentamicin on selected bacterial strains. *Med. Weter.* **2020**, *76*, 115–118. [CrossRef]
117. Yap, P.S.X.; Lim, S.H.E.; Hu, C.P.; Yiap, B.C. Combination of essential oils and antibiotics reduce antibiotic resistance in plasmid-conferred multidrug resistant bacteria. *Phytomedicine* **2013**, *20*, 710–713. [CrossRef] [PubMed]
118. Göger, G.; Çomoğlu, B.A.; İşcan, G.; Demirci, F. Evaluation of anticandidal effects of oils of commercial lavender (*Lavandula angustifolia* Miller) in combination with ketoconazole against some *Candida* Berkhout strains. *Trak. Univ. J. Nat. Sci.* **2020**, *21*, 13–19.
119. Prakash, A.; Baskaran, R.; Paramasivam, N.; Vadivel, V. Essential oil based nanoemulsions to improve the microbial quality of minimally processed fruits and vegetables: A review. *Food Res. Int.* **2018**, *111*, 509–523. [CrossRef]
120. Herculano, E.D.; de Paula, H.C.; de Figueiredo, E.A.; Dias, F.G.; Pereira, V.d.A. Physicochemical and antimicrobial properties of nanoencapsulated *Eucalyptus staigeriana* essential oil. *LWT Food Sci. Technol.* **2015**, *61*, 484–491. [CrossRef]
121. Donsì, F.; Annunziata, M.; Sessa, M.; Ferrari, G. Nanoencapsulation of essential oils to enhance their antimicrobial activity in foods. *LWT Food Sci. Technol.* **2011**, *44*, 1908–1914. [CrossRef]
122. Franklyne, J.; Mukherjee, A.; Chandrasekaran, N. Essential oil micro-and nanoemulsions: Promising roles in antimicrobial therapy targeting human pathogens. *Lett. Appl. Microbiol.* **2016**, *63*, 322–334. [CrossRef]
123. Bilia, A.R.; Guccione, C.; Isacchi, B.; Righeschi, C.; Firenzuoli, F.; Bergonzi, M.C. Essential oils loaded in nanosystems: A developing strategy for a successful therapeutic approach. *Evid. Based Complementary Altern. Med.* **2014**, *2014*, 1–14. [CrossRef]
124. Ciobanu, A.; Landy, D.; Fourmentin, S. Complexation efficiency of cyclodextrins for volatile flavor compounds. *Food Res. Int.* **2013**, *53*, 110–114. [CrossRef]
125. Cetin Babaoglu, H.; Bayrak, A.; Ozdemir, N.; Ozgun, N. Encapsulation of clove essential oil in hydroxypropyl beta-cyclodextrin for characterization, controlled release, and antioxidant activity. *J. Food Process. Preserv.* **2017**, *41*, e13202. [CrossRef]
126. Rakmai, J.; Cheirsilp, B.; Mejuto, J.C.; Torrado-Agrasar, A.; Simal-Gándara, J. Physico-chemical characterization and evaluation of bio-efficacies of black pepper essential oil encapsulated in hydroxypropyl-beta-cyclodextrin. *Food Hydrocoll.* **2017**, *65*, 157–164. [CrossRef]
127. Yuan, C.; Wang, Y.; Liu, Y.; Cui, B. Physicochemical characterization and antibacterial activity assessment of lavender essential oil encapsulated in hydroxypropyl-beta-cyclodextrin. *Ind. Crops Prod.* **2019**, *130*, 104–110. [CrossRef]
128. Das, S.; Gazdag, Z.; Szente, L.; Meggyes, M.; Horváth, G.; Lemli, B.; Kunsági-Máté, S.; Kuzma, M.; Kőszegi, T. Antioxidant and antimicrobial properties of randomly methylated β cyclodextrin–captured essential oils. *Food Chem.* **2019**, *278*, 305–313. [CrossRef] [PubMed]
129. Abrigo, M.; McArthur, S.L.; Kingshott, P. Electrospun nanofibers as dressings for chronic wound care: Advances, challenges, and future prospects. *Macromol. Biosci.* **2014**, *14*, 772–792. [CrossRef]

130. Rieger, K.A.; Schiffman, J.D. Electrospinning an essential oil: Cinnamaldehyde enhances the antimicrobial efficacy of chitosan/poly (ethylene oxide) nanofibers. *Carbohydr. Polym.* **2014**, *113*, 561–568. [CrossRef]
131. Zhang, W.; Ronca, S.; Mele, E. Electrospun nanofibres containing antimicrobial plant extracts. *Nanomaterials* **2017**, *7*, 42. [CrossRef]
132. Balasubramanian, K.; Kodam, K.M. Encapsulation of therapeutic lavender oil in an electrolyte assisted polyacrylonitrile nanofibres for antibacterial applications. *RSC Adv.* **2014**, *4*, 54892–54901. [CrossRef]
133. Wolny-Koładka, K.A.; Malina, D.K. Silver nanoparticles toxicity against airborne strains of *Staphylococcus* spp. *J. Environ. Sci. Health Part A* **2017**, *52*, 1247–1256. [CrossRef]
134. Wolny-Koładka, K.A.; Malina, D.K. Eco-friendly approach to the synthesis of silver nanoparticles and their antibacterial activity against *Staphylococcus* spp. and *Escherichia coli*. *J. Environ. Sci. Health Part A* **2018**, *53*, 1041–1047. [CrossRef]
135. Sofi, H.S.; Akram, T.; Tamboli, A.H.; Majeed, A.; Shabir, N.; Sheikh, F.A. Novel lavender oil and silver nanoparticles simultaneously loaded onto polyurethane nanofibers for wound-healing applications. *Int. J. Pharm.* **2019**, *569*, 118590. [CrossRef] [PubMed]
136. Haba, E.; Bouhdid, S.; Torrego-Solana, N.; Marqués, A.; Espuny, M.J.; García-Celma, M.J.; Manresa, A. Rhamnolipids as emulsifying agents for essential oil formulations: Antimicrobial effect against *Candida albicans* and methicillin-resistant *Staphylococcus aureus*. *Int. J. Pharm.* **2014**, *476*, 134–141. [CrossRef] [PubMed]
137. Predoi, D.; Iconaru, S.L.; Buton, N.; Badea, M.L.; Marutescu, L. Antimicrobial activity of new materials based on lavender and basil essential oils and hydroxyapatite. *Nanomaterials* **2018**, *8*, 291. [CrossRef] [PubMed]
138. Rashed, M.M.; Zhang, C.; Ghaleb, A.D.; Li, J.; Nagi, A.; Majeed, H.; Bakry, A.M.; Haider, J.; Xu, Z.; Tong, Q. Techno-functional properties and sustainable application of nanoparticles-based *Lavandula angustifolia* essential oil fabricated using unsaturated lipid-carrier and biodegradable wall material. *Ind. Crops Prod.* **2019**, *136*, 66–76. [CrossRef]
139. Predoi, D.; Groza, A.; Iconaru, S.L.; Predoi, G.; Barbuceanu, F.; Guegan, R.; Motelica-Heino, M.S.; Cimpeanu, C. Properties of basil and lavender essential oils adsorbed on the surface of hydroxyapatite. *Materials* **2018**, *11*, 652. [CrossRef]
140. Qiu, C.; Chang, R.; Yang, J.; Ge, S.; Xiong, L.; Zhao, M.; Li, M.; Sun, Q. Preparation and characterization of essential oil-loaded starch nanoparticles formed by short glucan chains. *Food Chem.* **2017**, *221*, 1426–1433. [CrossRef]

MDPI
St. Alban-Anlage 66
4052 Basel
Switzerland
Tel. +41 61 683 77 34
Fax +41 61 302 89 18
www.mdpi.com

Processes Editorial Office
E-mail: processes@mdpi.com
www.mdpi.com/journal/processes

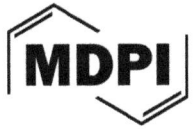